MOSBY'S
REVIEW FOR THE
PTCB
CERTIFICATION
EXAMINATION

MOSBY'S
REVIEW FOR THE
PTCB
CERTIFICATION
EXAMINATION

JAMES J. MIZNER Jr., BS Pharmacy, MBA, RPh
Pharmacy Technician Program Director
ACT College
Arlington, Virginia

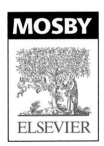

MOSBY
ELSEVIER

11830 Westline Industrial Drive
St. Louis, Missouri 63146

MOSBY'S REVIEW FOR THE PTCB CERTIFICATION EXAMINATION   ISBN-13: 978-0-323-03367-1
ISBN-10: 0-323-03367-9

ISBN-13: 978-0-323-03367-1
ISBN-10: 0-323-03367-9

Publisher: Michael Ledbetter
Executive Editor: Loren Wilson
Developmental Editor: Celeste Clingan
Publishing Services Manager: Pat Joiner
Project Manager: Jennifer Clark
Designer: Amy Buxton

Printed in the United States of America
Last digit is the print number: 9   8   7   6   5   4

Working together to grow
libraries in developing countries

www.elsevier.com | www.bookaid.org | www.sabre.org

ELSEVIER   BOOK AID
International   Sabre Foundation

Preface

Pharmacy technicians have become a major asset for both pharmacies and pharmacists in the world today. With an increasing population, longer life spans, patients taking multiple medications, and managed care playing a major role, pharmacies are seeing a major increase in processed prescriptions. A pharmacy cannot be successful in providing patient medications without knowledgeable pharmacy technicians assisting the pharmacist. State Boards of Pharmacy realize the importance of these pharmacy technicians in the drug delivery process and are committed to ensuring that pharmacy technicians possess the necessary skills to work in a pharmacy.

As of May 11, 2007, there are thirty-two State Boards of Pharmacies that recognize the Pharmacy Technician Certification Examination (PTCE) by the Pharmacy Technician Certification Board (PTCB) as the national certification examination for Pharmacy Technicians. These twenty-five states have state legislation requiring certification of all Pharmacy Technicians working in retail, a hospital, or any other specialized pharmacy setting. All states will require certification of technicians in the near future.

Mosby's Review for the PTCB Certification Examination; has been written to assist a pharmacy technician studying for the PTCB examination. *Mosby's Review for the PTCB Certification Examination;* is to be used to augment either a formalized pharmacy technician training program or on-the-job training, not replace it. The PTCB examination consists of three sections:

Assisting the Pharmacist

Maintaining Medication and Inventory Control Sections

Participation in the Administration and Management of Pharmacy Practice

The PTCB examination contains 100 multiple-choice questions; 90 questions are graded and 10 questions are evaluated for use in future examinations. At the time of the test, the student is unaware of the actual test questions and practice questions.

The PTCB has established competencies for each of these three sections. These competencies are the subtopics found in each section. After each section, the student will find multiple-choice review questions that have answers and rationales located in the back of the text. Also, Chapter 5 has four practice examinations with 140 questions each, also with answers and rationales in the back of the text. These practice exams can also be found on the CD-ROM attached to this text, along with two additional practice examinations and flashcards.

The pharmacy technician should use *Mosby's Review For the PTCB Certification Examination;* as a guide to determine which topics he or she may need additional assistance in while preparing for the examination. Good Luck!

James J. Mizner

Contents

4 PARTICIPATING IN THE ADMINISTRATION AND MANAGEMENT OF PHARMACY PRACTICE, *141*

Chapter 1

PTCE Test-Taking Skills

PREPARE FOR THE TEST

- Know exactly what you will be tested on. Review test outlines if available.
- Study all key topics that will appear on the examination.
- Spread out your review over a period of weeks. Focused reviews over time are more effective than "cramming."
- Outline your text and mark topics that need a more concentrated review.
- Try to predict questions that may be on the test and then test your skills in answering them.

ON THE DAY OF THE TEST

- Get enough sleep the night before the test. Make sure you have gotten adequate sleep the week before the test.
- Arrive early and choose a comfortable working area.
- Dress casually and comfortably. Take extra time planning appropriate clothes.
- Arrive prepared with necessary supplies (pencils, non-programmable calculator, admission ticket for the examination, and personal photo identification).

AS YOU TAKE THE TEST

- Listen, read, and follow the directions carefully.
- Look over the test before answering any questions. Scanning the test will provide you with key information about the scope and difficulty of the test.
- First complete the sections that are easiest for you.
- Answer the questions in order, but postpone questions that challenge you until later in the test. Answer the harder questions later.
- On your second pass through the test, ignore the answered questions and focus only on the questions you did not answer.
- Never leave a question unanswered; there is no penalty for guessing. (Time management is a key to success; it is to your advantage to answer all the items on the test.)
- Change your answers only when you are certain you made a mistake. Your first answer is usually the correct one.

TIPS FOR MULTIPLE-CHOICE QUESTIONS

- Remember that there is only one preferred answer, even though more than one answer may appear to be correct.
- Use the process of elimination when you do not know the answer. Eliminate the most obviously wrong answer first, then the second, and then make your best decision between the last two choices.
- If you are still unsure about which is the correct answer, select the longer or more descriptive answer of the remaining answer set.
- If the answer set presents a range of numbers, eliminate the highest and lowest, and then select from the middle range of numbers.
- Slow down when you see negative words in the question. Look for words such as *not, except*, etc. In this case, you need to identify the false statement instead of the true statement.

• Items that contain "absolutes" such as *always, never, must, all,* and *none* severely limit the meaning of the item. Statements that contain absolutes are usually incorrect.

PRETEST

1. Which of the following is not an example of an oral dosage form?
   a. Amoxicillin
   b. Depakote
   c. Nitrostat
   d. Synthroid

2. If an injectable drug is labeled 0.5 mcg/2 mL and the patient is to receive 0.125 mcg, how many milligrams should the patient receive?
   a. 0.5
   b. 1.0
   c. 1.5
   d. 2.0

3. If a patient is experiencing nausea and vomiting, which of the following dosage forms would be more effective?
   a. Capsule
   b. Oral solution
   c. Suppository
   d. Tablet

4. Which of the following is not a patient's right covered under HIPAA?
   a. The right to request an amendment to his or her health record.
   b. The right to obtain an accounting of any disclosures of his or her protected health information.
   c. The right to obtain a copy of his or her designated record set of protected health information.
   d. The right to receive compensatory and punitive damage for violations of HIPAA.

5. How many grams of NaCl are in 100 mL of NS solution?
   a. 0.009
   b. 0.09
   c. 0.9
   d. 9.0

6. Which of the following classes of antibiotics should not be taken with either fruit juices or colas?
   a. Macrolides
   b. Penicillins
   c. Quinolones
   d. Sulfas

7. How many milligrams of atropine sulfate are needed to make 30 mL of a 1:200 solution?
   a. 1.5
   b. 15
   c. 150
   d. 1,500

8. Which drug classification may cause rhinitis medicamentosa with repeated use?
   a. Antihistamines
   b. Corticosteroids
   c. Nasal decongestants
   d. Xanthine derivatives

9. Which of the following medications is not a combination product?
    a. Estratest
    b. Hyzaar
    c. Lotrel
    d. Remeron

10. Which route of administration has the quickest onset of action?
    a. IM
    b. IV
    c. PO
    d. PR

11. What is the weight in grams of 4 fl oz of orange peel with a specific gravity of 0.844?
    a. 84
    b. 103
    c. 112
    d. 142

12. Which of the following medications is not a proton pump inhibitor?
    a. Aciphex
    b. Concerta
    c. Prevacid
    d. Protonix

13. What type of drug is used to facilitate an examination or come to a conclusion regarding a condition or disease?
    a. Destructive agent
    b. Diagnostic agent
    c. Prophylactic agent
    d. Therapeutic agent

14. How many grams of fluorouracil will a 154-lb patient receive in 5 successive days at a dosage of 12 mg/kg/day?
    a. 0.42
    b. 0.84
    c. 4.2
    d. 8.4

15. An effervescent tablet has the following formula:

APAP	325 mg
CaCO3	280 mg
Citric acid	900 mg
Potassium bicarbonate	300 mg
Sodium bicarbonate	465 mg

How many grams would one tablet contain?
    a. 0.227
    b. 2.27
    c. 22.7
    d. 227

16. If a physician prescribes Keflex 250 mg qid × 10 days, how many milliliters of Keflex oral suspension containing 250 mg per 5 mL should be dispensed?
    a. 75
    b. 100
    c. 150
    d. 200

17. Which term refers to mistreatment of a patient based on age, gender, race, or sexual preference?
    a. Decorum
    b. Discrimination
    c. Harassment
    d. Innuendo

18. To which schedule does meperidine belong?
    a. II
    b. III
    c. IV
    d. V

19. What must be found on all controlled substance prescriptions?
    a. Pharmacy DEA number
    b. Physician's business license number
    c. Physician's DEA number
    d. Physician's license number

20. How many 250 mg capsules are needed to fill the following prescription: "Amoxicillin 500 mg tid for 10 d"?
    a. 20
    b. 40
    c. 60
    d. 80

21. Which of the following medications is not a calcium channel blocker?
    a. Diovan
    b. Isoptin
    c. Plendil
    d. Tiazac

22. Which disease is characterized by glycosuria, polydipsia, and polyuria?
    a. Addison disease
    b. Cushing disease
    c. Diabetes
    d. Hypertension

23. What should a pharmacy technician do if he or she observes a patient attempting to purchase Bayer aspirin while he or she is waiting for a prescription of warfarin to be filled by the pharmacy?
    a. Inform the patient of the interaction between aspirin and warfarin
    b. Inform the pharmacist of the situation and allow the pharmacist to counsel the patient
    c. Point out to the patient that the "house brand" of aspirin is just as effective as Bayer aspirin
    d. Refuse to sell the aspirin to the patient

24. What would a message of "NDC Not Covered" indicate to the pharmacy technician?
    a. The medication has been recalled by the FDA
    b. The patient's insurance plan does not cover the drug
    c. The medication is a controlled substance
    d. The medication is backordered by the wholesaler

25. How many capsules each containing 250 mg of chloramphenicol are needed to provide 50 mg/kg/day for 10 days for an adult weighing 187 lb?
    a. 17
    b. 82
    c. 170
    d. 822

26. If the dose of a drug is 150 mcg, how many doses can be prepared from 0.120 g?
    a. 8
    b. 80
    c. 800
    d. 8,000

27. What is the percentage strength of a 1:1,500 solution?
    a. 0.0006
    b. 0.0066
    c. 0.0666
    d. 0.6666

28. How should Nitrostat tablets be taken?
    a. PO
    b. PRT
    c. SQ
    d. SL

29. What type of information should be collected from the patient or representative before processing a prescription?
    a. Disease states of the patient
    b. Drug allergies
    c. Medications taken by the patient, whether prescription or OTC
    d. All of the above

30. Which of the following is an advantage of a parenteral drug?
    a. Difficult to reverse an overdose
    b. Rapid onset of action
    c. Possibility of injecting pathogens and pyrogens into the body
    d. Trauma to the body by the needle

31. What is the generic name for Celexa?
    a. Citalopram
    b. Phenylzine
    c. Selegine
    d. Tranylcypromine

32. Which oral antidepressant is also used as a topical preparation?
    a. Amitriptyline
    b. Doxepin
    c. Imipramine
    d. Nortriptyline

33. Rx: Hydrocortisone   1%
           Precipitated sulfur   20%
           Zinc oxide paste   ad 60 g

    How many grams of hydrocortisone and precipitated sulfur should be used in preparing this compound?
    a. Hydrocortisone   0.6 g;   Precipitated sulfur   12 g
    b. Hydrocortisone   2.86 g;   Precipitated sulfur   9.14 g
    c. Hydrocortisone   3 g;   Precipitated sulfur   9.60 g
    d. Hydrocortisone   6 g;   Precipitated sulfur   9.6 g

34. How many grams are in 30 gr?
    a. 0.2
    b. 2.0
    c. 20
    d. 200

35. What is the maximum number of refills allowed on a prescription of lorazepam if authorized by a physician?
    a. 0
    b. 5
    c. 12
    d. Unlimited

36. Why is it necessary to rotate medications on a shelf?
    a. To allocate shelf space effectively
    b. To ensure the medication with the shortest dating is dispensed before drugs with longer dating to reduce the possibility that the medication will expire before being dispensed.
    c. To prevent dust from accumulating on the shelf
    d. To prevent overstock from developing

37. How much time does a physician have to provide a written prescription for an "Emergency Prescription" for a Schedule II drug?
    a. 24 hr
    b. 48 hr
    c. 72 hr
    d. 96 hr

38. Which of the following reference books discusses the therapeutic equivalence of products?
    a. Drug Topics Blue Book
    b. Drug Topics Green Book
    c. Drug Topics Orange Book
    d. Drug Topics Red Book

39. Which form is used to inform a drug manufacturer of errors caused by commercial packaging and labeling?
    a. FDA Form 79
    b. Med Watch
    c. MERF
    d. USP-ISMP

40. What is the basic formula in calculating the price of a prescription?
    a. AAC + dispensing fee
    b. (AWP–% Discount) + dispensing fee
    c. Ingredient cost + dispensing fee
    d. MAC + dispensing fee

41. Which association represents the interests of chain drug stores?
    a. APHA
    b. NABP
    c. NACDS
    d. NCPA

42. What is the generic name for Serevent?
    a. Albuterol
    b. Beclomethasone
    c. Salmeterol
    d. Triamcinolone

43. What is the brand name for paroxetine?
    a. Effexor
    b. Paxil
    c. Prozac
    d. Zoloft

44. What is the drug of choice for status epilepticus?
    a. Carbamazepine
    b. Diazepam
    c. Phenytoin
    d. Primidone

45. A physician orders KCl 40 mEq to be added to D5W 1,000 mL and administered over 4 hr. The injection solution on hand is KCl 2 mEq/mL. How many milliliters of KCl should be added?
    a. 40
    b. 8
    c. 16
    d. 20

46. You have received a medication order to prepare 500 mL of a 1:500 solution. The pharmacy has in stock a concentrate of 80%. How much of the concentrate will you need to use?
    a. 1 mL
    b. 1.25 mL
    c. 498.75 mL
    d. 499 mL

47. What are the components of a total nutrient admixture solution?
    a. Amino acids-dextrose-lipids
    b. Amino acids-lipids
    c. Dextrose-proteins
    d. Dextrose-vitamins

48. What is the brand name for allopurinol?
    a. Anturane
    b. Colchicine
    c. Col-Probenecid
    d. Zyloprim

49. Which of the following drugs is not used for hyperlipidemia?
    a. Folic acid
    b. Questran
    c. TriCor
    d. Zocor

50. Inderal is to beta-blocker as Nasonex is to _____.
    a. ACE inhibitor
    b. H2 antagonist
    c. MAOI
    d. Topical corticosteroid

51. Which of the following drugs is not used to treat ADHD?
    a. Amitriptyline
    b. Amphetamine-dextroamphetamine
    c. Desipramine
    d. Methylphenidate

52. What is the generic name for Lodine?
    a. Diflunisal
    b. Etodolac
    c. Ibuprofen
    d. Oxaprozin

53. Which of the following drugs may be used prophylactically for influenza and to treat Parkinson's disease?
    a. Amantadine
    b. Bromocriptine
    c. Levodopa-carbidopa
    d. Selegiline

54. Nitroglycerin is to nitrate as nifedipine is to _____.
    a. ACE inhibitor
    b. Beta-blocker
    c. Calcium channel blocker
    d. Loop diuretic

55. Which of the following insulins has the longest duration of action?
    a. Humalog
    b. Lente
    c. Regular
    d. NPH

56. Which of the following pediculicides requires a prescription?
    a. Lindane
    b. Permethrin
    c. Both of them
    d. Neither of them

57. How many fluid ounces of a commercially available 17% solution of benzalkonium chloride should be used to prepare 1 gallon of 1:750 solution?
    a. 0.25
    b. 0.5
    c. 1.0
    d. 29.0

58. How many grams of hydrocortisone powder should be used to prepare 1 lb of a 0.25% hydrocortisone cream?
    a. 1.14
    b. 1.2
    c. 113.5
    d. 120

59. Which of the following medications is an angiotensin II receptor antagonist?
    a. Acebutolol
    b. Clonidine
    c. Losartan
    d. Terazosin

60. What is the net profit for a prescription that has an acquisition cost of $45.00, a dispensing cost of $3.75, and retails at $55.00?
    a. $3.75
    b. $6.25
    c. $10.00
    d. $13.75

61. Which of the following should not be mixed with Sandimmune?
    a. Carbonated beverages
    b. Chocolate milk
    c. Milk
    d. Orange juice

62. Which of the following is a prostaglandin E analog?
    a. Alginic acid
    b. Mesalamine
    c. Misoprostol
    d. Sucralfate

63. Rx: Codeine sulfate   15 mg/tsp
         Robitussin ad   120 mL

    How many 30-mg tablets of codeine sulfate should be used in preparing the prescription?
    a. 4
    b. 8
    c. 12
    d. 16

64. What is the meaning of the suffix "-dipsia"?
    a. Discharge
    b. Hardening
    c. Pain
    d. Thirst

65. What is the meaning of the abbreviation of "ut dict"?
    a. As directed
    b. As needed
    c. If there is need
    d. Ointment

66. Which pharmacy law is being violated if a pharmacy attempts to purchase medications from a secondary market in either Canada or Mexico?
    a. Drug Listing Act of 1972
    b. Durham-Humphrey Amendment
    c. Kefauver-Harris Amendment
    d. Prescription Drug Marketing Act of 1987

67. Which of the following drug classifications are not used to treat congestive heart failure?
    a. ACE inhibitors
    b. Angiotensin II antagonists
    c. Antiarrhythmics
    d. Beta-blockers

68. Which of the following is the generic name for Intron?
    a. Interferon alfa-2a
    b. Interferon alfa-2b
    c. Interferon beta-1a
    d. Interferon beta-1b

69. How many milliliters of 95% (v/v) alcohol and 30% (v/v) alcohol should be mixed to prepare 1,000 mL of a 50% (v/v) solution?
    a. 30%-307 mL; 95%-693 mL
    b. 30%-444 mL; 95% -556 mL
    c. 30%-556 mL; 95%-444 mL
    d. 30%-693 mL; 95%-307 mL

70. Which organization is responsible for accrediting pharmacy education programs?
    a. ACCP
    b. ACPE
    c. APhA
    d. ASHP

71. In what drug classification does estradiol belong?
    a. Antibiotic
    b. Beta-blocker
    c. Hormone
    d. NSAID

72. How many milligrams of epinephrine do you need to prepare 10 mL of a 1:250 epinephrine solution?
    a. 0.00004
    b. 0.04
    c. 40
    d. 400

73. Which of the following is not a required text in a pharmacy?
    a. A copy of the Controlled Substance Act
    b. NF
    c. PDR
    d. USP

74. How any tablets should be dispensed on the following prescription?
    Flagyl 250 2-week supply
    i tab po qid c food for 2 wk for both patient and partner. No alcohol
    a. 14
    b. 28
    c. 56
    d. 112

75. Which of the following medications is not used to treat angina?
    a. Isosorbide dinitrate
    b. Isosorbide mononitrate
    c. Lisinopril
    d. Nitroglycerin

76. What is the generic name for Augmentin?
    a. Amoxicillin-clavulanate
    b. Ampicillin-sulbactam
    c. Piperacillin-tazobactam
    d. Ticarcillin-clavulanate

77. Which of the following are the two most common floor stocks large-volume parenterals?
    a. D5W and 0.45 NS
    b. D5W and 0.9% NS
    c. D5W and sterile water for injection
    d. 0.9% NS and sterile water for injection

78. What is the gross profit for a prescription of 100 tablets of Zoloft 50 mg with an acquisition cost of $172.44/100 tablets, an AWP of $215.55/100 tabs, and a retail price of $226.50?
    a. −$10.95
    b. $10.95
    c. $43.11
    d. $54.06

79. Which of the following drugs is not a bronchodilator?
    a. Albuterol
    b. Ipratropium bromide
    c. Salmeterol
    d. Theophylline

80. Which of the following medications should be tapered off at discontinuation?
    a. Fexofenadine
    b. INH
    c. Prednisone
    d. SMZ-TMP

81. What group does Medicare not cover?
    a. Dialysis patients
    b. Disabled patients
    c. Infant patients
    d. Senior citizens

82. A 143-lb patient is to receive nitroprusside 50 mg in 250 mL of an IV solution. The patient is to receive 5 mcg/kg/min. How many mg/hr will the patient receive?
    a. 4.29
    b. 19.5
    c. 42.9
    d. 19,500

83. Which of the following insulin syringes is not available?
    a. 30 units
    b. 50 units
    c. 100 units
    d. 125 units

84. Which of the following products can be purchased as an exempt narcotic if all conditions outlined by the federal Controlled Substances Act are met?
    a. Phenobarbital
    b. Robitussin AC
    c. Stadol NS
    d. Tussionex

85. What is the maximum weighable amount for a Class A prescription balance?
    a. 0.6 g
    b. 6 g
    c. 60 g
    d. 15 g

86. Which term describes the range between the minimum effective concentration and minimum toxic concentration in a blood concentration curve?
    a. Concentration at site of action
    b. Duration of action
    c. Onset of action
    d. Therapeutic window

87. In what schedule is acetaminophen with codeine placed?
    a. II
    b. III
    c. IV
    d. V

88. What is the sensitivity of a Class A prescription balance?
    a. 0.6 mg
    b. 6.0 mg
    c. 60 mg
    d. 100 mg

89. You have been asked to prepare 1 L of a 2% (w/v) solution. You have a 100% stock solution in stock. How much diluent will be needed?
    a. 2.0 mL
    b. 20 mL
    c. 200 mL
    d. 980 mL

90. To which classification of medication does acyclovir belong?
    a. Analgesic
    b. Antibiotic
    c. Antifungal
    d. Antiviral

91. The average adult dose of Tylenol is 650 mg every 6 hr. If the patient is 5 years old and weighs 54 lb and if Tylenol is available in 160 mg/5 mL elixir, how many milliliters should be given to the patient using Clark's rule?
    a. 5.97
    b. 7.31
    c. 191
    d. 234

92. How many grams are in 600 mL of a 1:200 (w/v) solution of a drug?
    a. 0.03
    b. 0.3
    c. 3
    d. 30

93. How many grams of solute are in 1 L of 5% (w/v) solution?
    a. 0.5
    b. 5
    c. 50
    d. 5,000

94. Which type of syringe is used to administer a liquid medication to a patient?
    a. Adapt-a-Cap
    b. Hypodermic with Luer-Lok tip
    c. Hypodermic with Slip-Tip
    d. Oral syringe

95. What type of filter is used to prevent glass from entering the final solution when drawing from an ampoule?
    a. Depth filter
    b. Filter needle
    c. Filter straw
    d. Final filter

96. In what drug classification is quinapril?
    a. ACE inhibitor
    b. Alpha-blocker
    c. Beta-blocker
    d. Calcium channel blocker

97. To which drug classification does Singulair belong?
    a. Bronchodilator
    b. Corticosteroid
    c. Leukotriene inhibitor
    d. Xanthine derivative

98. Which of the following products is not a combination product?
    a. Bactrim DS
    b. Dyazide
    c. Estrace
    d. Prempro

99. What does VIPPS mean on an Internet pharmacy website?
    a. Value Incentive Pharmacy Practice Site
    b. Value Internet Pharmacy Practice Site
    c. Verified Internet Pharmacy Practice Site
    d. Verified Internet Preferred Provider Site

100. What is the percentage strength of an ointment if one mixes 10 g of hydrocortisone into Aquaphor to make 400 g?
    a. 0.003
    b. 0.03
    c. 0.3
    d. 3.0

101. You have been asked to prepare 20 mL of a drug dilution of 50 mg/mL from a stock solution of 2 g/5 mL. How many milliliters of diluent will be needed?
    a. 2.5
    b. 17.5
    c. 140
    d. 160

102. How much SWFI and D10W are required to make 250 mL of D6W?
    a. SWFI-100 mL; D10W-150 mL
    b. SWFI-167 mL; D10W-83 mL
    c. SWFI-83 mL; D10W-167 mL
    d. SWFI-150 mL; D10W-100 mL

103. What is the route of administration for heparin?
    a. IA
    b. IM
    c. IV
    d. Orally

104. Which of the following is not available as an ophthalmic dosage form?
    a. Ciprofloxacin
    b. Lansoprazole
    c. Latanoprost
    d. Timolol

105. Which of the following drugs does not cause stomach irritation?
    a. Acetaminophen
    b. Aspirin
    c. Corticosteroids
    d. NSAIDs

106. Maxzide is to tablet as Dyazide is to _____.
    a. Caplet
    b. Capsule
    c. Pill
    d. Tablet

107. Which type of medication does not require a prescription?
    a. Investigational medications
    b. Nonproprietary medications
    c. OTCs
    d. Proprietary medications

108. What is the meaning of "DX" on a patient's chart?
    a. Date of birth
    b. Diabetes
    c. Diagnosis
    d. Dispense

109. Rx: Amoxil 250 mg/5 mL
             i tsp tid × 10 days

    How much medication should be dispensed to the patient?
    a. 75 mL
    b. 100 mL
    c. 150 mL
    d. Cannot be determined

110. What is the saline content for a hypertonic saline solution?
    a. 0.2%
    b. 0.45%
    c. 0.9%
    d. 3.0%

111. How much would a patient pay for a prescription with a retail of $30.00 if he or she is to receive a 10% discount?
    a. $3.00
    b. $27.00
    c. $29.70
    d. $33.00

112. Which of the following is required when compounding a suspension?
    a. Emulsifying agent
    b. Flocculating agent
    c. Levigating agent
    d. Surface acting agent

113. What is a purchase order?
    a. A number assigned to a specific pharmacy
    b. A number used to identify an order
    c. A number assigned by the State Boards of Pharmacy
    d. A number that is the same on all orders from a given pharmacy

114. What is the name of a company that administers drug benefit programs?
    a. Employer
    b. HMO
    c. MAC
    d. PBM

115. Which of the following syringes is most likely to cause coring?
    a. 13 G
    b. 16 G
    c. 20 G
    d. 23 G

116. Which document do patients sign when they pick up a prescription covered by a third-party payer?
    a. Exempt narcotic book
    b. Patient register book
    c. Patient compliance book
    d. Signature log

117. Which of the following agencies is responsible for approving hospitals for Medicaid reimbursement?
    a. BOP
    b. DPH
    c. HCFA
    d. JCAHO

118. Which of the following medications is not taken prophylactically?
    a. Amoxicillin
    b. Chloroquine
    c. Propranolol
    d. INH

119. What is the infusion rate in milliliters per hour if 500 mL is infused over 4 hr?
    a. 100
    b. 125
    c. 500
    d. 2,000

120. The pharmacist has 15% (w/v) dextrose solution. How much dextrose is in a 1-L bag of this solution?
    a. 150 g
    b. 500 g
    c. 150 kg
    d. 300 g

121. How does air blow in a horizontal laminar flow hood?
    a. Away from the operator
    b. Down toward the work area
    c. Toward the operator
    d. Up toward the HEPA filter

122. What would be the route of administration for Mycelex troches?
    a. Buccal
    b. Oral
    c. Sublingual
    d. Topical

123. Which of the following is not a medical doctor?
    a. Chiropractor
    b. Ophthalmologist
    c. Psychiatrist
    d. Veterinarian

124. What condition can be treated by PTU and methimazole?
    a. Diabetes
    b. Estrogen replacement
    c. Hyperthyroidism
    d. Hypothyroidism

125. How many milligrams are in Nitrostat 1/150 gr?
    a. 0.65
    b. 0.4
    c. 0.325
    d. 0.1625

126. A patient has presented the following prescription to the pharmacy:
    Rx: Timoptic   .25% 15 mL
            Signa: i gtt ou bid

    Which of the following interpretations of the signa is correct?
    a. Instill one drop in each ear twice per day
    b. Instill one drop in each eye twice per day
    c. Instill one drop in left eye twice per day
    d. Instill one drop in left ear twice per day

127. What is the generic name for Zithromax?
    a. Azithromycin
    b. Clarithromycin
    c. Dirithromycin
    d. Erythromycin estolate

128. Which classification of drugs has interactions with many foods and OTC products?
     a. MAOIs
     b. MOAs
     c. SSRIs
     d. TCAs

129. What is the brand name for propoxyphene?
     a. Darvon
     b. Demerol
     c. Dilaudid
     d. Dolophine

130. What type of medication is infused using a PCA?
     a. Analgesics
     b. Antibiotics
     c. Antineoplastic agents
     d. TPN

131. Which antidote is used to treat an overdose of Lanoxin?
     a. Digibind
     b. Digitalis
     c. Digitoxin
     d. Digoxin

132. How many pounds would an 80-kg individual weigh?
     a. 36.36
     b. 120
     c. 176
     d. None of the above

133. Which of the following statements is true?
     a. Class A balances only have one pan to weigh powders
     b. There is no need to place weights on it because the weights are adjusted internally
     c. The weight goes on the right pan and the powder goes on the left pan
     d. The weight goes on the left pan and the powder goes on the right pan

134. Which type of pharmacy is located in a hospital and services patients within the hospital and ancillary areas?
     a. Clinical pharmacy
     b. Inpatient pharmacy
     c. Nursing pharmacy
     d. Outpatient pharmacy

135. What is the percentage of a 1:25 (w/v) solution?
     a. 0.04
     b. 0.4
     c. 4.0
     d. 40.0

136. Which pharmacy law prevents a prescription drug plan from requiring participants to use mail order pharmacy only?
     a. Any Willing Provider Law
     b. Freedom of Choice law
     c. Prescription Drug Equity Act
     d. Sherman Antitrust Amendments

137. Which of the following medications does not require a child-resistant container?
     a. APAP with codeine
     b. Hydrochlorothiazide
     c. Levothyroxine
     d. Nitroglycerin

138. On which schedule are anabolic steroids?
     a. II
     b. III
     c. IV
     d. V

139. To which drug classification does carbamazepine belong?
     a. Antibiotic
     b. Anticonvulsant agent
     c. Anti-Parkinson agent
     d. Antipsychotic agent

140. Which of the following is the generic name for Prozac?
     a. Fluoxetine
     b. Flunisolide
     c. Fluocinonide
     d. Fluticasone

Assisting the Pharmacist in Serving Patients

FEDERAL, STATE, OR PRACTICE SITE REGULATIONS, CODES OF ETHICS, AND STANDARDS PERTAINING TO THE PRACTICE OF PHARMACY

Ethics: a philosophy of doing the correct action. Good versus evil.

CODE OF ETHICS FOR PHARMACY TECHNICIANS

Preamble

Pharmacy technicians are health care professionals who assist pharmacists in providing possible care for patients. The principles of this code, which apply to pharmacy technicians working in any and all settings, are based on the application and support of the moral obligations that guide the pharmacy profession in relationships with patients, health care professionals, and society.

Principles

- A pharmacy technician's first consideration is to ensure the health and safety of the patient and to use knowledge and skills to the best of his or her ability in serving others.
- A pharmacy technician supports and promotes honesty and integrity in the profession, which includes a duty to observe the law, maintain the highest moral and ethical conduct at all times, and uphold the ethical principles of the profession.
- A pharmacy technician assists and supports the pharmacist in the safe, efficacious, and cost-effective distribution of health services and health care resources.
- A pharmacy technician respects and values the abilities of pharmacists, colleagues, and other health care professionals.
- A pharmacy technician maintains competency in his or her practice, and continually enhances his or her professional knowledge and expertise.
- A pharmacy technician respects and supports the confidentiality of a patient's records and discloses pertinent information only with proper authorization.
- A pharmacy technician never assists in the dispensing, promoting, or distribution of medications or medical devices that are not of good quality or do not meet the standards required by law.
- A pharmacy technician does not engage in any activity that will discredit the profession, and will expose, without fear or favor, illegal or unethical conduct in the profession.
- A pharmacy technician associates with and engages in the support of organizations that promote the profession of pharmacy through the utilization and enhancement of pharmacy technicians.

PHARMACY LAW

NOTE: This review book examines federal laws affecting the practice of law. Federal law takes precedence over state law unless the state law is stricter than the federal law, in which case the state law takes precedence. Every pharmacy technician must be aware of the state laws affecting the practice of pharmacy in his or her state.

PURE FOOD AND DRUG ACT 1906
Enacted in 1906 to prohibit the interstate transportation or sale of adulterated and misbranded food or drugs.

FOOD, DRUG AND COSMETIC ACT OF 1938 (FDCA 1938)
Food and Drug Administration (FDA) was created under this act and required that all new drug applications be filed with FDA. The FDCA 1938 clearly defined adulteration and misbranding of drugs and food products.

Adulteration
1. Consisting "in whole or in part of any filthy, putrid, or decomposed substance."
2. Ones "prepared, packed, or held under unsanitary conditions."
3. Prepared in containers "composed, in whole or in part, of any poisonous or deleterious substance."
4. Contains unsafe color additives.
5. Claims to be or represented as drugs recognized "in an official compendium," but differing in strength, quality or purity of the drugs.

Misbranding
1. Labeling that is "false or misleading in any particular."
2. Packaging that does not bear a label containing the name and place of business of the manufacturer, packer, or distributor or an accurate quantity of contents; conspicuously and clearly labeled with information by the act.
3. Fails to carry a "Warning—May be habit forming," if the product is habit forming.
4. Fails to "bear the established name of the drug, and in case it carries more than two or more active ingredients, the quantities of the ingredients, the amount of alcohol and also including—whether active or not—the established name and quantity of certain other substances described in the act."
5. Failure to label "adequate directions for use" or "adequate warnings against use in certain pathological conditions."
6. Are "dangerous to health when used in the dosage or manner or duration prescribed, recommended or suggested in the labeling."

DURHAM–HUMPHREY ACT OF 1951
An amendment to FDCA 1938 requiring all products to have adequate directions for use unless they contain the federal legend: "Caution: Federal law prohibits dispensing without a prescription."
1. Separated drugs into two categories: legend and nonlegend (OTC). A legend drug requires a prescription, while an over-the-counter (OTC) does not require a prescription. Prescription medications require the supervision of a physician.
2. Allows verbal prescriptions over the telephone
3. Allows refills to be called in from a physician's office

KEFAUVER-HARRIS AMENDMENT OF 1963
Kefauver-Harris requires that all medication on the market in the United States be pure, safe, and effective.

COMPREHENSIVE DRUG ABUSE PREVENTION AND CONTROL ACT OF 1970
The Drug Enforcement Agency (DEA) was created and placed under the supervision of the Department of Justice. Controlled Substances are placed in one of five schedules (classification or category) based on a potential for abuse and accepted medical use in the United States.

Schedule I
No accepted medical use in the United States and possesses an extremely high potential for abuse.

Examples of schedule I narcotics:
- Crack cocaine
- Crystal methamphetamine
- Ecstasy
- Hashish
- Hash oil

- Heroin
- LSD
- Marijuana
- Mescaline
- Opium
- PCP
- Peyote
- Psilocybin
- "Roofies"

Schedule II

Has a medical use, but has a high abuse potential with severe psychic or physical dependency (see Table 2-1).

Schedule III

Have accepted medical use and the abuse is potential less than Schedules I and II (see Table 2-2).

Schedule IV

Abuse potential is less than Schedule III, but may lead to limited physical or psychologic dependence.

Schedule V

Abuse potential is less than Schedule IV and includes exempt narcotics.

DEA Registration

Every facility that dispenses controlled substances must be registered with the DEA. The pharmacy registers with the DEA by submitting a DEA Form 224. The pharmacy must renew this registration every 3 years.

Ordering and Receipt

Schedule II

Schedule II medications are ordered by properly completing a DEA Form 222 (a triplicate order form). It must be signed by the individual in whose name the DEA registration is listed. A DEA Form 222 is valid only for 60 days. A DEA Form 222 must be completed either by typewriter, pen, or indelible pencil. Only one item per line, with a maximum of 10 different items per form are permitted. The number of lines ordered must be totaled on the bottom of the DEA Form 222. Unused forms must be kept secure in a location in the pharmacy. On receipt

TABLE **2-1 Examples of Schedule II Medications**

BRAND NAME	GENERIC NAME
Adderall	amphetamine/dextroamphetamine
Amytal	amobarbital
Cocaine	cocaine
Codeine	codeine
Demerol	meperidine
Dexedrine	dextroamphetamine
Dilaudid	hydromorphone
Dolophine	methadone
Duragesic	fentanyl
Morphine Sulfate	morphine
Numorphan	oxymorphone
OxyContin	oxycodone
Percocet	acetaminophen and oxycodone
Percodan	aspirin and oxycodone
Ritalin	methylphenidate
Seconal	secobarbital
Tylox	acetaminophen and oxycodone

TABLE **2-2** Examples of Schedule III-V Medications

BRAND	GENERIC	SCHEDULE
Ambien	zolpidem	IV
Anexsia	acetaminophen + hydrocodone	III
Ativan	lorazepam	IV
Bontril	phendimetrazine	III
Butisol	butabarbital	IV
Capital and codeine	acetaminophen + codeine	III
Cylert	pemoline	IV
Dalmane	flurazepam	IV
Darvocet	acetaminophen + propoxyphene	IV
Darvon	propoxyphene	IV
Empirin + Codeine	aspirin + codeine	III
Equanil	meprobamate	IV
Fastin	phentermine	IV
Fioricet + Codeine	acetaminophen + butalbital + caffeine + codeine	IV
Fiorinal	aspirin + butalbital + caffeine	IV
Fiorinal + Codeine	aspirin + butalbital + caffeine + codeine	IV
Halcion	triazolam	IV
Hycodan	hydrocodone	III
Hycomine Compound	hydrocodone + chlorpheniramine + phenylephrine + APAP + caffeine	III
Hycotuss	guaifenesin + hydrocodone	III
Klonopin	clonazepam	IV
Librium	chlordiazepoxide	IV
Lomotil	diphenoxylate + atropine	IV
Lorcet	acetaminophen + hydrocodone	III
Lortab	acetaminophen + hydrocodone	III
Noctec	chloral hydrate	IV
Phenobarbital	phenobarbital	IV
Restoril	temazepam	IV
Robitussin AC	guaifenesin + codeine	IV
Soma with Codeine	carisoprodol + codeine	III
Sonata	zaleplon	IV
Stadol	butorphanol	IV
Talwin	pentazocine	IV
Talwin NX	pentazocine-naloxone	IV
Tenuate	diethylpropion	IV
Tranxene	clorazepate	IV
Tussionex	chlorpheniramine + hydrocodone	III
Tylenol with Codeine	acetaminophen + codeine	III
Valium	diazepam	IV
Vicodin	acetaminophen + hydrocodone	III
Vicoprofen	ibuprofen + hydrocodone	III
Wygesic	acetaminophen + propoxyphene	IV
Xanax	alprazolam	IV

of medication, the number of packages must be recorded on a retained copy of 222, and dated and signed by the pharmacist (Figure 2-1). The pharmacist may not use ditto marks for the date or signature. The invoice or packing slip in addition to the completed DEA Form 222 must be retained in a secure location of the pharmacy for a minimum of 2 years.

Schedule III-V

Schedule III, IV, and V may be ordered by any method (written, fax, or verbal). After receipt, the invoice or packing slip must be dated, signed, stamped with a red C, and retained in a secure location in the pharmacy for a minimum of 2 years.

See Reverse of PURCHASER'S Copy for Instructions	No order form may be issued for schedule I and II substances unless a completed application form has been received. (21 CFR 1306-04).		OMB APPROVAL No. 1117-0010	
To: (*Name of Supplier*)	STREET ADDRESS		TO BE FILLED IN BY PURCHASER	
CITY and STATE	DATE	NATIONAL DRUG CODE		

L i n e No	No. of Packages	Size of Package	TO BE FILLED IN BY PURCHASER — Name of Items	NATIONAL DRUG CODE	No. of Packages Received	Date Received
1						
2						
3						
4						
5						
6						
7						
8						
9						
10						

◄ LAST LINE COMPLETED   (*MUST BE 10 OR LESS*)   SIGNATURE OF PURCHASER OR ATTORNEY OR AGENT

Date issued   DEA Registration No.   Name and Address of Registrant

Schedules

Registered no a   No. of the Order Form

DEA Form.222
(Oct. 1902)

U.S. OFFICIAL ORDER FORMS - SCHEDULES I & II
DRUG ENFORCEMENT ADMINISTRATION
PURCHASER'S Copy 3

Fig. 2-1 DEA 222 Sample Form.

Retention of DEA Records

Maintained for a minimum of 2 years, kept separately from other invoices, and kept readily retrievable. Readily retrievable refers to those that are separated from normal business records or easily identifiable by an asterisk, a red line, or visually identifiable. A red C must be stamped on Schedules III-V if they are filed with other invoices. They must be provided to a DEA representative within 72 hr after request.

Defective forms

A form is considered such if it is incomplete, illegible, or shows signs of alteration, erasure, or change. Must be kept for a minimum of 2 years and be readily retrievable.

Inventories

Initial Inventory

Complete and accurate inventory of all controlled substances before the opening of the first day of business for a pharmacy.

Biennial Inventory

Inventory taken every 2 years after initial inventory is taken. An exact count for Schedule II and estimated count for Schedule III-V must be performed. Records must be kept for a minimum of 2 years.

Perpetual Inventory

Shows controlled substances received by the facility, supplied to other locations, returned to pharmacy, and dispensed to patients. A perpetual inventory will show the actual number of units of a drug at a particular moment in time.

Return of controlled substances

Controlled substances can only be returned between DEA registrants. The DEA Form 222 is the official document for the transfer of Schedule II medications. Controlled substances cannot be returned from long-term care facilities because these facilities do not have a DEA number.

Destruction of outdated or damaged controlled substances

A DEA Form 41 must be submitted to DEA indicating the name, strength, and quantities of controlled substances, the date of destruction, the method of destruction, and witnesses present for the destruction. A retail pharmacy may submit one DEA Form 41 per year. Hospitals may have "blanket authorization."

Theft of controlled substances

After the discovery of a theft of controlled substances, the pharmacy must notify the nearest DEA diversion office, notify local police, and complete a DEA Form 106. The pharmacy must send the original copy of the DEA Form 106 to the DEA and retain one copy for its records.

Filling of controlled substances

Schedule II: Prescription can be either handwritten or computer generated but must be signed in ink by the physician with no allowable refills. A partial filling is allowed if the remaining quantity is available to the patient within 72 hr. A new prescription must be issued by the prescriber if additional quantities are to be provided after 72 hr. The pharmacist should notify the physician if the balance cannot be provided to the patient.

Emergency Filling of Schedule II Drugs

An oral prescription can be issued to a pharmacy under the following conditions:
1. Pharmacist must make a good faith attempt to identify the physician.
2. Limited to a quantity to treat the patient during this period.
3. Pharmacist must reduce order to writing.
4. Physician must write a prescription for this emergency quantity and the pharmacy must receive it within 7 days of the oral order.

Schedule II Drugs in Long-Term Care Facilities

A pharmacy may accept a facsimile of a Schedule II drug prescription for patients in a long-term care facility as the original written prescription and must be retained as such. A partial filling of Schedule II prescriptions for residents in a long-term care facility or patients diagnosed with a terminal illness is permitted. They may be filled partially for up to 60 days from the date of issue of the prescription, unless the prescription is discontinued sooner. A notation must be made on the prescription such as "long-term care facility patient" or "terminally ill patient." A failure to make this notation is a violation of federal law.

Schedule III-V

A prescription may be handwritten or computer generated by a physician's office, but must be signed by the physician in ink. The physician's office may telephone a schedule III-V prescription in to the pharmacy or fax one depending on state law. A patient may receive up to five refills within 6 months of the date the prescription was written if authorized. Partial fillings are permitted as long as refills are indicated on the prescription; do not exceed the total quantity prescribed by the physician; and no partial filling occurs after 6 months of the original date of the prescription.

Exempt Narcotics

Select cough and antidiarrhea prescription items can be purchased by an individual, if permitted by state law. The quantity dispensed must be in the original manufacturer's container and not exceed the quantity established by law. The purchaser must be at least 18 years of age and complete the Exempt Narcotic Book with the following information: date purchased, name of purchaser, address of purchaser, name of product and quantity purchased, price of transaction, and pharmacist's signature. There is a limit of one container in a 48-hr period.

POISON PREVENTION PACKAGING ACT OF 1970

The Poison Prevention Packaging Act of 1970 was enacted to reduce the accidental poisoning in children. The Act requires that most OTC and legend drugs be packaged in child-resistant containers. A child-resistant container is one that cannot be opened by 80% of the children younger than age 5, but can be opened by 90% of adults.

Exceptions for Child-Resistant Containers
- Single-time dispensing of product in noncompliant container as ordered by the prescriber.
- Single-time or blanket dispensing of product in noncompliant container as requested by patient or customer in a signed statement.
- One noncompliant size of the OTC product for elderly or handicapped patients provided that they contain the warning "This package for households without young children," or "Package Not Child Resistant."
- Drugs dispensed to institutionalized patients provided that these are to be administered by an employee of an institution.
- Medications not requiring child-resistant containers:
  Betamethasone with no more than 12.6 mg per package
  Erythromycin ethylsuccinate tablets in packages containing no more than 16 g
  Inhalation aerosols
  Mebendazole tablets with no more than 600 mg per package
  Methylprednisolone tablets with no more than 85 mg per package
  Oral contraceptives taken cyclically in the manufacturer's dispensing package
  Pancrelipase preparations
  Powdered anhydrous cholestyramine
  Powdered colestipol up to 5 g per packet
  Prednisone tablets with no more than 105 mg per package
  Sodium fluoride tablets with no more than 264 mg of sodium fluoride per package
  Sublingual and chewable isosorbide dinitrate, in dosages of 10 mg or less
  Sublingual nitroglycerin tablets

OCCUPATIONAL HEALTH AND SAFETY ACT (OSHA) OF 1970
OSHA ensures a safe and healthful workplace for all employees. The law was developed to ensure job safety and health standards for employees, maintain a reporting system for job-related injuries and illness, and reduce hazards in the workplace and to conduct audits to ensure compliance with the Act. Its impact on pharmacy is addressed to air contaminants, flammable and combustible liquids, eye and skin protection, and hazard communication standard. OSHA requires usage of Material Safety Data Sheets (MSDS) which are to be provided by the seller of a particular product to the purchaser. OSHA issues *Guidelines for Cytoxic (Antineoplastic) Drugs*.

DRUG LISTING ACT OF 1972
Each drug is assigned a specific 11-digit number to identify it. This number is known as an NDC (National Drug Code) number. The first five digits identify the manufacturer, the next four digits identify the drug product, and the final two digits represent the package size and packaging.

ORPHAN DRUG ACT OF 1983
Orphan drugs are medications for which there are fewer than 200,000 cases in the world. The law provides tax incentives and exclusive licensing for products of manufacturers to develop and market orphan medications.

DRUG PRICE COMPETITION AND PATENT-RESTORATION ACT OF 1984
Encourages the creation of both generic and new medications by streamlining the process for generic drug approval and by extending patent licenses.

PRESCRIPTION DRUG MARKETING ACT OF 1987
- Prohibits the reimportation of a drug into the United States by anyone except the manufacturer. Prohibits the sale or distribution of samples to anyone other than those licensed to prescribe them. *Currently being reconsidered by Congress.*
- Requires the following label to appear on all medications to be administered to animals, "Caution: Federal law restricts this drug to use by or on an order of a licensed veterinarian."

OMNIBUS BUDGET RECONCILIATION ACT OF 1987 (OBRA-87)

OBRA 87 established extensive revisions regarding Medicare and Medicaid Conditions of Participation regarding long-term care facilities and pharmacy. These include:
- resident's drug regimen must be free of unnecessary medications,
- antipsychotic drugs are not to be used unless the patient has a specific condition,
- patients requiring antipsychotic medication must be documented,
- patients receiving antipsychotic medications must receive gradual dose tapering,
- behavioral modification and drug holidays in order to see if the medication may be discontinued,
- residents are to be free of any significant medication errors,
- routine and emergency drugs must be provided to patients,
- long-term care facilities must have the services of a consultant pharmacist,
- medications must be labeled according to accepted professional principles,
- medications must be stored in locked compartments at the proper temperature according to both federal and state laws.

ANABOLIC STEROIDS CONTROL ACT OF 1990

Resulted in harsher penalties for the abuse of anabolic steroids and their misuse by athletes.

OMNIBUS BUDGET RECONCILIATION ACT OF 1990 (OBRA-90)

- Requires that manufacturers provide the lowest prices to any customer or Medicaid patient by rebating each state Medicaid agency the difference between their average price and the lowest price.
- Requires that an "offer to counsel" is made to every patient and drug utilization review is performed for every patient. A failure to do so may result in the loss of Medicaid funds.
- Authorizes government-sponsored demonstration projects relating to the provision of pharmaceutical care. Patient profiles are to be maintained for all patients

FDA SAFE MEDICAL DEVICES ACT OF 1990

Requires all medical devices be tracked and records maintained for durable medical equipment, such as infusion pumps.

AMERICANS WITH DISABILITIES ACT (ADA) 1990

ADA prevents discrimination of potential employees who may possess a disability. The business must make "a reasonable accommodation" for the potential employee.

RESOURCE CONSERVATION AND RECOVERY ACT

The Environmental Protection Agency (EPA) produced federal guidelines regarding the disposal of hazardous waste. Hazardous waste includes controlled substances. Flushing is no longer an acceptable method of destruction in many states.

FDA MODERNIZATION ACT

Federal drug legend ("Federal law prohibits the dispensing of this medication without a prescription") is now represented by the abbreviation "RX" on the container.

DIETARY SUPPLEMENT HEALTH AND EDUCATION ACT (DSHEA) OF 1994

Herbal products are dietary supplements rather than drugs. The manufacturers of supplements are allowed to make claims with regard to general health promotion, but not disease claims. According to the DSHEA, herbal products must:
1. be labeled as a dietary supplement
2. identify all ingredients by name
3. list the quantity of each ingredient
4. identify the plant and plant part from which the ingredient is derived
5. comply with any standards set by an official compendium
6. meet the quality, purity, and compositional specification

Guidelines are set to prevent adulteration and must follow Good Manufacturing Practices.

HEALTH INSURANCE PORTABILITY AND ACCOUNTABILITY ACT (HIPAA) OF 1996

- The purpose of the law was to improve portability and continuity of health coverage in the group and individual markets; combat waste, fraud, and abuse in health insurance and health care delivery; promote the use of medical savings accounts; improve access to long-term care services and coverage; and simplify the administration of health insurance.
- HIPAA requires that health care providers insure that patient confidentiality be maintained. HIPAA set boundaries on the use and the disclosure of protected health information and requires that patients be informed on how their protected information will be used. The information protected through HIPAA includes:
  1. Any information related to past, present, or future physical and mental health.
  2. Past, present, or future payments for health services received.
  3. Specific care the patient received, is receiving, or is willing to receive.
  4. Any information that can identify the patient as the individual receiving the care.
  5. Any information that someone could reasonably use to identify a patient as receiving care.
- There are two parts of HIPAA:
  Title I—Insurance Reform. Protects health insurance coverage for workers and families when they change or lose their jobs.
  Title II—Administrative Simplification. Established electronic transaction and Code Set Standards; required Health Information Privacy.

ACCUTANE 2002

All Accutane prescriptions must bear a yellow qualification sticker to be filled. The following conditions must be met:
- Two negative pregnancy tests with the first being used as a screening test and the second to confirm the results.
- A commitment to use two effective birth control methods for one month before, during, and one month after treatment has ceased.
- Sign a patient information/consent form about Accutane and its possible effects.
- Receive information and be encouraged to participate in the Accutane Survey.
- After the initial filling, female patients must have a negative pregnancy test and receive counseling before being issued a new prescription.
- Prescriptions must be filled within 7 days of receipt of the yellow qualification sticker.
- Phoned in prescriptions will not be honored, and requests for refills are not permitted.

ANY WILLING PROVIDER LAW

Allows any pharmacy to participate in a prescription drug benefit plan as long as the pharmacy agrees to the terms and conditions of the plan.

FREEDOM OF CHOICE LAW

Allows a member of a prescription drug plan to select any pharmacy for their pharmacy benefit as long as the pharmacy agrees to the terms and conditions of the plan.

FREEDOM OF CHOICE WITH REGARD TO LONG-TERM CARE

Long-term care residents may choose an outside pharmacy for their medications if the pharmaceutical service is not provided under their contract. A long-term care facility may refuse admission to a resident if the resident refuses to use the drug distribution system already in place. Long-term care facilities may establish policies to protect patients and require outside pharmacies to agree to policies.

PRESCRIPTION DRUG EQUITY LAW

Prohibits a prescription drug plan from requiring mail order prescription drug coverage without also providing non–mail order coverage.

MEDICARE DRUG, IMPROVEMENT, AND MODERNIZATION ACT OF 2003 (MPDIMA)

- Provides for a voluntary prescription drug benefit to Medicare beneficiaries
- Adds preventive medical benefits to senior citizens.

- Lowers the reimbursement rates for Medicare durable medical equipment.
- Creates a national competitive bidding program for durable medical equipment in 2007.
- Changes the way Medicare will pay for outpatient Part B drugs.
- Allows for a voluntary Medicare-approved discount card program to begin in June 2004.
- A new Medicare Part D prescription plan will be added in 2006 and will allow beneficiaries to enroll in either regional or national based insurance plans.

REGULATORY AGENCIES

Bureau of Alcohol, Tobacco, and Firearms (ATF)

- Sets regulations regarding the purchase of tax-free alcohol. Tax-free alcohol may be used in hospitals and clinics.

Centers for Medicare and Medicaid Service (CMS)

- Oversees Medicare and Medicaid; establishes conditions for a facility to be reimbursed for services rendered.

Drug Enforcement Agency (DEA)

- Enforces compliance with the Controlled Substance Act. This includes placing medications into the appropriate schedule, monitoring records and reports of controlled substances, registration of pharmacies, issuance of DEA Forms 222 and 41, and monitoring the destruction of controlled substances.

Environmental Protection Agency (EPA)

- Sets guidelines for the disposal of hazardous waste (includes disposal of controlled substances)

Food and Drug Administration (FDA)

- Assures that all pharmaceutical products are pure, safe, and effective. Reviews information supplied on MedWatch Forms. Can issue drug recalls if product is adulterated or misbranded (will perform post-recall audits to verify that manufacturers, wholesalers, pharmacists, and customers have been notified and appropriate action has occurred). Regulates the distribution of patient package inserts, repackaging of medications. Reviews new drug applications and investigational new drug applications.

Institutional Review Boards

- A board, committee, or other group designated by an institution to approve biomedical research in accordance with the FDA.

Joint Commission on Accreditation of Healthcare Organizations (JCAHO)

- Addresses quality of patient care and patient safety. Establishes standards and accredits the following health care providers: hospitals, home health care agencies, home infusion providers, long-term care pharmacies, ambulatory infusion pharmacies, home medical equipment and home oxygen providers, ambulatory surgical centers, community health centers, college and prison health care centers, nursing homes and subacute facilities, assisted living facilities, clinical laboratories, behavioral health organizations, alcohol and chemical dependency centers, health care networks, and preferred provider organizations. Accreditation is voluntary. JCAHO has been granted "deemed status" for participation in Medicare. This status states that the institution has met the Medicare Conditions of Participation and can receive Medicare funding. The institution does not need to meet annual Medicare surveys by state inspectors.

National Association of the Boards of Pharmacy (NABP)

- Composed of all State Boards of Pharmacy. Has no regulatory authority, but meets to discuss current trends and issues in pharmacy that affect the practice of pharmacy.

State Boards of Pharmacy (BOP)

- Regulatory state agency that oversees the practice of pharmacy in a given state. Clearly defines regulations affecting pharmacy, the roles, duties, and expectations of pharmacists and pharmacy technicians in that state. Has the ability to discipline pharmacies, pharmacists, and possibly pharmacy technicians for improper behavior.

PHARMACEUTICAL, MEDICAL, AND LEGAL DEVELOPMENTS THAT AFFECT THE PRACTICE OF PHARMACY

- American Society of Health System Pharmacists's "White Paper on Pharmacy Technicians"
- Computerization: method of processing, storing, and transferring prescriptions
- Online adjudication: method of billing insurance companies and ensuring payment for services
- Faxes: method of transmitting prescriptions/medication orders from a physician's office to a pharmacy
- Personal digital assistants (i.e., PDAs): method of transmitting prescriptions to a pharmacy.
- Medicare Drug, Improvement, and Modernization Act of 2003 (MDIMA)
- Drug Reimportation Reform: currently being examined
- Orphan Drug Law: promotes development of pharmaceutical products with small markets
- Reducing the amount of time a drug is covered by a patent, resulting in generic drugs becoming available earlier
- Revising the protocol for the development of AIDS medications
- Process for converting prescription medications to OTC status
- Allowing pharmacists to prescribe in specific situations
- Third-party health care providers
- Automation

STATE-SPECIFIC PRESCRIPTION TRANSFER REGULATIONS

- Technicians must be familiar with their state laws regarding the transfer of prescriptions between pharmacies. Federal law states that controlled substance prescriptions can only be transferred one time between pharmacies. Pharmacy technicians may assist the pharmacist in the transfer of prescriptions between pharmacies. A pharmacy technician may fax a copy of a prescription to another pharmacy under the supervision of a pharmacist.

THERAPEUTIC EQUIVALENCE

- According to the Orange Book, two drugs are therapeutically equivalent if they contain the same active ingredients, the same strength or concentration, the same dosage form, and the same route of administration. They must have the same clinical effect and safety profile.

THERAPEUTIC INTERCHANGE

- A substitution of one medication for another medication that is not generically equivalent but would provide the same therapeutic effect (i.e., substituting one macrolide antibiotic for another macrolide because of price) (Table 2-3).

EPIDEMIOLOGY

Epidemiology is defined as a medical science that deals with the incidence, distribution and control of a disease in a population. It includes the factors that may control the presence or absence of a disease.

RISK FACTORS FOR DISEASE

Age

- **Pediatric patients:** Organ systems may not be fully developed and immune system may not be fully in place.
- **Elderly:** Physiologic changes occur as one ages. These changes include auditory, gastrointestinal, pulmonary, cardiovascular, urinary, hormonal, and body composition changes. Absorption, distribution, metabolism, and elimination processes are affected by age. The elderly can be subdivided into three categories:
  Young-old: 65–74 years of age
  Middle-old: 75–84 years of age
  Old-old: 85 years of age and older

Gender

- An individual's gender may make them more prone to a disease condition or may affect how a drug may work in an individual. Hormone changes have been shown to have an effect on the development of a disease.

TABLE **2-3** **Therapeutic Equivalence Codes**

FDA CODE	DESCRIPTION
A	Drug products that are considered to be therapeutically equivalent to other pharmaceutically equivalent products
AA	Products not presenting bioequivalence problems in conventional dosage forms
AB	Products meeting necessary bioequivalence requirements
AO	Injectable oil solutions that are considered therapeutically equivalent to other pharmaceutically equivalent products
AP	Injectable aqueous solutions
AT	Topical products that are considered therapeutically equivalent to other pharmaceutically equivalent products
B Codes	Drug products that the Food and Drug Administration does not consider at this time to be therapeutically equivalent to other pharmaceutically equivalent products
BC	Controlled-release tablets, controlled capsules, and controlled-released injectables (controlled-release products for which such bioequivalence data are available have been coded AB)
BD	Active ingredients and dosage forms with documented bioequivalence problems
BE	Enteric-coated oral dosage forms (enteric-coated oral dosage forms for which bioequivalence data are available are coded AB)
BP	Active ingredients and dosage forms with potential bioequivalence problems
BR	Suppositories or enemas for systemic use
BS	Products having standard deficiencies
BT	Topical products
BX	Insufficient data: these products are presumed to be therapeutically not equivalent until adequate information becomes available for full evaluation for therapeutic equivalence

Genetic Factors

- A definitive link between heredity and disease has been shown. Many of the affective disorders may be passed from one generation to another generation. The possibility of developing either hypertension or diabetes is greatly increased in families, where there is a history of the disease. Hemophilia is another disease that is transmitted genetically.

Immune System

- An impaired immune system may make an individual more susceptible to bacterial or fungal infections. HIV and AIDS are examples of diseases that result from an impaired immune system.

Race

- Sickle cell anemia is a disease that targets individuals of African-American descent. African-American males have a higher predisposition toward hypertension, and attention deficit disorder (ADD)/attention deficit hyperactivity disorder (ADHD), and type I diabetes targets Caucasians.

SIGNS AND SYMPTOMS OF DISEASE STATES

Angina

- Chest pain is experienced because of an imbalance between oxygen supply and demand.

Anxiety

- A state of uneasiness characterized by apprehension and worrying about possible events.

Asthma

- Characterized by reversible small airway obstruction, progressive airway inflammation, and increased airway responsiveness from both endogenous and exogenous stimuli. Symptoms include wheezing, dyspnea, and coughing.

Bacterial Infections

- Occur when the body's immune system is unable to resist bacteria. Symptoms of a bacterial infection include a fever greater than 101°F and an increase in white blood cells (>12,000).

Benign Prostatic Hypertrophy
- An enlargement of the prostate of a male as he ages.

Bipolar Disease
- Depressive psychosis, alternating between excessive phases of mania and depression. Mania may be characterized by exhibiting three of the following symptoms: increased need for sleep, distractibility, elevated or irritable mood, excessive involvement in pleasurable activities with a potential for painful consequences, grandiose ideas, increase in activity, pressure to keep talking, and racing thoughts.

Bronchitis
- The lungs' defense mechanisms have been destroyed by cigarette smoke, occupational dusts, fumes, environmental pollution, or bacterial infection. Characterized by a cough that produces a purulent, green, or blood-soaked sputum.

Congestive Heart Failure
- The heart is unable to meet the metabolic needs of its tissues, resulting in the heart pumping less blood than it receives.

Constipation
- The result of low-fiber diets resulting in decreased colon content, increased colon pressure, and decreased propulsive motility.

Depression
- A psychiatric disorder that may be caused by changes in neurotransmitters (such as dopamine, norepinephreine, or serotonin) in the brain. Symptoms include a loss of interest in normal activities, low self-esteem, pessimism, self-pity, weight loss or gain, insomnia, loss of energy, feelings of worthlessness, feeling of guilt, or recurrent thoughts of death or suicide.

Diabetes
- **Gestational diabetes:** Occurs during the second and third trimester of pregnancy. Can be treated with exercise, diet, and insulin.
- **Type I diabetes:** An individual's body is unable to produce insulin and therefore he or she becomes insulin-dependent.
- **Type II diabetes (adult onset):** Individuals who have an impaired insulin secretion and are often insulin-resistant. Treatment includes weight reduction through diet and exercise.
- **Secondary diabetes:** Onset caused by taking various medications, such as oral contraceptives, beta-blockers, diuretics, calcium channel blockers, glucocorticoids, and phenytoin.

Drug-Induced Ulcers
- Ulcers caused by medication such as aspirin, anti-inflammatory agents, corticosteroids, potassium chloride, methotrexate, and iron.

Emphysema
- The destruction of alveoli, walls, or air sacs of the lungs, resulting in an obstruction of the airflow on expiration. May be caused by cigarette smoke, air pollution, occupational exposure, or genetic factors.

Epilepsy
- Abnormal electrical discharges in the cerebral cortex that may result in paroxysmal, recurring seizures.

Fungal Infections
- Infections caused by single-cell organisms that do not have chlorophyll, possess a cell wall, and reproduce by spores. Develop in individuals whose immune system has been compromised by disease, drug therapy, or poor nutrition.

Gastroesophageal Reflux Disease (GERD)

- Characterized by radiating burning or chest pain and the presence of an acid taste.

Hyperlipidemia

- An elevation of one or more lipoprotein levels. May be genetically determined.

Hypertension

- Systolic pressure (cardiac output) is greater than 140 mm Hg and the diastolic pressure (total peripheral resistance) is greater than 90 mm Hg. Disease does not have symptoms.

Hyperthyroidism (Graves Disease)

- An excessive secretion of thyroid hormone characterized by decreased menses, diarrhea, exophthalmos, flushing of the skin, heat intolerance, nervousness, perspiration, tachycardia, and possible weight loss.

Hypothyroidism

- A deficiency of thyroid hormone being secreted by the body, which may be attributed to an iodine deficiency, inflammation of the thyroid gland, or autoimmune destruction of the thyroid gland. Symptoms may include apathy; constipation; decreased heart rate; dry skin; nails or scalp; fatigue; enlarged thyroid; lowered voice pitch; myxedema; puffy face; reduced mental acuity; swelling of the eyelids; enlarged and thickened tongue; and possible weight gain.

Insomnia

- Characterized by the inability to sleep or remain asleep, which may caused by situations, medications, or psychiatric or medical conditions.

Manic Depression

- Mood of extreme excitement, excessive elation, hyperactivity, agitation, and increased psychomotor activity.

Myocardial Infarction

- The heart muscle is deprived of oxygen because of a reduced oxygen supply, and muscle cells die. May be caused by angina, excessive alcohol consumption, dyspnea on exertion, reduced pulmonary vital capacity, cigarette smoking, or atherosclerosis. Symptoms are described as burning tightness or squeezing of the chest, choking, and substernal pain radiating to the neck, throat, jaw, shoulders, and arms.

Obesity

- Individual's total body weight consists of greater fat than is considered normal. For males, it is 25% above the ideal body weight; for females, it is 35%.

Panic Disorders

- Intense anxiety characterized by a sense of fear, apprehension, or a premonition of serious illness or a life-threatening attack.

Schizophrenia

- Chronic psychotic disorder characterized by a retreat from reality, delusions, hallucinations, ambivalence, withdrawal, or regressive behavior.

Stroke

- An interruption of the oxygen supply to a specific area of the brain caused by a rupture or obstruction (clot) of the blood vessel resulting in a loss of consciousness. Complications may include retinopathy, neuropathy, vascular problems, neuropathy, or kidney damage.

Tuberculosis

- A disease affecting the lungs caused by *Mycobacterium tuberculosis* and spread via leukocytes and the lymph in the body. Tuberculosis is spread by respiratory droplets inhaled into the lungs of a person.

Ulcers

- Disorders of the upper gastrointestinal tract caused by excessive acid secretion. Ulcers may be categorized as gastric, which are local excavations of the gastric mucosa occurring more often in men from the Western hemisphere. Duodenal ulcers occur in the duodenum of the intestine and are usually caused by hypersecretion of acid. Stress ulcers develop from the breakdown of the natural mucosal resistance from severe physiologic stress caused by an illness.

Urinary Tract Infections

- Presence of bacteria in the urinary tract with localized symptoms. Symptoms include blood in the urine, fever, and burning sensation.

Viral Infections

- Diseases caused by agents smaller than bacteria, which are normally spread by direct contact, ingestion of contaminated food and water, or inhalation of airborne particles. May be acute, chronic, or slow in nature and the infection may be local or generalized. Symptoms are more severe than bacterial infections and include malaise, myalgia, headaches, chills, or fever.

DRUG INTERACTIONS

DRUG–DRUG INTERACTIONS

- One drug alters the action of another drug and includes addition, antagonism, potentiation, and synergism.
  Addition: The combined effect of two drugs. It is equal to the sum of the effects of each drug taken alone.
  Antagonism: One drug works against the action of another drug.
  Potentiation: One drug increases or prolongs the effect of another drug. The total effect is greater than the sum of the effects of each drug alone (e.g., Vistaril and Demerol).
  Synergism: The joint action of drugs in which their combined effect is more intense or longer in duration than the sum of the two drugs.

DRUG–DISEASE INTERACTIONS

- Various diseases may inhibit the absorption, metabolism, and elimination of different drugs. An example would be taking decongestants if the patient is either hypertensive or diabetic.

DRUG–NUTRIENT INTERACTIONS

- Poor nutrition may affect the metabolism of various drugs. An example of a drug–nutrient interaction occurs when warfarin and vitamin K are taken simultaneously.

DRUG–FOOD INTERACTIONS

1. Improved absorption occurs if the following drugs are taken with a fatty meal: ketoconazole, nitrofurantoin, and griseofulvin.
2. Decreased absorption occurs if the following drugs are taken with food: tetracycline, ciprofloxacin, etidronate, phenytoin, norfloxacin, zidovudine, levothyroxine, and didanosine.
3. Grapefruit juice affects the following drugs metabolized by cytochrome P450: calcium channel blockers, estrogens, cyclosporine, midazolam, and triazolam.
4. Warfarin interacts with food high in vitamin K such as romaine lettuce and spinach. Warfarin users should consult a cardiologist or internist for a list of these products.

DRUG-RELATED PROBLEMS

- An event or situation involving drug therapy that actually or potentially interferes with the optimum outcome. These drug-related problems include an untreated indication, improper drug selection, subtherapeutic dosage, failure to receive a drug, overdosage, and drug use without an indication.

EFFECTS OF PATIENT'S AGE ON DRUG AND NON-DRUG THERAPY

Neonates

- A child's organs are not fully developed until the child is 1 year old. Other factors affecting the amount of drug to be given to a child will depend on the child's age, weight, height, and body surface area.

Geriatrics

- Physiologic changes occur and include optic, auditory, gastrointestinal, pulmonary, cardiovascular, urinary, hormonal, and body composition changes. As an individual ages, the absorption, distribution, metabolism, and elimination will change, affecting the amount of drug and frequency of the dose. Other age-related factors include multiple health issues, lower body weight, and an increase in adverse drug reactions.

DRUG INFORMATION SOURCES INCLUDING PRINTED AND ELECTRONIC REFERENCE MATERIALS

- **Primary literature:** The original reports of scientific, clinical, technical, and administrative research projects.
- **Secondary literature:** General reference books based on primary literature. Includes abstracting services, bibliographic services, and specialized microfiche systems.
- **Tertiary literature:** Condensed works based on primary literature, which include monographs and textbooks.

Books

- **American Hospital Formulary Service Drug Information:** Provides information on uses, interactions, pharmacokinetics, and dosage and administration of drugs, both commercial and experimental.
- **Drug Topics Red Book:** A source of information concerning prices. Sections on emergency information, clinical reference guide, practice management and professional development, pharmacy and health care organizations, drug reimbursement information, manufacturer/wholesalers information, product identification, Rx product listing, OTC/non-drug products listing, and complementary/herbal product referencing. Drug Topics Red Book contains pricing information necessary for third party reimbursement.
- **Goodman and Gilman's: The Pharmacological Basis of Therapeutics:** The book examines the principles of pharmacokinetics as they relate to medications.
- **FDA: Approved Drug Products with Therapeutic Equivalence Evaluations (Orange Book):** Approved drugs for usage in the United States.
- **Drug Facts and Comparisons:** Provides information with regard to brand/generic names, orphan and investigational drugs, drug monographs, drug identification, and dosage calculations. Updated monthly.
- **Handbook on Injectable Drugs:** References the compatibility of various parenteral drugs.
- **Handbook of Non-Prescription Drugs:** OTC reference book.
- **Martindale, The Complete Drug Reference:** International reference book on medications.
- **Merck Index:** A source of chemical substance data.
- **Pharmaceutical Dosage Forms and Drug Delivery Systems:** Discusses dosage forms and delivery systems.
- **Physicians' Desk Reference (PDR):** Compilation of product inserts from the pharmaceutical manufacturers. Contains indexes of manufacturers and product category; generic and trade names; product identification guide; product information; diagnostic product information; and miscellaneous information.
- **Remington's Pharmaceutical Sciences:** Detailed book of the practice of pharmacy.
- **US Pharmacopoeia-National Formulary (USP-NF):** Official compendium of drug monographs setting official standards of pharmaceuticals.
- **USP Dictionary of USAN and International Drug Names**
- **USP Drug Information Vol. I—Drug Information for the Health Care Professional:** Describes medically accepted uses of medications, which include labeled and unlabeled uses of medications.
- **USP Drug Information Vol. II—Advice for the Patient:** This book assists the pharmacist in advising and counseling patients about their medication.
- **USP Drug Information Vol. III—Approved Drug Products and Legal Requirements:** Volume III discusses both state and federal requirements of a medication, which may be include storage and dispensing information.

Pharmacy Journals of Specific Pharmacy Organizations

- **AACP:** American Journal of Pharmaceutical Education
- **AAPS:** Pharmaceutical Research

- **AJHP:** American Journal of Health System Pharmacists
- **APhA:** Journal of American Pharmacists Association; Pharmacy Today
- **ASCP:** The Consultant Pharmacist
- **ASHP:** American Society of Health System Pharmacists
- **NCPA:** America's Pharmacist
- **NPTA:** Today's Technician

Pharmacy Magazines

- Chain Drug Store News
- Drug Topics
- Pharmacy Times
- The Script
- US Pharmacist

PHARMACOLOGY

Drug Nomenclature: Prefix + root word + suffix

ANTIBIOTICS

Sulfonamides: Bacteriostatic

Mechanism of action (MOA): Interfere with PABA and folic acid formation and thus destroy bacteria

Common indications: Urinary tract infections (UTIs), otitis media, ulcerative colitis, lower respiratory infections

Adverse reactions: Photosensitivity resulting in rashes or sunburns, nausea and vomiting, jaundice, blood complications, kidney damage

Special considerations: Avoiding direct sunlight or use sunscreens when exposed. Drink plenty of water to prevent crystallization in the urine. Trimethoprim/sulfamethoxazole infusions need to be stored at room temperature.

EXAMPLES OF SULFONAMIDES

GENERIC NAME	BRAND NAME	DOSAGE FORMS
sulfamethoxazole-trimethoprim	Bactrim or Septra	Oral suspension, tablet, IV
sulfasalazine	Azulfidine	Tablet, enteric-coated tablets, oral suspension
sulfisoxazole	Gantrisin	Tablet, oral suspension, ophthalmic ointment

PENICILLINS

MOA: Prevent bacteria from forming a cell wall

Common indications: Abscesses, meningitis, otitis media, pneumonia, respiratory infections, prophylaxis

Adverse reactions: Diarrhea, hives, rash, wheezing, anaphylaxis

Special considerations: Take on an empty stomach with water; avoid taking with colas or juices

Reconstitution concerns: Amoxicillin can be stored at room temperature but will last 14 days if refrigerated. Augmentin should be refrigerated and will last 10 days. Ampicillin will last 7 days if not refrigerated, but 14 days when refrigerated

EXAMPLES OF PENICILLINS

GENERIC NAME	BRAND NAME	DOSAGE FORMS
amoxicillin	Amoxil, Polymox	Capsule, oral suspension
ampicillin	Omnipen	Capsule, oral suspension
amoxicillin-clavulanate	Augmentin	Capsule, oral solution
dicloxacillin	Dynapen	Oral suspension, oral tablet, chewable tablet
penicillin	Veetids	Tablet, oral suspension

CEPHALOSPORINS

MOA: Prevent bacteria from forming a cell wall
Indications: Dental work, heart and pacemaker procedures, orthopedic surgery, pneumonia, upper respiratory and sinus infection
Adverse reactions: Share the same side effects as penicillins
Special considerations: 10% of population may have a cross-sensitivity to penicillin
Reconstitution concerns: Reconstituted cefaclor, cephalexin, and cefadroxil should be refrigerated and will last for 14 days. Cefuroxime suspension can be stored at either room temperature or refrigerated; will expire in 10 days. Loracarbef can be stored for 14 days at room temperature on reconstitution.

EXAMPLES OF CEPHALOSPORINS

GENERIC NAME	BRAND NAME	DOSAGE FORMS
cefaclor	Ceclor	Capsule, oral suspension, extended release Tablet
cefixime	Suprax	Oral suspension, tablet
cefpodoxime	Vantin	Oral suspension
cefadroxil	Duricef	Capsule, oral suspension, tablet
ceftibuten	Cedax	Oral suspension, capsule
cefuroxime	Ceftin or Zinacef	IM, IV, oral suspension, tablet
cephalexin	Keflex or Keftab	Capsule, oral suspension, tablet
cephradine	Velosef	Capsule

TETRACYCLINES

MOA: Inhibit protein synthesis in bacteria by binding ribosomes
Indications: Acne, chronic bronchitis, Lyme disease, walking pneumonia, prophylaxis for traveler's diarrhea
Adverse reactions: Gastrointestinal, such as nausea and vomiting; photosensitivity to the sun resulting in rashes and sunburns
Special considerations: May bind to antacids and dairy products and therefore decrease the effectiveness of antibiotic. Tetracyclines should be taken several hours apart from antacids and dairy products because of the possibility of chelation. They should not be taken by pregnant women because of possibility of dental birth defects. Children younger than age 9 should not be given tetracyclines. Taking expired tetracycline may result in toxicity and possibly death. Tetracycline injection that has been reconstituted is stable at room temperature for 12 hr. Doxycycline should be protected from light and reconstituted suspension can be stored at room temperature, but will expire in 14 days.

EXAMPLES OF TETRACYCLINES

GENERIC	BRAND	DOSAGE FORMS
doxycycline	Vibramycin	Capsule, IV, oral suspension, tablet
minocycline	Minocin	Capsule, IV, oral suspension, tablets
tetracycline	Achromycin, Sumycin	Capsule, oral suspension, topical

MACROLIDES

MOA: Inhibit protein synthesis by combining with ribosomes.
Indications: Pulmonary infections, chlamydia, *Haemophilus influenza*
Adverse reactions: May cause gastrointestinal distress
Special considerations: Patient should take macrolides with food. Clarithromycin may leave a metallic taste in one's mouth. The first dose of azithromycin is a loading dose, which is twice the normal daily dose
Reconstitution concerns: Reconstituted azithromycin injection is good for 24 hr when refrigerated; oral suspension will last 10 days if refrigerated. Clarithromycin does not need to be refrigerated after reconstitution, but will expire in 14 days. Erythromycin for IV injection must be used within 8 hr of reconstitution.

EXAMPLES OF MACROLIDES

GENERIC	BRAND	DOSAGE FORMS
azithromycin	Zithromax	Capsule, oral suspension
clarithromycin	Biaxin	Granules for oral suspension, film-coated tablet
dirithromycin	Dynabac	Enteric-coated tablet
erythromycin base	Eryc, E-mycin, Ery-tab	Capsule, tablet, enteric-coated tablet, film-coated tablet
erythromycin estolate	Ilosone	Capsule, oral suspension, tablet
erythromycin ethylsuccinate	EES	Oral suspension, tablet, chewable tablet
erythromycin stearate	Erythrocin	Film-coated tablet, IM, IV
erythromycin-sulfisoxazole	Pediazole	Oral suspension

QUINOLONES

MOA: Antagonize the enzyme responsible for collecting and replicating DNA; therefore causing DNA breakage and finally death
Indications: Bone and joint infections, dental work, infectious diarrhea, upper respiratory infections (URIs), and urinary tract infections (UTIs)
Adverse reactions: Nausea and vomiting, joint swelling, dizziness
Special considerations: Antacids interfere with absorption; potentiate the effect of theophylline products and may cause toxicity; phototoxicity; should not be prescribed to individuals younger than age 18 because of possible tendon damage; and should not be given to pregnant women. Ciprofloxacin injection should be protected from light. Ofloxacin injection needs to be protected from light.

EXAMPLES OF QUINOLONES

GENERIC	BRAND	DOSAGE FORMS
cinoxacin	Cinobac	Capsule
ciprofloxacin	Cipro	Tablet, oral suspension, ophthalmic, IM, IV
gatifloxacin	Tequin	Tablet, IM, IV
levofloxacin	Levaquin	IV, tablet
lomefloxacin	Maxaquin	Tablet
moxifloxacin	Avelox, Vigamox	Tablet
norfloxacin	Noroxin	Tablet
ofloxacin	Floxin, Ocuflox	Tablet, IV, ophthalmic

AMINOGLYCOSIDES

MOA: Inhibit bacterial protein synthesis by binding to ribosomal subunits
Indications: Life-threatening infections, sepsis, immunocompromised patients
Adverse reactions: Nephrotoxicity, ototoxicity, tinnitus, permanent deafness
Special considerations: Dosages need to be adjusted for each patient after first dose. Once per day dosing has tendency to reduce toxicities.

EXAMPLES OF AMINOGLYCOSIDES

GENERIC	BRAND	DOSAGE FORMS
gentamicin	Garamycin	Cream, IM, IV, ophthalmic
neomycin	Mycifradin	Tablet, solution, IM, cream, ointment
streptomycin	Streptomycin	IM, IV
tobramycin	Nebcin	IV, ophthalmic

MISCELLANEOUS ANTIBIOTICS

Clindamycin (Cleocin)
• Inhibits protein synthesis

- **Indications:** Acne, dental prophylaxis for penicillin-allergic patients, anaerobic pneumonia, bone infections, female genital infections
- **Adverse reactions:** Bloody diarrhea

Metronidazole (Flagyl)

- Destroys parts of the bacteria's DNA nucleus
- **Indications:** *Trichomonas* infections of vaginal canal, cervix, and male urethra; amebic dysentery, intestinal infections
- **Adverse reactions:** Metallic taste, diarrhea, rash, and "Antabuse-like reaction" when alcohol is consumed. An "Antabuse-like reaction" results in blurred vision, confusion, difficult breathing, the face becoming hot and scarlet, an intense throbbing in the head and neck, and chest pains
- **Special considerations:** Take with food and avoid any form of alcohol 1 day before, during, and 2 days after therapy with metronidazole.

Vancomycin (Vancocin)

Interferes with bacterial wall formation
Indications: Dialysis patients, endocarditis, and staph infections
Adverse reactions: Ototoxicity, nephrotoxicity, and neutropenia
Special considerations: Potential for overusage causing Centers for Disease Control and Prevention to issue specific guidelines for use. Patient needs to be kept hydrated.

ANTIFUNGALS

Fungus: A single-cell organism without chlorophyll, a cell wall is present, and reproduction occurs by spores. Fungal infections occur when immune system has been compromised
MOA: Prevent synthesis of ergosterol and inhibit fungal cytochrome P-450
Adverse reactions: Liver toxicities may develop; therefore liver function tests are recommended. Gastrointestinal distress may occur. Photosensitivity, rashes, and nausea are other common side effects
Special considerations: Antifungals may be used as either topical or systemic agent. Pulse dosing is recommended for nail fungal infections. Consuming a cola before taking itraconazole is recommended. Fatty meals should be taken with griseofulvin. Fluconazole suspension should be refrigerated and will expire in 14 days.

EXAMPLES OF ANTI-FUNGAL AGENTS

GENERIC	BRAND	DOSAGE FORMS
amphotericin B	Amphotec, Fungizone, Amphocin	Oral suspension, IV, topical
butenafine	Mentax	Topical cream
ciclopirox	Loprox	Topical
clotrimazole	Lotrimin	Oral troche, topical, vaginal
clotrimazole/betamethasone	Lotrisone	Cream
fluconazole	Diflucan	IV, tablet, oral suspension
griseofulvin	Grisactin, Fulvicin, Gris-Peg	Capsule, tablet, oral suspension
itraconazole	Sporanox	Capsule, oral suspension
ketoconazole	Nizoral	Tablet, topical cream, shampoo
miconazole	Monistat	Topical and vaginal
nystatin	Nilstat	Tablet, oral suspension, topical, vaginal
sertaconazole	Ertaczo	Cream
terbinafine	Lamisil	Tablet, topical cream, and solution
terconazole	Terazol	Vaginal cream and suppository

ANTIVIRALS

Indications: Cytomegalovirus retinitis, genital herpes, herpes simplex, herpes simplex keratitis, herpes zoster (shingles), influenza prophylaxis, organ transplants, varicella, chicken pox
Adverse reactions: Headaches, nausea, vomiting, diarrhea, constipation, renal disorders
Special considerations: Oral products should be taken with plenty of water. When acyclovir is reconstituted, the injection should be used within 12 hr.

EXAMPLES OF ANTIVIRALS

GENERIC	BRAND	DOSAGE FORMS
acyclovir	Zovirax	Capsule, tablet, oral suspension, IV, ointment
amantadine	Symmetrel	Capsule, syrup
famciclovir	Famvir	Tablet
rimantadine	Flumadine	Tablet, syrup
ribavirin	Virazole	Aerosol inhalant
valacyclovir	Valtrex	Caplet
zanamivir	Relenza	Inhalant

ANTIRETROVIRALS

Indications: Limits the progression of the retrovirus that causes HIV, which may progress to AIDS

NUCLEOSIDE REVERSE TRANSCRIPTASE INHIBITORS (NRTIS)

MOA: Inhibit the release of neuraminidase, a viral enzyme, to prevent the spread of the virus to healthy cells. NRTIs bind and inhibit the action of neuraminidase. This results in the formation of a defective proviral nucleus, which is unable to become part of the host cell's nuclei
Adverse reactions: Nausea, vomiting, peripheral neuropathy

EXAMPLES OF NRTIs

GENERIC	BRAND	DOSAGE FORMS
abacavir	Ziagen	Solution, tablet
didanosine	Videx, Videx EC	Capsule, tablet, powder
emtricitabine	Emtriva	Tablet
lamivudine	Epivir	Tablet, solution
stavudine	Zerit	Capsule, powder
tenofovir	Viread	Tablet
zalcitabine	Hivid	Tablet
zidovudine	Retrovir	Capsule, syrup, IV
zidovudine-lamivudine	Combivir	Tablet
zidovudine-lamivudine-abacavir	Trizivir	Tablet

NON-NUCLEOSIDE TRANSCRIPTASE INHIBITORS (NNRTIS)

MOA: Inhibit the action of neuraminidase by preventing the formation of the proviral DNA
Adverse reactions: Dizziness, headache, rashes, nightmares, hallucinations, and hepatotoxicity
Special considerations: Drug interactions are common; can induce or inhibit the cytochrome P-450 systems; resistance to one NNRTI results in resistance to the others.

EXAMPLES OF NRTIs

GENERIC	BRAND	DOSAGE FORMS
delavirdine	Rescriptor	Capsule, tablet
efavirenz	Sustiva	Capsule
nevirapine	Viramune	Capsule, tablet

PROTEASE INHIBITORS

MOA: Prevent the cleavage of certain HIV protein precursors, which are necessary for the replication of new viruses
Adverse reactions: Redistribution of body fat ("protease paunch," humped back), facial atrophy, breast enlargement, hyperglycemia, hyperlipidemia

EXAMPLES OF PROTEASE INHIBITORS

GENERIC	BRAND	DOSAGE FORMS
fosamprenavir	Lexiva	Tablet
indinavir	Crixivan	Capsule
lopinavir-ritonavir	Kaletra	Solution, capsule
nelfinavir	Viracept	Powder, tablet
ritonavir	Norvir	Solution, capsule
saquinavir	Invirase	Capsule

ANTIHISTAMINES, ANTITUSSIVES, DECONGESTANTS, AND EXPECTORANTS

Antihistamines

MOA: Block the release of histamine (H1) in the respiratory system
Indications: Treatment of allergies, insomnia, rashes, hay fever, dizziness, prophylaxis for drug reactions and allergies
Adverse reactions: Drowsiness, anticholinergic reactions such as drying up of body fluids, possible hyperactivity in children
Special considerations: Antihistamines have synergistic effect with alcohol.

EXAMPLES OF ANTIHISTAMINES

GENERIC	BRAND	DOSAGE FORMS
azelastine	Astelin	Spray
brompheniramine	Dimetapp	Tablet, caplet, syrup
cetirizine	Zyrtec	Tablet
chlorpheniramine	Chlor-Trimeton	Tablet, capsule
clemastine	Tavist	Tablet, syrup
cyproheptadine	Periactin	Tablet, syrup
diphenhydramine	Benadryl	Capsule, tablet, topical, elixir, IV
fexofenadine	Allegra	Tablet
hydroxyzine HCl	Atarax	Tablet, capsule, syrup, IM, IV
hydroxyzine pamoate	Vistaril	Capsule, syrup
loratadine	Claritin	Tablet, syrup
meclizine	Antivert, Bonine	Tablet, capsule, chewable tablet
promethazine	Phenergan	Tablet, syrup, suppository, IM, IV

Antitussives

MOA: Depression of the cough center or suppression of nerve receptors in respiratory system
Indications: Cough suppression
Adverse reactions: CNS depression, nausea, light-headedness
Special considerations: Dextromethorphan interacts with MAO inhibitors; benzonatate should be swallowed, but not chewed.

EXAMPLES OF ANTITUSSIVES

GENERIC	BRAND	DOSAGE FORMS
benzonatate	Tessalon Perles	Capsule
codeine	Codeine	Tablet, elixir
dextromethorphan	Benylin, Delsym, Hold, Robitussin DM	Syrup, lozenges
diphenhydramine	Benadryl	Capsule, tablet, syrup
hydrocodone-homatropine	Hycodan	Syrup, tablet

Decongestants

MOA: Stimulation of the alpha-adrenergic receptors, resulting in consideration the dilated arteries within the nasal mucosa

Indications: Temporary relief of nasal congestion from the common cold, sinusitis, and upper respiratory allergies
Adverse reactions: CNS stimulation, increased blood pressure, increased heart rate, insomnia, anxiety, tremor, rhinitis medicamentosa, and headache
Special considerations: Decongestants should be avoided if patient has diabetes, heart disease, hypertension, hyperthyroidism, prostatic hypertrophy, and Tourette's syndrome.

EXAMPLES OF DECONGESTANTS

GENERIC	BRAND	DOSAGE FORMS
oxymetazoline	Afrin	Nasal drops
phenylephrine	Neo-Synephrine Neo-Synephrine II	Nasal drops and spray, IV
pseudoephedrine	Sudafed	Capsule, tablet, oral solution

Expectorants

MOA: Decrease thickness of mucus by decreasing the viscosity of the liquid
Indications: To remove mucus from both lungs and airway passages when coughing
Adverse reactions: Nausea and vomiting, drowsiness, and gastrointestinal distress
Special considerations: Patient should consume plenty of water while taking medication.

EXAMPLES OF EXPECTORANTS

GENERIC	BRAND	DOSAGE FORMS
guaifenesin	Robitussin, Humibid	Capsule, caplet, liquid, tablet

AFFECTIVE DISORDERS

Anxiety: A state of uneasiness characterized by apprehension and worry about possible events
Indications: To control anxiety contributed from either exogenous or endogenous stress
Adverse reactions: May cause either physical or psychologic dependence, drug accumulation, birth defects if taken during early pregnancy, muscle relaxation, sedation, and depression
Special considerations: Many agents used to treat anxiety are controlled substances; therefore, federal and state controlled substance laws must be obeyed. Antianxiety agents should be tapered on discontinuation.

EXAMPLES OF ANTIANXIETY AGENTS

GENERIC	BRAND	DOSAGE FORMS	CONTROLLED SUBSTANCE
alprazolam	Xanax	Tablet	Yes
amoxapine	Asendin	Tablet	No
buspirone	BuSpar	Tablet	No
chlordiazepoxide	Librium	Capsule, injection	Yes
clorazepate	Tranxene	Capsule, tablet	Yes
diazepam	Valium	Tablet, injection	Yes
lorazepam	Ativan	Tablet, IM, IV	Yes
meprobamate	Equanil	Tablet	Yes
oxazepam	Serax	Capsule, tablet	Yes

DEPRESSION

Characterized by feelings of pessimism, worry, intense sadness, loss of concentration, slowing of mental process, problems with eating and sleeping.

Selective Serotonin Reuptake Inhibitors (SSRIs)

MOA: Block the reuptake of serotonin
Adverse reactions: Nervousness, insomnia, nausea, diarrhea, loss of weight, decreased libido, and ejaculatory disturbances

Indications: Major depression, obsessive-compulsive behavior, anxiety
Special considerations: Delay of onset for SSRIs is 10–21 days; avoidance of alcohol should be avoided. This drug interacts with phenytoin

EXAMPLES OF SSRIs

GENERIC	BRAND	DOSAGE FORMS
citalopram	Celexa	Tablet, liquid
duloxetine	Cymbalta	Capsule
escitalopram	Lexapro	Tablet
fluoxetine	Prozac	Capsule, liquid
fluvoxamine	Luvox	Tablet
paroxetine	Paxil	Tablet
sertraline	Zoloft	Tablet
venlafaxine	Effexor	Tablet, timed-release capsule

Tricyclic Antidepressants (TCA)

MOA: Block reuptake of norepinephrine or serotonin
Indications: Depression, nocturia (bedwetting) in children
Adverse reactions: Cardiotoxic in high doses, postural hypotension in the elderly, drowsiness and anticholinergic effects
Special considerations: Noticeable results may not occur for several weeks.

EXAMPLES OF TCAs

GENERIC	BRAND	DOSAGE FORMS
amitriptyline	Elavil	Tablet, injection
desipramine	Norpramin	Tablet
doxepin	Sinequan, Zonalon	Capsule, oral liquid, cream
imipramine	Tofranil	Capsule, tablet, injection
maprotiline	Ludiomil	Tablet
nortriptyline	Pamelor, Aventyl	Capsule, oral solution
protriptyline	Vivactil	Tablet

Monoamine Oxidase (MAO) Inhibitors

MOA: Inhibit enzymes, which break down catecholamine
Indications: Atypical depression
Adverse reactions: Possible hypertension
Special considerations: If physician changes therapy MAO inhibitor should be discontinued for 2 weeks before new therapy begins. Patient should avoid certain foods containing tyramine (aged cheeses, certain wines, and certain yeast products); MAO inhibitors should not be taken if patient is taking ephedrine, amphetamine, methylphenidate, levodopa, or meperidine.

EXAMPLES OF MAO INHIBITORS

GENERIC	BRAND	DOSAGE FORMS
phenelzine	Nardil	Tablet
selegiline	Eldepryl	Tablet
tranylcypromine	Parnate	Tablet

BIPOLAR DISORDER

Is a depressive psychosis, alternating between excessive phases of mania and depression.
MOA: Not known
Adverse reactions: Bloating and abdominal distress, bloody stools, acne, leucocytosis, hand tremor, increased body weight, polyuria, polydipsia, nocturia, and abnormal development of fetus during pregnancy

Special considerations: Blood levels must be established for patients taking lithium and should be in the range of 0.6–0.8 mg/mL. Salt content must be monitored and alcohol avoided. Carbamazepine interacts with benzodiazepines, cimetidine, corticosteroids, cyclosporine, diltiazem, doxycycline, erythromycin, ethosuximide, isoniazid, MAO inhibitors, oral contraceptives, phenytoin, propoxyphene, theophylline, thyroid medications, TCAs, valproic acid, verapamil, and warfarin.

EXAMPLES OF BIPOLAR AGENTS

GENERIC	BRAND	DOSAGE FORMS
carbamazepine	Tegretol	Tablet, chewable tablet, suspension
divalproex	Depakote	Tablet
lithium	Eskalith, Lithonate	Capsule, tablet
valproic acid	Depakene	Capsule, syrup, IV

PSYCHOSIS

A chronic psychotic disorder manifested by a retreat from reality, delusions, hallucinations, ambivalence, withdrawal, and bizarre or regressive behavior.

Indications: Used to reduce the symptoms associated with psychosis, such as hallucinations, delusions, and thought disorders

Adverse reactions: Sedation, anticholinergic responses, postural hypotension, excessive tanning, hyperglycemia, lack of menses, nonreversible bone marrow depression, dystonia, akathisia, and pseudoparkinsonism. The following drugs may minimize the side effects: dimenhydrinate, benztropine, diphenhydramine, trihexyphenidyl

Special considerations: Gains in reducing symptoms may take anywhere from 6 to 12 weeks. Discontinuing medication may lead to relapse of symptoms. Thioridazine has a ceiling dose of 800 mg/day and promazine should not exceed 1,000 mg/day.

EXAMPLES OF ANTIPSYCHOTIC AGENTS

GENERIC	BRAND	DOSAGE FORMS
clozapine	Clozaril	Tablet
fluphenazine	Prolixin	Tablet, liquid, IM, IV
haloperidol	Haldol	Tablet, liquid, IM
loxapine	Loxitane	Capsule, liquid, IM
olanzapine	Zyprexa	Tablet
prochlorperazine	Compazine	Tablet, capsule, liquid, suppository, IM, IV
promazine	Sparine	Tablet, IM
risperidone	Risperdal	Tablet, liquid
thioridazine	Mellaril	Tablet, liquid
thiothixene	Navane	Capsule, IM
trifluoperazine	Stelazine	Tablet, liquid, IM
ziprasidone	Geodon	Capsule, injection

CNS DISORDERS

Convulsions/Epilepsy

Neurologic disorder defined as paroxysmal, recurring seizures. Involves disturbances of neuronal electrical activity. Seizures can be partial, generalized (grand mal, petit mal, myoclonic, and atonic), or status epilepticus.

MOA: Blocks the firing of neurotransmitters, resulting in a raised the level of depolarization

Adverse reactions: Sedation and loss of cognitive processes

Special considerations: Monotherapy is preferred over polytherapy unless patient is not responding to monotherapy. A large number of drug interactions may occur with anticonvulsants because of induction or inhibition. Divalproex should be taken with water, not with carbonated drinks.

EXAMPLES OF ANTICONVULSANT AGENTS

GENERIC	BRAND	DOSAGE FORMS
carbamazepine	Tegretol	Tablet, chewable tablet, suspension
clonazepam	Klonopin	Tablet
divalproex	Depakote	Tablet
fosphenytoin	Cerebyx	IV
gabapentin	Neurontin	Capsule, suspension
lamotrigine	Lamictal	Tablet
oxcarbazepine	Trileptal	Oral liquid, tablet
phenobarbital	Luminal	Tablet, solution, IM, IV
phenytoin	Dilantin	Tablet, capsule, suspension, IV
primidone	Mysoline	Tablet, suspension
valproic acid	Depakene	Capsule, syrup, IV
zonisamide	Zonegran	Capsule

Parkinson's Disease

A group of disorders resulting from the pathologic alterations of the basal ganglia.
Adverse reactions: Nausea, vomiting, cardiac arrhythmias, drowsiness, postural hypotension, insomnia, constipation, diarrhea
Special considerations: Therapy is aimed at symptomatic relief. Numerous side effects may occur, resulting in a continual change of therapy. Alcohol should be avoided.

EXAMPLES OF ANTIPARKINSON AGENTS

GENERIC	BRAND	DOSAGE FORMS
amantadine	Symmetrel	Capsule, syrup
benzotropine	Cogentin	Tablet, IM, IV
bromocriptine	Parlodel	Tablet, capsule
entacapone	Comtan	Tablet
levodopa	Larodopa	Tablet
levodopa-carbidopa	Sinemet	Tablet
pergolide	Permax	Tablet
ropinirole	ReQuip	Tablet
selegiline	Eldepryl	Tablet
trihexyphenidyl	Artane	Capsule, elixir, tablet

Attention Deficit Disorders (ADD)

Characterized by hyperactivity, impulsivity, and distractibility.
Special considerations: Schedule II drugs with high potential for abuse. Patients taking methylphenidate should have complete blood counts performed periodically. Caffeine should be avoided because of its ability to decrease the effectiveness of the medication.

EXAMPLES OF ADD AGENTS

GENERIC	BRAND	DOSAGE FORMS
amphetamine-dextroamphetamine	Adderall	Tablet
atomoxetine	Strattera	Capsule
clonidine	Catapres	Tablet, transdermal patch
desipramine	Norpramin	Tablet
dexamethylphenidate	Foscalin	Tablet
imipramine	Tofranil	Capsule
methylphenidate	Ritalin, Concerta	Tablet, timed-release tablet
pemoline	Cylert	Tablet

Multiple Sclerosis (MS)

An autoimmune disease in which the myelin sheaths around nerves degenerate. Loss of muscles and eyesight.
Adverse reactions: Photosensitivity

Special considerations: Products require special storage. Copaxone is given daily, Betaseron is administered every other day, and Avonex is administered once weekly.

EXAMPLES OF MS AGENTS

GENERIC	BRAND	DOSAGE FORMS
glatiramer acetate	Copaxone	Injection, SC
interferon beta-1a	Avonex	Single-dose vial, SC
interferon beta 1-b	Betaseron	Injection, SC
mitoxantrone	Novantrone	IV
tizanidine	Zanaflex	Tablet

Alzheimer's Disease

Degenerative disease of the brain leading to dementia; depression and agitation may occur during the course of the disease.
Adverse reactions: Nausea, vomiting, and diarrhea
Special considerations: There are no drugs that can reverse the cognitive abnormalities of Alzheimer's disease.

EXAMPLES OF AGENTS USED TO TREAT ALZHEIMER'S DISEASE

GENERIC	BRAND	DOSAGE FORMS
donepezil	Aricept	Tablet
gingko	Gingko	Tablet
memantine	Namenda	Tablet
rivastigmine	Exelon	Capsule, oral liquid

RESPIRATORY AGENTS

Asthma

An inflammation in the lungs that causes the airways to constrict and is characterized by wheezing, dyspnea, and cough.

Bronchodilators

MOA: Cause the B2 receptors to relax the smooth muscles, resulting in a decrease of bronchospasms
Indications: Airway obstruction, chronic obstructive pulmonary disease, reversible bronchospasms associated with bronchitis and emphysema
Adverse reactions: CNS stimulation, which may result in nervousness, tremors, anxiety, nausea, palpitations, tachycardia, arrhythmias
Special considerations: Patients may overmedicate themselves to control their asthma. Ipratropium solution needs to be protected from light. Salmeterol needs to be stored at room temperature, protected from freezing temperatures and direct sunlight. A salmeterol canister should be stored with the nozzle end down.

EXAMPLES OF BRONCHODILATORS

GENERIC	BRAND	DOSAGE FORMS
albuterol	Proventil HFA, Ventolin	Aerosol, capsule, solution, syrup, tablet, inhaler
bitolterol	Tornalate	Inhaler, inhalation solution
epinephrine	Primatene and Bronkaid Mist, Adrenalin	Aerosol, SC, IM, IV
formoterol fumarate	Foradil	Capsule
ipratropium	Atrovent	Inhaler, nasal spray
ipratropium-albuterol	Combivent	Aerosol
pirbuterol	Maxair	Inhaler
salmeterol	Serevent	Inhaler, inhalant disks
terbutaline	Brethine	Injection, tablet
tiotropium	Spiriva	Powdered capsule placed in a handihaler

Xanthine derivatives

MOA: Reverse bronchospasm associated with antigens and irritants. Improve contractility of diaphragm
Indications: Used to treat lung disease that is unresponsive to other medications. Used as a bronchodilator in reversible airway obstruction caused by asthma, chronic bronchitis, or emphysema
Special considerations: Blood levels need to be maintained at 8 mcg/mL to 20 mcg/mL. Theophylline may interact with macrolide and fluoroquinolone antibiotics.

EXAMPLES OF XANTHINE DERIVATIVES

GENERIC	BRAND	DOSAGE FORMS
aminophylline	Truphylline	Tablet, liquid, IM, IV
theophylline	Theo-Dur, Slo-Phyllin	Capsule, tablet, solution

Leukotriene inhibitors

MOA: Block the effects of leukotrienes, resulting in blocking of tissue inflammatory responses such as edema
Indications: Prophylaxis and long-term treatment of asthma
Adverse reactions: Headache
Special considerations: Patients using Singulair must be older than 6 years of age.

EXAMPLES OF LEUKOTRIENE INHIBITORS

GENERIC	BRAND	DOSAGE FORMS
montelukast	Singulair	Tablet
zafirlukast	Accolate	Tablet
zileuton	Zyflo	Tablet

Corticosteroids

MOA: Stimulate adenylate cyclase and inhibit inflammatory cells
Adverse reactions:
  Inhaled corticosteroids: oral candidiasis, irritation and burning of the nasal mucosa, hoarseness, and a dry mouth
  Oral corticosteroids: facial hair on females, breast development in males, "buffalo hump" or "moon face," edema, weight gain, and easy bruising
Special considerations: Long-term oral dosing needs to be tapered off to avoid nightmares.

EXAMPLES OF CORTICOSTEROIDS

GENERIC	BRAND	DOSAGE FORMS
beclomethasone	Beclovent, Vanceril, Vancenase	Inhaler
budesonide	Rhinocort	Inhaler
dexamethasone	Decadron	Solution, tablet
flunisolide	AeroBid	Inhaler
fluticasone	Flovent, Flonase	Inhaler
fluticasone/salmeterol	Advair	Inhaler
methylprednisolone	Medrol	Tablet
triamcinolone	Azmacort	Inhaler

Mast cell stabilizers

MOA: Inhibit inflammatory cells
Indications: Prophylaxis, has no usage for an acute attack
Adverse reactions: Patients using cromolyn may experience an unpleasant taste after inhalation, hoarseness, dry mouth, and stuffy nose.

Special considerations: Airway passages must be open before use; therefore, a bronchodilator is used first in conjunction with mast cell stabilizers. Patient compliance is an obstacle because of dosing four times per day.

EXAMPLES OF MAST CELL STABILIZERS

GENERIC	BRAND	DOSAGE FORMS
cromolyn	Intal, NasalCrom	Inhaler
nedocromil	Tilade	Inhaler

Emphysema

Characterized by the destruction of the tiny alveoli, walls, or air sacs of the lungs. Major risk factors include cigarette smoking, air pollution, occupational exposure, and genetic factors.

Bronchitis

An obstruction of the airflow during expiration. May be caused by cigarette smoke, exposure to occupational dusts, fumes, environmental pollution, and bacterial infection. Characterized by a cough that produces a purulent, green, or blood-soaked sputum. The lungs' defense mechanism has been destroyed and there is excessive mucus expectoration with at least 30 mL of sputum 24 hr for 3 months. Mucolytics are used for its treatment

Cystic Fibrosis

A fatal disease involving the gastrointestinal and respiratory systems. An increased secretion of viscous mucus resulting in hypoxia.

Mucolytic agents

MOA: Break apart glycoprotein, resulting in a reduction of viscosity, easier movement and removal of secretions
Adverse reactions: Mucomyst has an unpleasant odor and taste that may cause noncompliance
Comments: Mucomyst has an unpleasant taste and odor, resulting in patient noncompliance

EXAMPLES OF MUCOLYTIC AGENTS FOR THE TREATMENT OF CYSTIC FIBROSIS

GENERIC	BRAND	DOSAGE FORMS
acetylcysteine	Mucomyst	Solution
dornase alfa	Pulmozyme	Solution

Tuberculosis

A slow, progressive respiratory disease with symptoms of weight loss, fever, night sweats, malaise, and loss of appetite. A major issue with tuberculosis is patient compliance because of the length of therapy and number of medications a patient may be taking. Asymptomatic patients will receive isoniazid daily for 12 months; patients with clinical symptoms are treated with at least two medications.
Special considerations: Patients should avoid alcohol

EXAMPLES OF TUBERCULOSIS AGENTS

GENERIC	BRAND	DOSAGE FORMS
ciprofloxacin	Cipro	IM, IV, suspension, tablet
ethambutol	Myambutol	Tablet
isoniazid (INH)	Laniazid, Nydrazid	Tablet
isoniazid-pyrazinamide-rifampin	Rifater	Tablet
isoniazid-rifampin	Rifamate	Tablet
rifampin	Rifadin	Capsule, IV
rifapentine	Priftin	Tablet

Smoking

Smoking increases the risk of heart disease, chronic obstructive pulmonary disease, and stroke. Acute risks include shortness of breath, aggravation of asthma, impotence, infertility, and increased serum carbon monoxide concentration. Smoking cessation results in a reduced risk of lung, laryngo esophageal, oral, pancreatic, bladder and cervical cancer, and coronary artery disease.

EXAMPLES OF SMOKING CESSATION AGENTS

GENERIC	BRAND	DOSAGE FORMS
bupropion	Zyban	Tablet
nicotine	Habitrol, Nicoderm, Nicotrol, Nicorette, Nicotrol NS	Transdermal patch, gum, spray

GASTROINTESTINAL AGENTS

Antacids

MOA: Neutralize stomach acid to prevent reflux
Adverse effects: Constipation and diarrhea
Special considerations: Increased frequency of dosing resulting in poor patient compliance; reduces the effectiveness of tetracycline; is available as OTC.

EXAMPLES OF ANTACIDS

GENERIC	BRAND	DOSAGE FORMS
aluminum hydroxide	Amphojel	Tablet, liquid
aluminum hydroxide-magnesium hydroxide	Maalox. Mylanta	Tablet, liquid
magnesium hydroxide	Milk of Magnesia (MOM)	Tablet, liquid
magnesium trisulcate	Gelusil	Tablet

H2 Antagonists

MOA: Block gastric acid and pepsin secretion from histamine, gastrin, certain foods, caffeine, and cholinergic stimulation through competitive inhibition at H2 receptors of the gastric parietal cells
Adverse effects: Constipation, drowsiness
Special considerations: Bedtime dose is extremely important in therapy. Drug interactions include aspirin, alcohol, caffeine, cough/cold preparations. Available as an OTC in lower doses. Famotidine IV should be stored at room temperature; reconstituted oral suspension can be stored at room temperature and will expire in 30 days.

EXAMPLES OF H2 ANTAGONISTS

GENERIC	BRAND	DOSAGE FORMS
cimetidine	Tagamet (OTC available)	Tablet, liquid, IM, IV
nizatidine	Axid (OTC available)	Tablet, capsule
ranitidine	Zantac (OTC available)	Tablet, liquid, IM, IV, oral solution
famotidine	Pepcid (OTC available)	Tablet, suspension, IM, IV

Proton Pump Inhibitors

MOA: Inhibit the parietal cell adenosine triphosphate (ATP) pump
Indications: GERD, erosive esophagitis; taken with other agents in treatment of *Helicobacter pylori*
Adverse reactions: Diarrhea, dehydration
Special considerations: Capsules may be opened up and placed in apple sauce if patient has difficulty swallowing.

EXAMPLES OF PROTON PUMP INHIBITORS

GENERIC	BRAND	DOSAGE FORMS
esomeprazole	Nexium	Capsule
lansoprazole	Prevacid	Capsule, oral powder packets
omeprazole	Prilosec	Capsule
pantoprazole	Protonix	Tablet, IV
rabeprazole	Aciphex	Tablet

Coating Agents

MOA: Form a protective coat over ulcer against gastric acid, pepsin, and bile salts

EXAMPLES OF COATING AGENTS

GENERIC	BRAND	DOSAGE FORMS
alginic acid	Gaviscon	Tablet, chewable tablet, liquid
sucralfate	Carafate	Tablet, liquid suspension

ANTI-INFLAMMATORY AGENTS

Indications: Crohn's disease and ulcerative colitis
Adverse reactions: Nausea, vomiting, and headache
Special considerations: Sulfasalazine is contraindicated in patients allergic to "sulfas" and aspirin. Will bind to iron tablets. Patient needs to be kept hydrated, and the drug should be taken after meals. Will stain urine orange-yellow and permanently stain soft contact lenses yellow.

EXAMPLES OF ANTI-INFLAMMATORY AGENTS

GENERIC	BRAND	DOSAGE FORMS
mesalamine	Rowasa. Asacol, Pentasa	Suppository, enema, tablet, capsule
sulfasalazine	Azulfidine	Tablet, liquid

ANTIDIARRHEALS

Adverse reactions: Constipation, respiratory depression, drowsiness
Special considerations: Diarrhea may lead to dehydration of the individual and may mask more serious conditions, including malabsorption of drugs and nutrients.

EXAMPLES OF ANTIDIARRHEALS

GENERIC	BRAND	DOSAGE FORMS
attapulgite	Kaopectate	Liquid, tablet
bismuth subsalicylate	Pepto Bismol	Tablet, caplet, liquid
diphenoxylate with atropine	Lomotil	Tablet, liquid
loperamide	Imodium, Imodium AD (OTC)	Caplet, capsule, liquid

CONSTIPATION

Emollients/Lubricants/Saline Laxatives

MOA: Emollient laxatives—draw water into colon resulting in bowel evacuation
Adverse reactions: Nausea, vomiting, and diarrhea

EXAMPLES OF EMOLLIENTS/LUBRICANTS LAXATIVES/SALINE LAXATIVES

GENERIC	BRAND	DOSAGE FORMS
dioctyl calcium sulfosuccinate	Surfak	Tablet, capsule, liquid
docusate sodium	Colace	Tablet, capsule, microenema
lactulose	Cephulac	Solution
mineral oil	Mineral Oil	Solution
magnesium hydroxide	Milk of Magnesia (MOM)	Liquid
sodium phosphate	Fleet Phospho-Soda	Liquid

Stimulant Laxatives

MOA: Increase gut activity from mucosal stimulation
Adverse reactions: Diarrhea, allergic reactions such as hives and peripheral swelling

EXAMPLES OF STIMULANT LAXATIVES

GENERIC	BRAND	DOSAGE FORMS
bisacodyl	Dulcolax	Tablet, suppository
senna	Senokot	Tablet, syrup, granules

Bulk-Forming Laxatives

MOA: Increase fiber in the diet, resulting in intestinal peristalsis
Special considerations: Considered the safest to use; patient should drink plenty of water.

EXAMPLES OF BULK-FORMING LAXATIVES

GENERIC	BRAND	DOSAGE FORMS
methylcellulose	Citrucel, Fibertrim	Tablet, powder
psyllium hydrophilic mucilloid	Metamucil	Powder

Bowel Evacuant Laxatives

MOA: Increase osmolarity of bowel fluids
Indications: Bowel cleansing before gastrointestinal examination
Special considerations: Patient should fast for at least 3 hr before administration. Eight ounces should be taken every 10 minutes until 4 L is consumed.
Example: Polyethylene glycol-electrolyte solution (PEG); also known as GoLYTEly or NuLytely

ANTIEMETICS

MOA: Inhibit the impulse going from the chemo-trigger zone to the stomach
Indications: Used to treat side effect of nausea, which may be associated with various medications
Adverse reactions: Drowsiness
Special considerations: Phenothiazines may cause hypotension and must be used cautiously in children because of the potential of overdosage resulting in seizures. Promethazine suppositories need to be refrigerated and protected from light.

EXAMPLES OF ANTIEMETICS

GENERIC	BRAND	DOSAGE FORMS
chlorpromazine	Thorazine	Tablet, capsule
dimenhydrinate	Dramamine	Tablet, chewable tablet, oral solution
granisetron	Kytril	Tablet, IV
hydroxyzine HCl	Atarax	Tablet, syrup, IM, IV
meclizine	Antivert, Bonine (OTC)	Tablet
metoclopramide	Reglan	Tablet, syrup, IM, IV

EXAMPLES OF ANTIEMETICS—Cont'd

GENERIC	BRAND	DOSAGE FORMS
ondansetron	Zofran	Tablet, IV
prochlorperazine	Compazine	Tablet, capsule, syrup, IV, suppository
promethazine	Phenergan	Tablet, syrup, IM, IV, suppository
thiethylperazine	Torecan	Tablet, suppository, IM, IV
trimethobenzamide	Tigan	Capsule, IM, suppository

ANTIFLATULENTS

MOA: Reduce surface tension resulting in gas bubbles being released more easily
Indications: Flatulence, gastric bloating, and postoperative gas pains
Example: Simethicone (Gas X, Mylicon, Phazyme)

OBESITY DRUGS

Obesity: Males: 25% of total body weight over ideal body weight. Females: 35% of total body weight over ideal body weight
Adverse reactions: CNS stimulation, dizziness, fatigue, insomnia, dry mouth, nausea, abdominal discomfort, constipation, hypertension, palpitations, and arrhythmias
Special considerations: All are controlled substances, except Xenical. One must follow both federal and state controlled substance regulations regarding processing, filling, and record keeping.

EXAMPLES OF DRUGS USED TO TREAT OBESITY

GENERIC	BRAND	DOSAGE FORMS
diethylpropion	Tenuate	Tablet
mazindol	Mazanor	Tablet
phentermine	Fastin, Ionamin	Capsule
orlistat	Xenical	Capsule
sibutramine	Meridia	Capsule

URINARY SYSTEM DRUGS

Diuretics: Maintain balance of water, electrolytes, acids and bases in the body

Thiazide Diuretics

MOA: Promote sodium and water excretion in the urine, resulting in lower sodium levels in blood vessels and a reduction in vasoconstriction
Indications: Adjunctive therapy in cardiovascular diseases, such as hypertension
Adverse reactions: Hypokalemia, hypomagnesemia, hyperuricemia, hyperglycemia, hypercalcemia, photosensitivity
Special considerations: Patients may be advised to take potassium supplements or to add bananas or oranges to their diet.

EXAMPLE OF THIAZIDE DIURETICS

GENERIC	BRAND	DOSAGE FORMS
hydrochlorothiazide	Hydrodiuril, Esidrix	Tablet

Loop Diuretics

MOA: Inhibit reabsorption of sodium and chloride in the ascending loop of Henle and distal renal tubules resulting in urinary excretion of water
Indications: Adjunctive therapy in cardiovascular diseases, hypertension
Adverse reactions: Low levels of sodium, chloride, magnesium, calcium, and potassium
Comments: Diuretics should be taken early in the day to avoid nocturia (frequent urination during the night). Discolored furosemide tablets or solution should be discarded.

EXAMPLES OF LOOP DIURETICS

GENERIC	BRAND	DOSAGE FORMS
bumetanide	Bumex	Tablet, injection
ethacrynic acid	Edecrin	Injection
furosemide	Lasix	Tablet, oral solution, IM, IV
torsemide	Demadex	Tablet, IV

Potassium-Sparing Diuretics

MOA: Exchange of sodium excreted in urine to returning potassium to the body
Indications: Adjunctive therapy in cardiovascular issues, hypertension
Adverse reactions: Hyperkalemia, arrhythmias, gynecomastia in males
Special considerations: Should be avoided in patients taking angiotensin-converting enzyme (ACE) inhibitors due to potassium sparing effect.

EXAMPLES OF POTASSIUM-SPARING DIURETICS

GENERIC	BRAND	DOSAGE FORMS
amiloride	Midamor	Tablet
spironolactone	Aldactone	Tablet
triamterene	Dyrenium	Capsule

Combination Diuretic Products

Adverse reactions: Hyperkalemia, patients taking Maxzide may experience a change in their urine color to blue-green
Special considerations: Should not be given to patients on ACE inhibitors.

EXAMPLES OF COMBINATION DIURETIC PRODUCTS

GENERIC	BRAND	DOSAGE FORMS
bisoprolol-hydrochlorothiazide	Ziac	Tablet
triamterene-hydrochlorothiazide	Dyazide, Maxzide	Capsule, tablet

Alpha-Blockers Used in the Treatment of Prostatic Disease

MOA: Relax smooth muscles, especially in the prostatic tissue, resulting in a reduction of urinary symptoms
Adverse reactions: Headache, orthostatic hypotension, and dizziness

EXAMPLES OF ALPHA-BLOCKERS

GENERIC	BRAND	DOSAGE FORMS
alfuzosin	Uroxatral	Tablet
doxazosin	Cardura	Tablet
dutasteride	Avodart	Capsule
finasteride	Proscar	Tablet
prazosin	Minipress	Capsule
tamsulosin	Flomax	Tablet
terazosin	Hytrin	Capsule, tablet

URINARY TRACT AGENTS

Urex or Hiprex (Methenamine)

Bactericidal agent used to treat urinary tract infections. Citrus products and antacids should be avoided when taking this medication. Sulfonamides are contraindicated

Pyridium or Azo-Standard (Phenazopyridine)

Local anesthetic that should be taken with an antibiotic for 2 days.

Elmiron (Pentosan Polysulfate Sodium)

Oral preparation for interstitial cystitis.

Ditropan (Oxybutynin)

Antispasmodic used to decrease frequent urination.

Detrol (Tolterodine)

Used to treat frequent urination with strong anticholinergic effects.

CARDIOVASCULAR AGENTS

Arrhythmias

Contractions of ventricle and atria are not synchronized. Premature contractions include tachycardia, atrial flutter, and atrial fibrillation.

Membrane-stabilizing agents used in the treatment of arrhythmias

MOA: Slow the movement of ions into the cardiac cells, resulting in a reduction of the action potential
Adverse reactions: Nausea, vomiting, dizziness
Special considerations: Procainamide and quinidine are extremely similar and have been interchanged in therapy. Lidocaine is drug of choice for emergency IV therapy.

EXAMPLES OF MEMBRANE-STABILIZING AGENTS

GENERIC	BRAND	DOSAGE FORMS
disopyramide	Norpace	Capsule
flecainide	Tambocor	Tablet
lidocaine	Xylocaine	IV
procainamide	Pronestyl	Tablet, capsule, IM, IV
mexiletine	Mextil	Tablet
propafenone	Rythmol	Tablet
quinidine	Quinaglute	Tablet, IM, IV

Inhibitors of neurotransmitter release and reuptake used in the treatment of arrhythmias

MOA: Prevent the release of various transmitters and prolong the action potential
Adverse reactions: Hypotension, bradycardia, mental depression, and decreased sexual ability
Special considerations: IV amiodarone must be mixed in a glass container with D5W.

EXAMPLES OF INHIBITORS OF NEUROTRANSMITTER RELEASE AND REUPTAKE

GENERIC	BRAND	DOSAGE FORMS
amiodarone	Cordarone	Tablet, IV
sotalol	Betapace	Tablet

Calcium channel blockers used in the treatment of arrhythmias

MOA: Prevent movement of calcium ions through slow channels, resulting in a reduction through the AV node, SA node action, and relax coronary artery smooth muscle
Adverse reactions: Bradycardia, hypotension, heart block, cardiac failure, constipation, headache, and dizziness
Comments: Diltiazem must be stored in a light-resistant container.

EXAMPLES OF CALCIUM CHANNEL BLOCKERS

GENERIC	BRAND	DOSAGE FORMS
diltiazem	Cardizem	Capsule, tablet, IM, IV
verapamil	Isoptin, Calan, Verelan	Tablet, capsule, IV

Congestive Heart Failure (CHF)

The pumping ability of the heart is unable to meet the metabolic needs of the body's tissue, resulting in the heart pumping less blood than it receives and finds blood accumulating in the chambers of the heart.

Antiarrhythmics used in the treatment of congestive heart failure

Lanoxin is the drug of choice since it increases the force of contraction; increases the effective refractory period of the AV node; and affects the SA node through direct stimulation.
Adverse reactions: Nausea, vomiting, and arrhythmias
Special considerations: Concern for digoxin toxicity. A symptom of digoxin toxicity is seeing a greenish-bluish halo.

ACE inhibitors used in the treatment of congestive heart failure

MOA: Inhibit the conversion of angiotensin I to angiotensin II. Lower quantities of angiotensin II increase plasma renin activity and reduce aldosterone secretion
Adverse reactions: A dry, unproductive cough; dizziness occurs during the first few days of therapy; angioedema and possible postural hypotension
Special considerations: ACE inhibitors have a potassium-sparing effect; therefore, one must be aware of possibility of hyperkalemia. Should be avoided in patients receiving lithium.

EXAMPLES OF ACE INHIBITORS

GENERIC	BRAND	DOSAGE FORMS
benazepril	Lotensin	Tablet
captopril	Capoten	Tablet
enalapril	Vasotec	Tablet, IV
fosinopril	Monopril	Tablet
lisinopril	Prinivil, Zestril	Tablet
perindopril	Aceon	Tablet
quinapril	Accupril	Tablet
ramipril	Altace	Capsule
trandolapril	Mavik	Tablet

Angiotensin II Antagonists used in the treatment of congestive heart failure

MOA: Block the action of angiotensin II at its receptors
Adverse reactions: Angioedema and cough

EXAMPLES OF ANGIOTENSIN II ANTAGONISTS

GENERIC	BRAND	DOSAGE FORMS
candesartan	Altacand	Tablet
irbesartan	Avapro	Tablet
losartan	Cozaar	Tablet
olmesartan	Benicar	Tablet
telmisartan	Micardis	Tablet
valsartan	Diovan	Capsule

Myocardial Infarction (MI)

The heart muscle does not receive enough oxygen because of a reduced blood supply, and muscle cells die. MI can be prevented through behavior modifications, which include eliminating smoking, controlling diabetes, reducing hypertension through diet and modification, exercising three times per week, reducing calories to meet ideal weight, decreasing alcohol consumption, reducing cholesterol/triglycerides, and aspirin therapy if appropriate. Beta-blockers are used and should be tapered accordingly after the occurrence of MI.

Beta-blockers used in the treatment of MI

MOA: Block response to beta-stimulation, resulting in a reduction in the heart rate, myocardial contractility, blood pressure, and myocardial demand
Adverse reactions: Heart depression, bronchoconstriction, impotence, fatigue, depression, and bradycardia
Special considerations: Discontinuation should be tapered to reduce likelihood of angina.

EXAMPLES OF BETA-BLOCKERS

GENERIC	BRAND	DOSAGE FORMS
acebutolol	Sectral	Capsule
atenolol	Tenormin	Tablet, IV
betaxolol	Kerlone	Tablet
carvedilol	Coreg	Tablet
esmolol	Brevibloc	IV
metoprolol	Lopressor	Tablet, IV
nadolol	Corgard	Tablet
propranolol	Inderal	Tablet, capsule, IV, IM
sotalol	Betapace	Tablet

Angina Pectoris

An imbalance between the oxygen supply and oxygen demand in the body.

Nitrates used in the treatment of angina

MOA: Relaxes vascular smooth muscle resulting in lower venous return and cardiac filling and therefore decreased tension in cardiac walls. Coronary vessels are dilated
Adverse reactions: Orthostatic hypotension, flushing
Comments: Nitroglycerin inhalant is flammable. Nitroglycerin injection needs to be protected from light. Medication should not be stopped abruptly, but tapered.

EXAMPLES OF NITRATES

GENERIC	BRAND	DOSAGE FORMS
isosorbide dinitrate	Isordil, Dilatrate-SR, Sorbitrate	Tablet, capsule, sublingual tablet
isosorbide mononitrate	Imdur	Tablet
nitroglycerin	Nitrobid, Nitro-Dur, Nitrostat, Transderm Nitro	Spray, tablet, capsule, ointment, injection, IV, transdermal patch

Calcium channel blockers used in the treatment of angina

MOA: Inhibit calcium ions from entering "slow channels" of the vascular smooth muscle and the myocardium, resulting in relaxation of the coronary smooth muscle and coronary vasodilation and a decrease in oxygen demand
Adverse reactions: Constipation, drowsiness
Special considerations: Should be taken with food; caffeine should be limited in quantity. Nifedipine liquid-filled capsules need to be protected from light.

EXAMPLES OF CALCIUM CHANNEL BLOCKERS

GENERIC	BRAND	DOSAGE FORM
amlodipine	Norvasc	Tablet
diltiazem	Cardizem	Capsule, tablet, IV
felodipine	Plendil	Tablet

EXAMPLES OF CALCIUM CHANNEL BLOCKERS—Cont'd

GENERIC	BRAND	DOSAGE FORMS
isradipine	DynaCirc	Capsule
nicardipine	Cardene	Capsule, injection
nifedipine	Procardia, Adalat	Capsule, IV
verapamil	Calan, Isoptin, Verelan, Covera HS	Tablet, capsule, IV

Beta-blockers used in the treatment of angina

MOA: Slow the heart rate, resulting in a decreased myocardial contractility and lowered blood pressure, resulting in a decrease in oxygen demand

Adverse reactions: Bradycardia

Special considerations: May mask symptoms of hypoglycemia and hyperthyroidism. Medication should be tapered off when discontinuing therapy.

EXAMPLES OF BETA-BLOCKERS

GENERIC	BRAND	DOSAGE FORMS
atenolol	Tenormin	Tablet, IV
metoprolol	Lopressor, Toprol XL	Tablet, IV
nadolol	Corgard	Tablet
propranolol	Inderal	Capsule, tablet, solution, IV

Hypertension

Diuretics used in the treatment of hypertension

MOA: Reduce total peripheral resistance

Adverse reactions: Possible hypokalemia depending on agent used

Special considerations: Should be taken early in the day to eliminate the possibility of nocturia.

EXAMPLES OF DIURETICS

GENERIC	BRAND	DOSAGE FORMS
chlorothiazide	Diuril	Tablet, IM, IV
furosemide	Lasix	Tablet, oral solution, IM, IV
hydrochlorothiazide	Esidrix, Hydrodiuril	Tablet
spironolactone	Aldactone	Tablet
triamterene-hydrochlorothiazide	Dyazide, Maxzide	Capsule, tablet

Calcium channel blockers used in the treatment of hypertension

MOA: Dilate arterioles, resulting in a reduction of total peripheral resistance, energy consumption, and oxygen requirement

Adverse reactions: Drowsiness

EXAMPLES OF CALCIUM CHANNEL BLOCKERS

GENERIC	BRAND	DOSAGE FORMS
amlodipine	Norvasc	Tablet
bepridil	Vascor	Tablet
diltiazem	Cardizem	Capsule, tablet, IV
felodipine	Plendil	Tablet
isradipine	DynaCirc	Capsule
nicardipine	Cardene	Capsule, injection
nifedipine	Procardia, Adalat	Capsule, IV
verapamil	Calan, Isoptin, Verelan, Covera HS	Tablet, capsule, IV

ACE inhibitors used in the treatment of hypertension

MOA: Block angiotensin-converting enzymes to prevent the conversion of angiotensin I to angiotensin II, resulting in a reduction in total peripheral resistance and improving elasticity of arteries

EXAMPLES OF ACE INHIBITORS

GENERIC	BRAND	DOSAGE FORMS
benazepril	Lotensin	Tablet
captopril	Capoten	Tablet
enalapril	Vasotec	Tablet, IV
fosinopril	Monopril	Tablet
lisinopril	Prinivil, Zestril	Tablet
quinapril	Accupril	Tablet
perindopril	Aceon	Tablet
ramipril	Altace	Capsule
trandolapril	Mavik	Tablet

Angiotensin II-receptor antagonists used in the treatment of hypertension

MOA: Binds to angiotensin II-receptors and block vasoconstrictive effects of the arteries

EXAMPLES OF ANGIOTENSIN II-RECEPTOR ANTAGONISTS

GENERIC	BRAND	DOSAGE FORMS
losartan	Cozaar	Tablet
valsartan	Diovan	Capsule

Beta-blockers used in the treatment of hypertension

MOA: Block beta-receptor response to adrenergic response, resulting in decreased heart rate, myocardial contractibility, blood pressure, and myocardial response

EXAMPLES OF BETA-BLOCKERS (CARDIO-SELECTIVE)

GENERIC	BRAND	DOSAGE FORMS
acebutolol	Sectral	Capsule
atenolol	Tenormin	Tablet, IV
metoprolol	Lopressor, Toprol XL	Tablet, IV

EXAMPLES OF BETA-BLOCKERS

GENERIC	BRAND	DOSAGE FORMS
carvedilol	Coreg	Tablet
labetalol	Normodyne, Trandate	Tablet, IV
nadolol	Corgard	Tablet
propranolol	Inderal	Capsule, tablet, solution, IV
timolol	Blocadren	Tablet

CNS agents used in the treatment of hypertension

MOA: Stimulate alpha 2 adrenergic responses in the brain and reduce sympathetic outflow from the vasomotor center in the brain, resulting in decreased heart rate, cardiac output, and total peripheral resistance
Adverse reactions: Drowsiness, fatigue, depression, fluid retention

EXAMPLES OF CNS AGENTS

GENERIC	BRAND	DOSAGE FORMS
clonidine	Catapres	Tablet, patch, IV
guanfacine	Tenex	Tablet, liquid
methyldopa	Aldomet	Tablet, oral suspension, IV

Peripheral acting agents used in the treatment of hypertension

MOA: Block alpha stimulation to peripheral nerves, resulting in vasodilation and hypotension
Adverse reactions: Hypotension

EXAMPLES OF PERIPHERAL ACTING AGENTS

GENERIC	BRAND	DOSAGE FORMS
doxazosin	Cardura	Tablet
prazosin	Minipress	Capsule
terazosin	Hytrin	Capsule

Vasodilators used in the treatment of hypertension

MOA: Reduce arteriole smooth muscle, resulting in lower peripheral resistance
Adverse reactions: Tachycardia, palpitations, flushing, and headache

EXAMPLES OF VASODILATORS

GENERIC	BRAND	DOSAGE FORMS
fenoldopam	Corlopam	IV
hydralazine	Apresoline	Tablet
minoxidil	Loniten	Tablet

Combination products used in the treatment of hypertension

MOA: An additive effect to lower blood pressure and reduce the number of side effects
Special considerations: Fewer side effects because medications are in lower dosages.

EXAMPLES OF COMBINATION PRODUCTS

GENERIC	BRAND	DOSAGE FORMS
enalapril-hydrochlorothiazide	Vaseretic	Tablet
losartan-hydrochlorothiazide	Hyzaar	Tablet
trandolapril-verapamil	Tarka	Tablet

ANTICOAGULANT THERAPY

MOA: Prevent proper clot formation while maintaining adequate coagulation
Adverse reactions: Bleeding, urine may turn red-orange; feces may turn red or black
Special considerations: Warfarin injection must be protected from light. Patient should avoid foods rich in vitamin K if they are taking warfarin. Many drug interactions occur with warfarin. Mephyton is given to treat an overdose of warfarin. Blood clotting must be monitored through prothrombin time or INR testing. Heparin is to be given either IV or SC, never IM. Protamine sulfate is used to treat overdoses of heparin.

EXAMPLES OF ANTICOAGULANTS

GENERIC	BRAND	DOSAGE FORMS
argatroban	Argatrobin	Injection
bivalirudin	Angiomax	IV

EXAMPLES OF ANTICOAGULANTS—Cont'd

GENERIC	BRAND	DOSAGE FORMS
dalteparin	Fragmin	SC
enoxaparin	Lovenox	SC
fondaparinux	Arixtra	Injection
heparin	Heparin	IV, IC
lepirudin	Refludan	IV
tinzaparin	Innohep	SC
warfarin	Coumadin	Tablet

HYPERLIPIDEMIA

An elevation of one or more of the lipoprotein levels.
Blood cholesterol levels per 100 mL of blood
- 240 mg: at risk
- less than 200 mg: desirable
- 135 mg: more desirable

Blood low-density lipoprotein levels per 100 mL of blood
- 160 mg: high risk
- 139–159 mg: borderline risk
- less than 139 mg: desirable

HMG-CoA Reductase Inhibitors Used in the Treatment of Hyperlipidemia

MOA: Inhibit the enzyme that catalyzes the rate-limiting step in cholesterol synthesis
Adverse reactions: GI upset, headache, muscle pain, and fever
Special considerations: Liver function tests should be conducted every 6 months.

EXAMPLES OF HMG-COA REDUCTASE INHIBITORS

GENERIC	BRAND	DOSAGE FORMS
atorvastatin	Lipitor	Tablet
fluvastatin	Lescol	Capsule
lovastatin	Mevacor	Tablet
pravastatin	Pravachol	Tablet
rosuvastatin	Crestor	Tablet
simvastatin	Zocor	Tablet

Fibric Acid Derivatives Used in the Treatment of Hyperlipidemia

MOA: Unknown
Adverse reactions: Headache, nausea, vomiting, diarrhea, skin rash, alteration in liver and kidney function

EXAMPLES OF FIBRIC ACID DERIVATIVES

GENERIC	BRAND	DOSAGE FORMS
clofibrate	Atromid S	Capsule
fenofibrate	TriCor	Capsule
gemfibrozil	Lopid	Tablet, capsule

Bile Acid Sequestrants Used in the Treatment of Hyperlipidemia

MOA: Form a nonabsorbable complex with bile acids in the intestine
Adverse reactions: Nausea and vomiting

EXAMPLES OF BILE ACID SEQUESTRANTS

GENERIC	BRAND	DOSAGE FORMS
cholestyramine	Questran	Powder
colesevelam	WelChol	Tablet
colestipol	Colestid	Tablet, granule

NARCOTIC/OPIOID ANALGESICS

Narcotics/opioids: May provide analgesia, sedation, euphoria, or dysphoria during pain management

MOA: Narcotic/opioid analgesics that interact with specific receptor sites and have an effect on the central nervous system (CNS). The body produces endorphins, enkephalins, and dynorphins. These susbstances are released by the brain after the release of stimuli caused by pain. An increase in the level of pain results in an increase in the release of these substances. There is a decrease in the nerve transmission to the CNS, resulting in a decrease in the sensation of pain. Narcotic/opioid analgesics respond to the same receptors as endorphins, enkephalins, and dynorphins

Adverse reactions: Respiratory depression, constipation, mental confusion, nausea, and vomiting

Special considerations: Have a potential for tolerance and addiction. All opiates are controlled substances and one must adhere to both federal and state laws regarding processing, dispensing and maintaining proper records of controlled substances. Increased fluid intake is recommended along with stool softeners to combat constipation.

EXAMPLES OF NARCOTICS/OPOIDS

GENERIC	BRAND	DOSAGE FORMS	CONTROLLED SUBSTANCE SCHEDULE
acetaminophen with codeine	Tylenol with Codeine	Capsule, tablet, IM, IV, SC, elixir	III
butorphanol	Stadol, Stadol NS	Nasal spray, IM	IV
codeine	Codeine	Tablet, IM, oral solution	II
fentanyl	Duragesic	Transdermal patch, IV	II
hydrocodone	Hycodan	Tablet, syrup	III
hydrocodone-acetaminophen	Lortab, Vicodin	Tablet, expectorant, elixir	III
hydromorphone	Dilaudid	Tablet, syrup, liquid, IM, IV, SC, suppository	II
meperidine	Demerol	Tablet, syrup, IM, IV, SC	II
methadone	Dolophine	Oral concentrate, oral solution, tablet	II
morphine	MS Contin	Tablet	II
oxycodone	OxyContin	Capsule, liquid, tablet	II
oxycodone-acetaminophen	Percocet, Tylox	Tablet, capsule	II
oxycodone-aspirin	Percodan	Tablet	II
pentazocine	Talwin	Tablet, IM, IV, SC	IV
pentazocine-naloxone	Talwin NX	Tablet	IV
propoxyphene-acetaminophen	Darvocet N	Tablet	IV
propoxyphene HCl	Darvon	Capsule	IV

NON-NARCOTIC ANALGESICS

Nonsteroidal Anti-Inflammatories (NSAIDs)

Indications: Antipyretic, analgesic, and anti-inflammatory agent

MOA: Inhibit prostaglandin synthesis, preventing the sensitization of the pain receptors

Adverse reactions: Stomach irritation, drowsiness, nausea, abdominal cramps, jaundice, and rash

EXAMPLES OF NSAIDS

GENERIC	BRAND	DOSAGE FORMS
diclofenac	Voltaren, Cataflam	Tablet, ophthalmic drops
diflunisal	Dolobid	Tablet
etodolac	Lodine	Tablet, capsule
fenoprofen	Nalfon	Tablet, pulvule
flurbiprofen	Ansaid, Ocufen	Tablet, ophthalmic drops
ibuprofen	Motrin, Advil, Nuprin	Tablet, liquid, drops, chewable tablets
indomethacin	Indocin	Capsule, IV, suppository
ketorolac	Toradol	Tablet, IM, IV
nabumetone	Relafen	Tablet
naproxen	Anaprox, Naprosyn	Tablet, caplet
oxaprozin	Daypro	Caplet
piroxicam	Feldene	Capsule

Aspirin

Indications: Analgesic, antipyretic, anti-inflammatory, antirheumatic
MOA: Reduce fever by increasing blood flow to the skin and inhibiting prostaglandin synthesis
Adverse reactions: Stomach ulceration, anemia, prolonged pregnancy and labor, tinnitus, dizziness, headache and mental confusion
Special considerations: Should not be given to children who have been exposed to chickenpox; may result in Reye's syndrome. Should not be given to patients who are taking warfarin.

Acetaminophen

Indications: Analgesic and antipyretic
MOA: Mechanism has not been established
Adverse reactions: May increase bleeding in patients taking warfarin; may damage liver and therefore should not be given to patients who are suffering from liver disease or are alcoholics

Selective 5-HT receptor agonists

MOA: Stimulate serotonin receptors in the cerebral and temporal arteries, which will cause vasoconstriction, which inhibits neural transmission, resulting in excessive vasodilation of the cranial arteries
Adverse reactions: Tingling warm sensation, chest discomfort, dizziness, and vertigo
Comment: Sumatriptan injection needs to be protected from light.

EXAMPLES OF SELECTIVE 5-HT RECEPTOR AGONISTS

GENERIC	BRAND	DOSAGE FORMS
almotriptan	Axert	Tablet
eletriptan	Relpax	Tablet
frovatriptan	Frova	Tablet
naratriptan	Amerge	Tablet
rizatriptan	Maxalt	SL tablet, tablet
sumatriptan	Imitrex	SC, tablet, nasal spray, IM
zolmitriptan	Zomig	Tablet

THYROID HORMONES

Hypothyroidism

Iodine deficiency disease in children results in cretinism. The symptoms in adults include apathy, decreased heart rate, and depression; symptoms in a child include short stature, a thick tongue, and possible enlarged thyroid, lowered voice pitch, myxedema, puffy face, reduced mental acuity, and weight gain.
MOA: Thyroid replacement therapy
Adverse reactions: Cardiotoxicity and hyperthyroidism
Special notation: Patient should undergo TSH tests. Levothyroxine injection needs to be used promptly after reconstitution.

EXAMPLES OF HYPOTHYROID AGENTS

GENERIC	BRAND	DOSAGE FORMS
levothyroxine	Synthroid, Levothroid, Levoxyl	Tablet, injection
liothyronine	Cytomel	Tablet
liotrix	Thyrolar	Tablet
thyroid	Armour Thyroid	Tablet

Hyperthyroidism (Grave's Disease)

An excessive secretion of thyroid hormones that may be caused by thyroid nodules, an excessive iodine intake, or a tumor causing overproduction of thyroid-stimulating hormones. Symptoms include decreased menses, diarrhea, exophthalmos, heat intolerance, nervousness, perspiration, tachycardia, and possible weight loss

MOA: Therapy includes hormone replacement or surgery

Adverse reactions: Fever, sore throat, unusual bleeding or bruising, headache, or malaise

EXAMPLES OF HYPERTHYROID AGENTS

GENERIC	BRAND	DOSAGE FORMS
methimazole	Tapazole	Tablet
propylthiouracil	PTU	Tablet
radioactive iodine		Capsule, oral solution

HORMONE REPLACEMENT THERAPY

Estrogen Replacement Therapy

Relieves symptoms of estrogen deficiency. The deficiency results in symptoms of vasomotor instability, drying and atrophy of vaginal mucosa, insomnia, irritability, and mood changes

MOA: Suppress follicle-stimulating hormone secretion, which blocks follicular development and ovulation

Adverse reactions: Nausea, bloating, weight gain, breast tenderness, and possible breakthrough bleeding

Comments: All estrogen products should be dispensed with a patient package insert. Conjugated estrogen therapy is cyclical. Estraderm and Vivelle are applied twice weekly, whereas Climara is applied weekly.

EXAMPLES OF ESTROGENS

GENERIC	BRAND	DOSAGE FORMS
conjugated estrogen	Premarin	Tablet, cream
conjugated estrogen-medroxyprogesterone	Prempro, Premphase	Tablet
diethylstilbestrol (DES)		Tablet, IM
estradiol	Estrace	Tablet, transdermal, cream, IM
	Estraderm	IM, tablet, transdermal
	Vivelle, Climara	Transdermal system
estradiol-norethindrone	Activella, Combipatch	Tablet, transdermal patch
estradiol-norgestimate	Ortho-Prefest	Tablet
estropipate	Ogen	Tablet, cream
ethinyl estradiol-norethindrone acetate	Estinyl	Tablet

Progestins

Indications: Treatment of menstrual dysfunction, such as uterine bleeding, amenorrhea, dysmenorrhea, and endometriosis

MOA: Inhibit luteinizing hormone secretion by means of a negative feedback on the hypothalamic anterior pituitary axis

Adverse reactions: Weight gain, depression, fatigue, acne, and hirsutism

EXAMPLES OF PROGESTINS

GENERIC	BRAND	DOSAGE FORMS
levonorgestrel	Norplant	Implant
medroxyprogesterone	Amen, Cycrin, Provera	Tablet
norethindrone	Micronor	Tablet

Oral Contraceptives

Normally are a combination of progestin and estrogen.

MOA: Suppress ovulation by interfering with production of hormones that regulate the menstrual cycle and alter the cervical mucus

Adverse reactions: Potential for heart attack, stroke, and thromboembolic disease. Other side effects include nausea, weight gain, breast tenderness, and depression

Comments: Oral contraceptives must be dispensed with a patient package insert.

EXAMPLES OF ORAL CONTRACEPTIVES

GENERIC	BRAND	DOSAGE FORMS
Biphasic		
estradiol cypionate-medroxyprogesterone	Lunelle	Injection
ethinyl estradiol-desogestrel	Cyclessa, Desogen, Kariva, Mircette, Ortho-Cept	Tablet
ethinyl estradiol-drospirenone	Yasmin	Tablet
ethinyl estradiol-ethynodiol diacetate	Demulen	Tablet
ethinyl estradiol-etonogestrel	NuvaRing	Ring
ethinyl estradiol-levonorgestrel	Levlen, Tri-Levlen, Triphasil	Tablet
ethinyl estradiol-norelgestromin	Ortho Evra	Patch
ethinyl estradiol-norethindrone	Estrostep Fe, femhrt, Loestrin Fe, Ovcon	Tablet
ethinyl estradiol-norgestimate	Ortho Tri-Cyclen, Ortho Tri-Cyclen Lo	Tablet
ethinyl estradiol-norgestrel	Lo/Ovral, Low-Orgestrel, Ovral	Tablet
Emergency Contraceptives		
levonorgestrel	Plan B	Tablet
norgestrel	Ovrette	Tablet
Progestin		
norgestrel	Ovrette	Tablet
Parenteral		
estradiol cypionate-medroxyprogesterone	Lunelle	Injection
medroxyprogesterone	Depo-Provera	Injection
Implant		
levonorgestrel	Norplant	Capsule

EXAMPLES OF ORAL CONTRACEPTIVE INTERACTIONS

CLASS	DRUGS	TYPE OF INTERACTION
Antibiotics	Erythromycin, griseofulvin, penicillin, rifampin, tetracycline	May decrease effectiveness of oral contraceptive from interference of enterohepatic cycling of estrogen resulting in a fluctuation of hormone levels
Anticonvulsants	Tegretol, Dilantin, Mysoline, phenobarbital	Decrease contraceptive action from increased metabolism of hormones
Antifungals	Diflucan, Nizoral, Sporanox	May decrease effectiveness of oral contraceptives
Benzodiazepines	Dalmane, Halcion, Librium, Valium, Xanax	Metabolism of benzodiazepine may be decreased, resulting in an increase of side effects
Bronchodilator	Theophylline	Increased side effects of theophylline resulting from decreased theophylline metabolism
Corticosteroids	Hydrocortisone, methylprednisolone, prednisolone, prednisone	Increased effects from inhibition of metabolism by oral contraceptives
Lipid-lowering agents	Atromid S	Decreased oral contraceptive effect
Tricyclic antidepressants	Elavil, Tofranil	Increased side effects of tricyclic antidepressants

BONE DISEASE AGENTS

Fosamax (Alendronate) and Fosamax with Vitamin D

Biphosphate approved for osteoporosis. Inhibits bone reabsorption by osteoclasts. It should be taken 30 minutes before first meal, beverage, or medication of the day. The medication should be taken with 6–8 oz of water to avoid esophageal burning. The patient should not lie down for at least 30 minutes after taking medication.

Miacalcin (Calcitonin-Salmon)

A nasal spray for estrogen replacement therapy. One should alternate nostrils each day. Patient may experience local nasal side effects.

Evista (Raloxifene)

Inhibits estrogen receptors.

CORTICOSTEROIDS

Addison's Disease

A deficiency of glucocorticoids and mineralocorticoids that is treated with corticosteroids. Symptoms of Addison's disease include debilitating weakness, weight loss, hyperpigmentation of the skin, reduced blood pressure, low sodium and glucose levels, and hyperkalemia.

Cushing's Disease

Overproduction of steroids or caused by excessive administration of corticosteroids over an extended period. Symptoms include a protruding abdomen and fat over the shoulder blades.

Indications: Inhibit inflammation

Adverse reactions: Stomach irritation, hypertension from sodium retention, slow wound healing, thinning of skin, peptic ulcer disease, increased infections, reduced white blood cell function, truncal obesity, moon face, buffalo hump, hyperglycemia, hypokalemia, osteoporosis, alterations in mood, manic-depressive behavior, and cataracts

EQUIVALENCY OF CORTICOSTEROIDS COMPARED WITH THE DAILY SECRETION OF HYDROCORTISONE (20 MG)

CORTICOSTEROID	BRAND NAME	EQUIVALENCY (MG)	ANTI-INFLAMMATORY POTENCY
betamethasone	Diprolene	0.6	25.0
cortisone	Cortone	25.0	0.8
dexamethasone	Decadron	0.75	30.0
hydrocortisone	Hydrocortisone	20.0	1.5
methylprednisolone	Medrol	4.0	5.0
prednisolone	Pediapred	5.0	4.0
prednisone	Deltasone	5.0	3.0
triamcinolone	Aristocort	4.0	5.0

SIDE EFFECTS OF CORTICOSTEROIDS

TYPE OF EFFECT	SIDE EFFECT
Cardiovascular	Hypertension
Dermatologic	Impaired wound healing, thinning of the skin, petechiae, purpura
Gastrointestinal	Peptic ulcer disease, pancreatitis
Immune system	Infections and reduction of white blood cell function
Metabolic	Redistribution of fat deposits, acne, hirsutism, growth suppression, hyperglycemia, hypokalemia, sodium and water retention
Musculoskeletal	Osteoporosis and vertebral compression
Neuropsychiatric	Alterations in mood; manic-depressive, psychotic, suicidal, or schizophrenic tendencies
Ophthalmic	Cataracts and glaucoma

HYPOGLYCEMIC AGENTS

Diabetes

Type I diabetes: Body is unable to produce insulin and individual is insulin dependent
Type II diabetes: Impaired insulin secretion
Gestational diabetes: Diabetes resulting from pregnancy
Secondary diabetes: Diabetes caused by other medications

Oral hypoglycemic agents

First-generation sulfonylureas: Increases insulin release
Second-generation sulfonylureas: Promotes release of insulin from the beta cells of the pancreas; increases insulin sensitivity and lowers blood glucose levels
Comment: Adjunct to exercise and diet.

Enzyme inhibitors

Inhibits intestinal wall enzymes that convert saccharides into glucose, resulting in lowering of postprandial hyperglycemia
Adverse reactions: Abdominal pain, diarrhea, and flatulence
Contraindications: Patients with cirrhosis, inflammatory bowel disease, colon ulceration, and intestinal obstruction

Biguanides

Decreases intestinal absorption of glucose and improves insulin sensitivity.
MOA: Decreases intestinal absorption of glucose and improves insulin sensitivity
Adverse reactions: Nausea, metallic aftertaste, and weight loss
Comment: Needs to be titrated upward over a period of weeks.

Glitazones

Improves cellular response to glucose.
MOA: Improves cellular response to insulin
Adverse reactions: Increased plasma volume and elevated high-density lipoprotein levels

EXAMPLES OF HYPOGLYCEMIC AGENTS

GENERIC	BRAND	AGENT TYPE	DOSAGE FORMS
acarbose	Precose	Enzyme inhibitor	Tablet
glimepiride	Amaryl	Second-generation sulfonylureas	Tablet
glipizide	Glucotrol, Glucotrol XL	Second-generation sulfonylureas	Tablet
glyburide	DiaBeta Glynase, Micronase	Second-generation sulfonylureas	Tablet
metformin	Glucophage	Biguanide	Tablet
miglitol	Glyset	Enzyme inhibitor	Tablet
nateglinide	Starlix	Meglitinide	Tablet
repaglinide	Prandin	Meglitinide	Tablet
pioglitazone	Actos	Glitazone	Tablet
rosiglitazone	Avandia	Glitazone	Tablet
Combination Products			
glipizide-metformin	Metaglip		Tablet
glyburide-metformin	Glucovance		Tablet
rosiglitazone-metformin	Avandamet		Tablet

Injectable hypoglycemic agents

Comments: Humulin insulin can be stored at room temperature for 1 month. Regular insulin can only be used in IVs.

EXAMPLES OF INJECTABLE HYPOGLYCEMIC AGENTS

GENERIC	BRAND	DURATION OF ACTION
Insulin injection	Regular Iletin I	Rapid
	Regular Iletin II	Rapid
	Novolin R	Rapid
Isophane insulin	NPH Iletin I	Intermediate
	Humulin N	Intermediate
Isophane insulin suspension and insulin injection	Humulin 70/30	Intermediate
Isophane insulin suspension and insulin injection	Humulin 50/50	Intermediate
Insulin zinc suspension	Lente I	Intermediate
	Humulin L	
Insulin zinc suspension; extended lente	Humulin Ultralente	Long-acting
Insulin analog injection	Humalog	Rapid
Insulin glargine	Lantus	Long-acting

TOPICAL, OPHTHALMICS, AND OTICS

Psoriasis

Patches of red, scaly skin, usually on the elbows and knees. May be caused by illness, injury, or emotional stress
MOA: Regulates skin cell production and proliferation

EXAMPLES OF AGENTS TO TREAT PSORIASIS

GENERIC	BRAND	DOSAGE FORMS	SPECIAL CONSIDERATIONS
acitretin	Soriatane	Capsule	
alefacept	Amevive	Injection	
calcipotriene	Dovonex	Cream, Ointment	Patient should wash hands after each application
coal tar	Tegrin	Shampoo	
methotrexate	Rheumatrex	Tablet, IM, IV	May inhibit normal cell growth
pimecrolimus	Elidel	Cream	
tacrolimus	Protopic	Ointment	

Acne Vulgaris

MOA: Remove keratinocytes in the sebaceous follicle. They loosen the horny cells at the mouth of the ducts, resulting in easy sloughing
Special considerations: Hands should be washed after each application.

EXAMPLES OF AGENTS TO TREAT ACNE VULGARIS

GENERIC	BRAND	DOSAGE FORMS	SPECIAL CONSIDERATIONS
adapalene	Differin	Gel	Water based—causes less irritation than Retin-A
azelaic acid	Azelex	Cream	Thin film should be applied to affected area twice per day
clindamycin-benzoyl peroxide	BenzaClin	Gel	
furfuryladenine	Kinerase	Cream	Alternative to Retin-A or Renova; causes less irritation
tretinoin	Retin-A	Cream, gel, lotion	Avoid exposure to sun; hands should be washed after each use; may cause severe irritation
tretinoin	Renova	Cream	Has a more moisturizing effect than Retina-A

Actinic Keratoses

MOA: Antiproliferative agents for skin cancer
Special considerations: May cause transient burning of the skin.

EXAMPLES OF AGENTS TO TREAT ACTINIC KERATOSES

GENERIC	BRAND	DOSAGE FORMS	SPECIAL CONSIDERATIONS
fluorouracil	Efudex	Cream, solution	Proper hand washing should be followed; avoid direct sunlight; needs to be disposed of properly because it is an antineoplastic agent
masoprocol	Actinex	Cream	Area needs to be washed and massaged in properly; should be used for 4 weeks

Topical Fungi

MOA: Prevent the synthesis of ergosterol, which is needed for fungal cell membranes. Inhibit fungal cytochrome 450

Special considerations: Pulse dosing is effective in treating fungal infections in toe and finger nails.

EXAMPLES OF TOPICAL ANTIFUNGAL AGENTS

GENERIC	BRAND	DOSAGE FORMS	SPECIAL CONSIDERATIONS
amphotericin B	Fungizone	Cream, lotion, ointment, injection	Used to treat patients with a progressive fungal infection
butenafine	Mentax	Cream	Used to treat athlete's foot, jock itch, and ringworm; used daily for 4 weeks
clotrimazole	Lotrimin, FemCare, Mycelex	Cream, lotion, vaginal, troche	Available OTC / Available OTC
econazole	Spectazole	Cream	
griseofulvin	Fulvicin	Tablet, capsule, oral suspension	Fungal infections of the hair, skin, and nails; avoid exposure to sun; take with a fatty meal
miconazole	Monistat	Cream, vaginal, IV, spray	OTC; used to treat vulvovaginal candidiasis
nystatin	Mycolog, Mycostatin	Cream, ointment, oral suspension, capsule	Commonly used to treat children with candidiasis; patients are told to swish and swallow
oxiconazole	Oxistat	Cream, lotion	
sertaconazole	Ertaczo	Cream	
sulconazole	Exelderm	Cream	
terbinafine	Lamisil	Cream, tablet	Taken orally once per day for 6 wk for fingernails and for 12 wk for toenail infections; may be pulse dosed
tolnaftate	Tinactin	Liquid, powder, cream, solution	OTC

Topical Corticosteroids

MOA: Able to penetrate the skin and are able to suppress the hypothalamic-pituitary axis

Special considerations: Creams and ointments should not be considered interchangeable. A thin layer should be applied sparingly to the affected area. Ointments are more potent than creams. Superpotent corticosteroids should not be used for more than 2 weeks and patients should not receive more than 50 g in 1 week.

EXAMPLES OF TOPICAL CORTICOSTEROID AGENTS

GENERIC	BRAND	DOSAGE FORMS
betamethasone 0.05%	Diprolene	Cream, gel, ointment
clobetasol 0.05%	Temovate	Cream, ointment
desoximetasone 0.25%	Topicort	Cream, ointment
diflorasone 0.05%	Florone	Ointment
fluocinonide 0.05%	Lidex	Cream, ointment, solution
halobetasol 0.05%	Ultravate	Cream, ointment
mometasone 0.1%	Elocon	Ointment

EXAMPLES OF TOPICAL ANTIBIOTICS

GENERIC	BRAND	DOSAGE FORMS
bacitracin-neomycin-polymyxin B	Triple Antibiotic	Ointment
clindamycin	Cleocin T	Cream, gel, lotion, solution
erythromycin	T-stat, ATS, Eryderm	Gel, roll-on, solution
metronidazole	MetroGel, MetroCream	Gel, cream
mupirocin	Bactroban	Ointment
neomycin-polymyxin B	Neosporin	Ointment
silver sulfadiazine	Silvadene	Cream
tetracycline	Topicycline	Solution

Glaucoma

Chronic disorder characterized by abnormally high internal eye pressure that destroys the optic nerve and may cause loss of vision. Three types of glaucoma exist: open-angle glaucoma, narrow-angle, and secondary glaucoma.

Glaucoma agents

MOA: Reduce intraocular pressure
Special consideration: Drug treatment cannot cure the disease, but can control it.

EXAMPLES OF OPHTHALMIC AGENTS USED IN TREATMENT OF GLAUCOMA

GENERIC	BRAND	DOSAGE FORMS	COMMENTS
apraclonidine	Iopidine	Solution	
betaxolol	Betoptic	Solution, suspension	
brimatoprost	Lumigan	Solution	
brimonidine	Alphagan	Solution	Reduces fluid production in the eye
brinzolamide	Azopt	Solution	Should not be taken with carbonic anhydrase inhibitors
dipivefrin	Propine	Solution	
dorzolamide	Trusopt	Solution	Bitter taste may occur after administration
latanoprost	Xalatan	Solution	May cause light colored eyes to turn brown; should be stored in the refrigerator
timolol	Timoptic	Solution	
travoprost	Travatan	Solution	
unoprostone	Rescula	Solution	

EXAMPLES OF OTHER OPHTHALMIC AGENTS

GENERIC	BRAND	DOSAGE FORMS	CLASSIFICATION
ciprofloxacin	Ciloxan	Solution	Antibiotic
cromolyn sodium	Crolom	Solution	Mast cell stabilizer
dexamethasone	Ak-Dex	Ointment	Corticosteroid
diclofenac	Voltaren	Solution	NSAID
flurbiprofen	Ocufen	Solution	NSAID
gentamicin	Garamycin	Solution	Antibiotic
ketorolac	Acular	Solution	NSAID
naphazoline	Naphcon	Solution	Decongestant
ofloxacin	Ocuflox	Solution	Antibiotic
sulfacetamide-prednisolone	Blephamide	Ointment, solution, suspension	Corticosteroid
sulfacetamide sodium	Bleph-10	Ointment, solution	Antibiotic
tobramycin-dexamethasone	TobraDex	Ointment, solution	Corticosteroid
trifluridine	Viroptic	Solution	Antiviral
vidarabine	Vira-A	Ointment	Antiviral

EXAMPLES OF OTIC AGENTS

GENERIC	BRAND	DOSAGE FORMS	CLASSFICATION
antipyrine-benzocaine	Auralgan	Solution	Analgesic
carbamide peroxide	Auro, Debrox	Solution	Wax dissolver
neomycin-polymyxin B-hydrocortisone	Cortisporin	Suspension, solution	Antibiotic
triethanolamine-polypeptide-oleate condensate	Cerumenex	Solution	Wax dissolver

CHEMOTHERAPY AGENTS

Alkylating Agents

MOA: Bind irreversible cross-links in DNA, resulting in cells unable to reproduce

Adverse reactions: Myelosuppression

Antibiotics

MOA: Inhibit DNA-dependent RNA synthesis; delay or inhibit mitosis

Adverse reactions: Cardiotoxicity

Antimetabolites

MOA: Blend into normal cell constituents, causing them to become nonfunctional, or prevent the normal function of a key enzyme

Adverse reactions: Nausea, vomiting, and diarrhea

Nitrogen Mustards

MOA: Bind irreversible cross-links in DNA and RNA, preventing normal nucleic acid function

Plant Alkaloids

MOA: Prevent formation of spindle fibers

EXAMPLES OF CHEMOTHERAPY AGENTS

GENERIC	BRAND	DOSAGE FORMS	CLASSFICATION
bleomycin	Blenoxane	IV, IM, SC	Antibiotic
busulfan	Myleran	Tablet	Alkylating
chlorambucil	Leukeran	Tablet	Nitrogen mustard
cisplatin	Platinol	IV, tablet	Alkylating
cyclophosphamide	Cytoxan	Tablet, injection	Alkylating
cytarabine	Cytosar-U	SC, IM, IV	Antimetabolite
daunorubicin	Cerubidine	IV	Antibiotic
doxorubicin	Adriamycin	IV	Antibiotic
epirubicin	Ellence	IV	Antimetabolite
etoposide	VePesid	Capsule, IV	Plant alkaloid
fluorouracil	Efudex	Cream, IV, topical solution	Antimetabolite
hydroxyurea	Hydrea	Capsule	Antimetabolite
lomustine	CEENU	Capsule	Alkylating
melphalan	Alkeran	IV	Nitrogen mustard
mercaptopurine	Purinethol	Tablet	Antimetabolite
methotrexate	Rheumatrex	IM, IV, tablet	Antimetabolite
mitomycin C	Mutamycin	IV	Antibiotic
temozolomide	Temodar	Capsule	Antibiotic
thioguanine	Tabid	Tablet	Antimetabolite
thiotepa	Immunex	IV	Nitrogen mustard
valrubicin	Valstar	Injection into the bladder	Antimetabolite
vinblastine	Velban	IV	Plant alkaloid
vincristine	Oncovin	IV	Plant alkaloid

HORMONES

MOA: Inhibit synthesis of adrenal steroids

EXAMPLES OF HORMONE AGENTS

GENERIC	BRAND	DOSAGE FORMS	TARGET
aminoglutethimide	Cytadren	Tablet	Breast, prostate
flutamide	Eulexin	Capsule	Prostate
goserelin	Zoladex	Implant, SC	Prostrate, endometriosis, metastatic breast cancer
leuprolide	Lupron Depot	SC	Prostrate carcinoma, endometriosis
megestrol	Megace	Suspension, tablet	Breast, endometrial
tamoxifen	Nolvadex	Tablet	Breast

EXAMPLES OF BIOLOGIC RESPONSE MODIFIERS

GENERIC	BRAND	DOSAGE FORMS	ADVERSE EFFECTS
aldesleukin	Proleukin	IV	
interferon alfa-2a	Roferon	IM, IV, SC	Weight loss, metallic taste, nausea, vomiting, and abdominal cramps
interferon alfa-2b	Intron	IM, IV, SC	Changes in mental status, sore throats, fever, fatigue, and unusual bleeding
interferon beta-1a	Avonex	IM	Myalgia, fever, chills, malaise, and fatigue
interferon beta-1b	Betaseron	SC	Myalgia, fever, chills, malaise, and fatigue

HUMAN GROWTH HORMONES

MOA: Stimulates the growth of linear bone, skeletal muscle, and organs

EXAMPLES OF HUMAN GROWTH HORMONES

GENERIC	BRAND	DOSAGE FORMS	SPECIAL CONSIDERATIONS
somatrem	Protropin	IM, SC	Refrigerate; sodium retention and increased blood glucose
somatropin	Humatrope, Nutropin	IM, SC	Used in children; drug should not be shaken; may cause both hypoglycemic and hyperglycemic responses

VITAMINS, ELECTROLYTES, AND NUTRITIONAL SUPPLEMENTS

Vitamins

Essential organic constituents found in many food products and necessary for normal metabolic functions. May be either water soluble or fat soluble. Fat-soluble vitamins accumulate in large stores, primarily in the liver. Deficiencies may lead to disease after periods of restricted intake. Excessive intake may result in toxicity. Water-soluble vitamins are easily eliminated by the kidney on a daily basis.

EXAMPLES OF WATER-SOLUBLE VITAMINS

VITAMIN	GENERIC	INDICATIONS	SOURCES
B1	Thiamine	Coenzyme in carbohydrate metabolism Beriberi	Pork, liver, kidney, whole cereal, grains, beans, and yeast
B2	Riboflavin	Maintains integrity of mucous membranes and metabolic energy pathways	Milk, liver, kidney, cereals, and green, vegetables
B3	Nicotinic acid	Involved in fat synthesis, electron transport, and protein metabolism; deficiencies result in diarrhea, dementia, and dermatitis; prevents pellagra	Liver, yeast, lean meats, peanuts, beans
B5	Pantothenic acid	Deficiencies may result in fatigue, headache, sleepiness, nausea, GI pain, and disturbances of coordination	Vegetables, cereals, yeast, and liver
B6	Pyridoxine	Coenzyme in amino acid and fatty acid metabolism	All plants and animals

EXAMPLES OF WATER-SOLUBLE VITAMINS—Cont'd

VITAMIN	GENERIC	INDICATIONS	SOURCES
B9	Folic acid	Needed for the production of healthy red blood cells	Liver and fresh green vegetables
B12	Cyanocobalamin	Intrinsic factor for the production of red blood cells; deficiency is seen in pernicious anemia	Animal tissue
Biotin		Deficiency is characterized by dermatitis and anorexia	Yeast, egg yolk, vegetables, nuts, and cereals
C	Ascorbic acid	Maintaining normal cell membrane permeability promotes wound healing and has anti-inflammatory ability; prevents scurvy	Green plants, tomatoes, citrus fruits

EXAMPLES OF FAT-SOLUBLE VITAMINS

VITAMIN	GENERIC	INDICATIONS	SOURCE
A	Retinol	Prevents keratomalacia	Milk, butter, cheese, liver, and fish oils
D2	Ergocalciferol	Prevents rickets in small children and prevents osteomalacia in adults	Butter, milk, cheese, egg yolk, and fish oils
D3	Cholecalciferol		
E	Tocopherols	Antioxidant for unsaturated fatty acids; deficiency is characterized by irritability, edema, and hemolytic anemia	Soybean oil, wheat germ, rice germ, nuts, corn, butter, eggs, and green leafy vegetables
K	Phytonadione	Formation of prothrombin	Leafy green vegetables, wheat bran, and soybean

Minerals

- Calcium–needed for proper muscle and nerve function; necessary for proper bone and tooth formation; prevention of osteoporosis
- Chromium–aids in metabolism of sugars
- Copper–needed for proper blood formation
- Iodine–needed for proper thyroid function
- Iron–needed for red blood cell formation
- Magnesium–needed for muscle function
- Potassium–needed for heart and nerve function: cellular homeostasis
- Sodium–needed for nerve and muscle formation; cellular homeostasis
- Sulfur–needed for energy production and cellular function
- Zinc–needed for proper immune function

RELATIVE ROLE OF DRUG AND NONDRUG THERAPY

EXAMPLES OF HERBAL MEDICATIONS

NAME	INDICATIONS
Aloe vera	Wound and burn healing
American ginseng	Energy, stress, immune system builder
Basil	Reducing gas
Bilberry	Eye and vascular disorders
Black cohosh	Menopause, premenstrual syndrome, mild depression, arthritis
Cascara sagrada	Laxative
Cat's claw	Anti-inflammatory, antimicrobial, antioxidant, immunosupportive
Catnip tea	Diarrhea
Cayenne	Eliminates chills and discomfort from colds; promotes the healing of ulcers
Chamomile	Calming agent, sedative
Chasteberry	Premenstrual syndrome
Chondroitin	Osteoarthritis

Continued

EXAMPLES OF HERBAL MEDICATIONS—Cont'd

NAME	INDICATIONS
Cinnamon	Gas, diarrhea, upset stomach
Cramp bark	Menstrual cramping
Cranberry	Urinary tract infection
Dandelion	Water retention associated with premenstrual syndrome
Dill	Gas and indigestion
Dong quai	Anemia, energy (females), menopause, dysmenorrheal, premenstrual syndrome
Echinacea	Boost immune system
Evening primrose oil	Premenstrual syndrome
Fennel	Stomach cramps and gas
Feverfew	Headaches; prophylaxis for migraine
Ginger	Antiemetic, anti-inflammatory, gastrointestinal distress
Glucosamine	Osteoarthritis and rheumatoid arthritis
Goldenseal	Boosts immune system
Grapeseed	Antioxidant, allergies, circulation
Green tea	Anticancer, antioxidant, lowers cholesterol
Hop tea	Sleeping aid
Isoflavones	Cancer prevention, decreased bone loss, lower cholesterol, menopausal symptoms
Kava	ADD, ADHD, anxiety, sedation
Lomatium	Antiviral agent for the flu, immunostimulant
Lungwort	Upper respiratory infections
Marshmallow root	Scratchy throat, ulcers, colitis
Melatonin	Insomnia
Milk thistle	Antioxidant, liver disease
Panax	Energy, stress, immune system builder
Passionflower	Tranquilizer
Peppermint	Upset stomach
Saw palmetto	Benign prostatic hyperplasia
Siberian ginseng	Athletic performance, stress, immune builder
Skullcap	Tension headaches, irritability and anxiety associated with premenstrual syndrome, stress
Slippery elm bark	Sore throats
St. John's wort	Improves immune system
Valerian	Sedative, analgesic, nervous tension
White willow bark	Aspirin substitute (analgesic, antipyretic, and anti-inflammatory)
Wild yam	Female vitality

LIFESTYLE/BEHAVIORAL MODIFICATIONS AND THEIR IMPACT ON SPECIFIC DISEASE STATES

ASTHMA

Remove factors from life that may trigger attacks such as pets, dust, and smoke-filled areas. Yearly flu shots are recommended.

DIABETES

Type II or adult-onset diabetes can be modified through weight reduction; oral contraceptives may cause gestational diabetes; secondary diabetes may be caused by oral contraceptives, beta-blockers, diuretics, calcium channel blockers, glucocorticoids, and phenytoin.

HYPERLIPIDEMIA

Modify types of fat consumed, especially saturated fat.

HYPERTENSION

Modify detrimental lifestyle factors by lowering sodium intake; reducing consumption of calories to reduce weight; increasing regular aerobic activity; lowering alcohol consumption; eliminating nicotine usage; and lowering stress levels.

OBESITY

Weight loss occurs when calories consumed are fewer than calories expended. Strategies include changing the amount of protein, carbohydrates, and fat consumed in daily diet; keeping records of what is eaten; restricting cues that stimulate eating; eating smaller portions; avoid skipping meals; avoid eating late at night.

SMOKING CESSATION

Set a date to stop; inform family and close associates of decision to stop smoking; remove cigarettes and other tobacco products from environment; avoid areas where smoking occurs; if attempts have failed in the past, look for causes and make plans on dealing with these situations; may be difficult at first to stop, but remain persistent.

STROKE

Modify smoking behavior, coronary artery disease, diabetes, alcohol intake, hyperlipidemia, hypertension, obesity, and physical inactivity.

PRACTICE SITE POLICIES AND PROCEDURES REGARDING PRESCRIPTIONS OR MEDICATION ORDERS

- **ASAP Order:** An order that is not as urgent as a STAT order, but should be given special preference in filling
- **PRN Orders:** Medications on an as-needed basis in a hospital
- **Standing Order:** Receiving a specific drug at a specific time each day in a hospital
- **STAT Order:** An order requiring a medication to be filled within 15 minutes in a hospital

INFORMATION TO BE OBTAINED FROM PATIENT/PATIENT'S REPRESENTATIVE

Information collected from either the patient or their representative by the pharmacy technician is maintained on a patient profile. Every patient has a profile. This information is necessary for the pharmacist to ensure that the patient receives the proper medication and to reduce potential adverse effects.

This information includes:
- **Patient information:** Name, sex, address, and age of patient. The telephone number of the patient is highly recommended
- **Billing information:** Who is responsible for payment of prescription; whether it is the patient or a third-party provider. The third-party provider information includes a group number and subscriber number (i.e., Social Security number) and the individual's relationship to the cardholder
- **Disease states or health conditions:** Specific medications can have an adverse effect on a disease state or condition; drug–disease interactions
- **Medications patient is taking:** Either prescription or OTC medications. Information is used to prevent drug–drug interactions
- **Drug allergies:** Any medication allergies the patient is known to possess. This information is necessary to ensure that the patient does not receive a medication that can have an adverse effect on the patient

REQUIRED PRESCRIPTION ORDER REFILL INFORMATION

Information required for refilling a prescription includes patient's name, patient's home telephone number, and prescription number. Some systems require the name, strength, and quantity of medication. Pharmacies may be able to locate a prescription by reviewing the patient's profile.

FORMULA TO VERIFY THE VALIDITY OF A PRESCRIBER'S DEA NUMBER

DEA Number

A DEA number consists of two letters and seven numbers assigned to a physician. A physician is required to have a DEA number if he or she wishes to write prescriptions for controlled substances. Institutions, such as hospitals and pharmacies, are required to have a DEA number if controlled substances are dispensed from these locations.

Verifying a DEA Number

- The first letter is either an A, B, F, or M.
- The second letter is the first letter of the physician's last name when they apply for a DEA number

- Add the numbers in the first, third, and fifth positions together
- Add the numbers in the second, fourth, and sixth positions together. Multiply the sum by two
- Add both sums of numbers together. The number in the last column farthest from the right should be the same as the seventh digit of the DEA number. For example, what should be the seventh digit in Dr. Andrew Shedlock's DEA number, if it begins with BS452589_____?

Add $4 + 2 + 8 = 14$
Add $5 + 5 + 9 = 19$; multiply 19 by 2 and get 38
Add 14 to 38 and get 52; the last number should be a 2; therefore, the correct
DEA number for Dr. Andrew Shedlock is BS4525892

TECHNIQUES FOR DETECTING FORGED OR ALTERED PRESCRIPTIONS

Types of Fraudulent Prescriptions

a. Legitimate prescription pads are stolen from physicians' offices and are written for fictitious patients
b. Drug abusers may alter the physician's prescription to obtain larger quantities of medications
c. Drug abusers may have prescription pads from legitimate physicians printed with a different callback number that is answered by an accomplice to verify the prescription
d. Drug abuser will call in prescriptions and give their own telephone number as a callback number
e. Computers may be used to create prescriptions for nonexistent physicians or to copy legitimate physicians' prescriptions

Signs Indicating That a Prescription Was Not Issued for a Legitimate Medical Purpose

a. Prescriber writes significantly more prescriptions or in larger quantities compared with other practitioners in the area
b. The patient appears to be returning too frequently. For example, a prescription that should last for a month is being refilled biweekly or more frequently
c. The prescriber writes prescriptions for antagonistic drugs, such as stimulants and depressants simultaneously
d. The patient is presenting prescriptions written in the names of other people
e. A number of people appear simultaneously or within a short time bearing similar prescriptions from the same physician
f. "Strangers," individuals who are not regular residents of the community, show up with prescriptions from the same physician

Characteristics of Forged Prescriptions

a. Prescription looks "too good"; the prescriber's handwriting is too legible
b. Quantities, directions, or dosages differ from usual medical usage
c. Prescription does not comply with the acceptable standard abbreviations or appears to be textbook presentation
d. Prescription appears to be photocopied
e. Directions written in full with no abbreviations
f. Prescriptions written in different color inks, pens, or different handwriting

PREVENTION TECHNIQUES

a. Know the prescriber and his or her signature
b. Know the prescriber's DEA registration number
c. Know the patient. Check the date of when the prescription was written
d. If there is a discrepancy, the patient must have a plausible reason before the medication is dispensed
e. Anytime there is doubt, request proper identification
f. If you believe that you have a forged, altered, or counterfeited prescription, do not dispense it. Contact the local police
g. If you discover a pattern of prescription abuses, contact the state board of pharmacy or the local DEA office

Knowledge of Techniques for Detecting Prescription Errors

- Verify the patient information is correct, including their birth date, home address, and telephone. Some patients with very common names may appear several times in the pharmacy system. Choosing the incorrect patient may result in an incorrect drug utilization review. Incorrect patient information may lead to incorrect billing to an insurance carrier
- Make sure that the dose is appropriate for the age of the patient
- Check the label on the stock bottle and the NDC number in the computer against the original for confirmation of the order. If it does not seem right, bring it to the attention of the pharmacist
- Pull the appropriate medication from the shelf. Take the label with you when you are retrieving the medication. Do not make assumptions about dosage forms; creams and ointments are different; capsule and spansules are not the same; dosage forms with CR, XL, and SA are not the same as normal tablets or capsules
- Place stock bottles back on shelf on the prescription being verified by the pharmacist. Extra bottles and clutter on the counter can contribute to errors
- Place correct auxiliary label on top of container so the pharmacist can check it before placing it on the bottle for dispensing
- If counting medication out manually, count in multiples of fives

EFFECTS OF PATIENT'S DISABILITIES ON DRUG AND NONDRUG THERAPY

- As patients age, their eyesight may begin to deteriorate. This may increase the possibility of misreading the label and not taking their medication properly
- As patients age, their hearing may decline and they may not properly hear questions being asked and thus provide incorrect information to the pharmacy or not thoroughly understand how they are to take their medication
- An individual's dexterity may worsen as he or she ages and may cause difficulty in removing the lid of the container, resulting in the possibility of missed doses
- As individuals age, they may experience several conditions resulting in additional medications to be taken. The possibility of side effects will increase. Treatment of these side effects may result in additional side effects
- An individual's mental sharpness may decrease, resulting in missed doses from forgetfulness

TECHNIQUES, EQUIPMENT, AND SUPPLIES FOR DRUG ADMINISTRATION

- Home infusion supplies include IV starter kits, CVC starter kits, catheters, IV tubing, extension tubing, IV connectors, IV filters, injection caps, syringes and needles, IV poles, sterile dressings, antibacterial cleansing solutions, sharps containers, infectious waste containers, tape, masks, gloves, batteries (for battery-operated infusion kits), chemotherapy spill kits
- Infusion pumps
- Insulin syringes: 30, 50, 100 units/mL
- Oral syringes: May be used for pediatric medications.
- Radiopharmaceuticals (nucleotide and carrier drugs, such as MAA, MDP, Choletec, Cardiolite, Techniscan)
- Vaginal inserters/vaginal creams and suppositories

MONITORING AND SCREENING EQUIPMENT

Pharmacy technicians should be familiar in the usage of various types of monitoring and screening equipment. These may include:
- AIDS testing kits: Detect HIV antibodies in the blood
- Air purifiers: Remove dust, pollen, spores, secondhand smoke, and other irritants from room air
- Blood-glucose monitors (glucometer): Used to determine glucose in the blood
- Blood pressure monitors: Used to determine blood pressure of an individual
- Echocardiogram: Used to measure the functionality of the heart valves
- Electrocardiogram: Used to measure cardiac rates and rhythms
- Nebulizers: Generate very fine particles of liquid in a gas and are used in providing inhalation therapy
- Oxygen therapy: Supplemental oxygen is used to treat both respiratory and nonrespiratory clinical disorders
- Peak flow meter: Used to measure and manage asthma in an individual
- Phototherapy: Used in the treatment of neonatal jaundice; consists of an illuminator, fiber optic cable, and fiber optic panel
- Pneumograms: Two-channel recording of heart rate and respiration in the monitoring of apnea

- Pregnancy testing kits: Used to diagnose pregnancy based upon the ability to detect human chorionic gonadotropin (HCG) in the urine
- Sphygmomanmeter: Used to measure vital capacity
- Steam vaporizers: Provide relief for upper respiratory illness, such as colds and sinusitis
- Thermometers: Used to measure body temperature and will be of one three types—oral, rectal, or stubby. Basal thermometers are used to determine whether or not a women is ovulating

MEDICAL AND SURGICAL APPLIANCES AND DEVICES

- Bedpans: Used for the collection of feces
- Breast pumps: Allows women to continue breastfeeding their baby when they return to work. They may be either manual or electrical
- Bulb syringes: A nonsterile irrigation method for the nose, ear, wounds, or vagina
- CADD-Plus pump: Infusion pump for antibiotics
- CADD Prizm PCS pump/patient controlled analgesias (PCA)
- CADD-TPN: Infusion pump for total parenteral nutrition
- Cane: A walking device that provides a means to transfer weight off the weak limb and provide balance over the supporting limbs
- Catheters: Used to collect urine from a patient unable to urinate naturally
- Commode: A portable toilet used when a patient is unable to ambulate from the bed to the bathroom
- Crutches: Provide support for the patient's wrist and elbow; provide more support than a cane
- Cushions and supplies for pressure sores:
- Elastometric balloon system: Pressurized balloon and is infused by deflating the device
- Electric heating pads: Used to apply dry heat to an individual and does not result in the leaking or spilling of hot water on an individual. The temperature is kept constant
- Enema Syringes: Used for irrigating with water, salt solution, soap suds, or special medications
- Enteral feeding tubes include: Nasogastric tube (NG), nasoduodenal tube (ND), nasojejunal tube (NJ), percutaneous endoscopic tube (PEG), and percutaneous endoscopic jejunostomy tube (PEJ)
- Gravity infusion system: Medication in a minibag is infused by means of gravity. Patient controls the number of drops
- Hospital beds: May be either manual or electrical; fixed or variable height and may come with a mattress, safety rails, bed handles, alternating pressure pads and trapeze bars
- Hot water bottles: A method of applying dry heat to an area. They should have a cover to prevent the skin from becoming burned
- IV push system: manually depressing syringe
- Moist heat packs: Known as hydrocollators. Can be heated either by boiling water or being placed in a microwave. They are reusable and can be stored in the freezer when not in use
- Ostomy appliance for solid waste: Known as a colostomy bag
- Ostomy appliance for urine and semisolids: Used for urinary diversions and ileostomies.
- Patient lifter: May be either hydraulic or a screw type lifter. Enables a patient to be lifted up and down into a chair
- Syringe infusion system: Medication is infused by a special syringe pump
- Traction: May be either flexion or hyperextension. Can be used for cervical or pelvic traction
- Transcutaneous electrical nerve stimulation (TENS): Delivers electrical signals throughout the skin to control pain
- Urinals: Use to collect urine. Male and female urinals differ in shape
- Vacuum constriction device: A nonsurgical solution to impotence in men. The penis is placed in a patented vacuum cylinder, which generates blood flow in the penis resulting in an erection
- Walker: Provides steadier support than a cane but it requires good arms, wrists, and hands
- Wheelchairs: Should be individualized for the patient based on the patient's physical limitations and lifestyle. A wheelchair should provide good body alignment

PROPER STORAGE CONDITIONS

All medications have specific storage conditions determined by the manufacturer, which include the type of container (such as a light-resistant container) and temperature. The following definitions indicate the proper temperature at which a drug is to be properly stored.

Cold: Not to exceed 8°C (46°F)

Cool: Any temperature between 8 and 15°C (46–59°F)

Room temperature: Any temperature between 15 and 30°C (59–86°F)

Warm: Any temperature between 30 and 40°C (86–104°F)

Excessive heat: Any temperature above 40°C (104°F)

Specific packaging requirements include:

- **Light-resistant container:** Protects contents from the effects of light through the use of special materials or by an opaque covering
- **Tamper-resistant packaging:** Sealed in a manner that would alert an individual that the package had been opened
- **Tight container:** Protects contents from contamination by liquids, solids, or vapors during normal shipping, handling, storage, and distribution
- **Hermetic container:** The container is impermeable to air under normal handling, shipment, storage, and distribution
- **Single-unit container:** The container holds a specific quantity of drug for a single dose
- **Single-dose container:** Single-unit container intended for parenteral administration only
- **Unit-dose container:** A single-unit container for articles intended for administration other than the parenteral route as a single dose, directly from the container

AUTOMATED DISPENSING TECHNOLOGY

Automated Dispensing Systems

A drug storage device or cabinet that electronically dispenses medications in a controlled fashion and track medication use. Automatic dispensing allows a nurse to obtain medication for inpatients at the point of use. The systems require user identifiers and passwords and internal electronic devices track nurses accessing the system, track the patients for whom medications are administered, and provide usage to the hospital's financial office for the patients' bills. The system may be centralized or decentralized.

Robotics

Using machinery that increases productivity in the pharmacy and results in fewer prescription errors.

Outpatient Dispensing System

- Baker cells: Can accurately count and dispense up to 600 tablets per minute. A flexible, lockable system that can adapt to various space requirements and can be expanded if necessary. Can interface with pharmacy host system.

Inpatient Dispensing Systems

- **AcuDose-Rx** (HBOC/McKesson): A decentralized medication distribution center. Operational after a physician's order has been entered into the patient's profile. Authorized users choose the patient's profile and select the appropriate drug.
- **Baxter ATC-212:** The system uses a microcomputer to pack unit-dose tablets and capsules for oral administration. It is installed at the pharmacy. Medications are stored in calibrated canisters that are designed specifically for each medication. The canisters are assigned a numbered location intending to reduce mixup errors upon dispensing. A order is sent to the microcomputer and a tablet is dispensed from a particular canister. The drug is ejected into a strip-packing device in which it is labeled and hermetically sealed.
- **McLaughlin Dispensing System:** Includes a bedside dispenser, a programmable magnetic card, and a pharmacy computer. It is a locked system that is loaded with the medications for a specific patient. At the correct dosing time, the bedside dispenser drawer unlocks automatically to allow a dose to be removed and administered to the patient. A light above the patient's door illuminates at the appropriate dosing time.
- **MedCarousel:** A medication and storage system and retrieval system for hospital pharmacies with vertically rotating shelves and is bar code scannable.
- **Physician's Order Entry System:**
   Med Direct: An automated system for communicating medication ordering for managing documents.
   OmniLink Rx: An advanced patient safety solution for the management of handwritten physician orders; it simplifies the communication of orders from remote nursing stations to the pharmacy. Improves communication between nursing and pharmacy, resulting in improved efficiency and productivity.

- **PYXIS Medstation, Medstation RX, and Medstation Rx:** This is an automated dispensing device kept on the nursing unit. The Medstation interfaces with the pharmacy computer. Physician orders are entered into the pharmacy computer and then transferred to the Medstation where patient profiles are displayed to the nurse who accesses the medications for verified orders. Each nurse is provided with a password that must be used to access the Medstation. Charges are made automatically for drugs dispensed by the unit.
- **Robot RX:** A centralized, robotic drug distribution system that automates storage, dispensing, returning, restocking, and crediting bar-coded inpatient medications.
- **SafetyPak:** An automated bar code medication packaging system. Can be used for unit-dose and multidose oral solid medications. Automates the replenishment of decentralized cabinets and the filling of individual patient medication bins.

PACKAGING REQUIREMENTS

The packaging is determined by the manufacturer's specification to ensure the effectiveness and shelf life of the drug. The packaging will be affected by how a medication is to be stored in the pharmacy. A pharmacy technician must be familiar with the packaging of each medication. The packaging conditions take into consideration temperature, humidity, light, and incompatibilities with other medications and various types of packaging materials.

All medications, whether prescription or OTC, are subject to the Poison Prevention Act of 1970. Exceptions to this law include:
- Single time dispensing of product in noncompliant container as ordered by the physician
- Single-time or blanket dispensing of product in noncompliant container as requested by patient or customer in a signed statement
- One noncompliant size of OTC product for elderly or handicapped patients provided that they contain the warning "This package for households without young children," or "Package Not Child Resistant"
- Drugs dispensed to institutionalized patients provided that these are to be administered by an employee of the institution

SPECIFIC DRUGS
- Betamethasone with no more than 12.6 mg per package
- Erythromycin ethylsuccinate tablets in packages containing no more than 16 g
- Inhalation aerosols
- Mebendazole tablets with no more than 600 mg per package
- Methylprednisolone tablets with no more than 85 mg per package
- Oral contraceptives taken cyclically in manufacturer's dispensing package
- Pancrelipase preparations
- Powdered anhydrous cholestyramine
- Powdered colestipol up to 5 g per packet
- Prednisone tablets with no more than 105 mg per package
- Sodium fluoride tablets with no more than 264 mg of sodium fluoride per package
- Sublingual and chewable isosorbide dinitrate, in dosages of 10 mg or less
- Sublingual nitroglycerin tablets

NDC NUMBER COMPONENTS

Each drug is assigned a specific 11-digit number to identify it. The first five numbers identify the manufacturer, the next four numbers identify the drug product, and the final two numbers represent the package size and packaging. If a medication is reformulated, it will be given a new NDC number. If a drug manufacturer purchases another drug company, the NDC number will also change.

PURPOSE FOR LOT NUMBERS AND EXPIRATION DATES

Lot numbers are assigned by the drug manufacturer to identify a given batch of medication. Expiration dates are assigned by the manufacturer, and ensure the amount of time a product will be pure, safe, and effective to be used by a patient. The expiration date is the last day of a particular month of a given year. Both of these pieces of information are used in the recall of a drug whether by the manufacturer or the FDA

INFORMATION FOR PRESCRIPTION OR MEDICATION ORDER LABEL(S)

A prescription is filled in an outpatient pharmacy for a patient. A medication order is filled for an individual who has been assigned a bed in a hospital or long-term care facility.

Required Prescription Label Information
- Date when the prescription was filled
- Serial (prescription) number of the prescription
- Name and address of the pharmacy
- Name of the patient
- Name of the prescribing physician
- All directions for use on the prescription
- Generic or brand name of the prescription
- Strength of the medication
- Name of the drug manufacturer
- Quantity of the drug
- Expiration date of the drug
- Initials of the licensed pharmacist
- Number of refills allowed

Auxiliary (Ancillary) Labels

Provide additional information, such as special instructions, warnings, or storage conditions to the patient. They may provide information on the administration of the drug.

Required Medication Order Label Information
- Name and location of patient
- Trade/generic name of drug
- Strength of drug
- Quantity of drug
- Expiration date of medication
- Lot number of medication

REQUIREMENTS REGARDING PATIENT PACKAGE INSERTS

A patient package insert is an informational leaflet written for the lay public describing the benefits and risks of medications.

Information Found on a Package Insert
- Description
- Clinical pharmacology
- Indications and usage
- Contraindications
- Warnings
- Precautions
- Adverse reactions
- Drug abuse and dependence
- Overdosage
- Dosage and administration
- How supplied
- Date of the most recent revision of the labeling

A pharmacy is required to provide patient package inserts to all patients receiving metered dose inhalers, oral contraceptives, estrogen, progesterone, and Accutane.

SPECIAL DIRECTIONS AND PRECAUTIONS FOR PATIENT/PATIENT'S REPRESENTATIVE REGARDING PREPARATION AND USE OF MEDICATIONS

The following information can be given to a either the patient or the patient's representative. This information may be considered as counseling and therefore it is the pharmacist's responsibility rather than a pharmacy technician's:

- Name of medication
- Dosage form
- Dosage
- Route of administration
- Duration of therapy
- Action to be taken if a dose is missed
- Common or severe side effects
- Interactions and contraindications of the medication (to include food)
- Self-monitoring of medication
- Proper storage of medication
- Special directions

TECHNIQUES FOR ASSESSING A PATIENT'S COMPLIANCE WITH PRESCRIPTION OR MEDICATION ORDER

- Calculate how many days the prescriptions should last (i.e., days supply = quantity dispensed/quantity taken each day)
- If the patient is seeking a refill early or the prescription is lasting longer than it should last, the pharmacist should seek information from the patient. If the directions have changed, a new prescription should be issued from the physician
- The pharmacist should ascertain the reason for possible noncompliance of the patient in an empathetic manner. The patient may have received professional samples from the physician, or the patient may admit he or she has been experiencing financial difficulties, resulting in noncompliance
- Pharmacists should attempt to persuade physicians not to use "as directed," for directions to the patient
- If the patient has forgotten to take their medication, the pharmacist should work with the patient to find a way to solve the issue
- Finally, the pharmacist should emphasize the importance of compliance to the patient in a caring and understanding manner

ACTION TO BE TAKEN IN THE EVENT OF A MISSED DOSE

Patients need to check with the pharmacist regarding what to do if they forget a dose. Situations vary depending on the medication and frequency of dosing. Providing this information is part of counseling and can only be done by a pharmacist.

MEDICATION DISTRIBUTION

REQUIREMENTS FOR MAILING MEDICATIONS

The US Post Office will not allow the mailing of controlled substances with the exception of the Veterans Administration. Other postal services (such as FedEx or UPS) are not governed by these regulations, but the outside label of the package is to be unmarked so it cannot be identified. Medications mailed from a drug manufacturer must be sent by registered mail with a return request form.

DELIVERY SYSTEMS FOR DISTRIBUTING MEDICATIONS

Drug Distribution System

A safe and economical method of distributing a medication. A drug distribution system includes the packaging that holds the medication during the transfer of the drug from the pharmacy to the patient.

- **Centralized dispensing:** A system of distribution in which all functions—processing, preparation, and distribution—occur in the main area. Medications are transported to the floors on a daily basis at predetermined times. Multiple deliveries may be needed for certain intravenous preparations for stability issues. The pharmacist is responsible for visually checking the work of the technicians. Centralized dispensing has greater management control.

- **Decentralized dispensing (satellite pharmacy):** A system of distribution in which all functions (processing, preparation, and distribution) occur on or near the nursing unit. A decentralized pharmacy may service multiple nursing units. An advantage of a decentralized pharmacy is the pharmacist-physician-nurse-patient relationship.
- **Floor stock system:** A storage of medication on the patient care units of a hospital. The nursing staff is responsible for all aspects of preparation and administration of medications. Disadvantages of this system include:
  1. Increased potential for medication errors—pharmacist does not review medication orders
  2. Increased drug inventory is needed because of multiple inventories. Poor inventory control
  3. Storage and control problems due to limited storage on nursing floors
  4. Greater possibility of drug diversion and misappropriation of medications
- **Individual prescription system:** Medications are dispensed in a multiple dose vials. A 3-5 day supply is provided by the pharmacy. Time management issues occur.
- **Unit-dose:** Provides the medication in its final "unit of use." Improves productivity and reduces errors during ordering, distribution, storage, and administration of the medication. Advantages of unit dose include: a reduction in medication errors, improved drug control, a decrease in the overall cost of medication distribution, improved medication billing and decreased medication credits, and a reduction in drug inventories Variations in the unit dose system include a modified unit-dose system and a blended unit-dose system.

Modified unit dose: Combines unit-dose medications blister packaged (punch cards, bingo cards or blister cards) instead of being placed in a box. Packaged in quantities of 30, 60, or 90.

Blended unit dose: Combines unit of use with non-unit dose drug distribution system.

- **Multiple medication package:** All medications for a specific administration time are packaged together.
- **Modular cassette:** combination of drawer exchange with unit dose (7-day system).

Dumbwaiter: An in-house elevator used to transport medications and supplies. Major disadvantage of dumbwaiters is that they move vertically only.

Robotics: A mobile, computerized mechanical device programmed to move throughout the hospital and deliver medications. In certain situations, robotics can be programmed to scan and pick medications for specific patients.

Pneumatic tube: A method of sending medication orders through the hospital by placing them in a tube and sending them to a dispatcher who then forwards them to a specific location.

REQUIREMENTS FOR DISPENSING INVESTIGATIONAL DRUGS

- Investigational drugs are dispensed for a controlled study only, which is sponsored by a drug manufacturer or agency. The FDA may allow dispensing of a particular drug for a particular situation when all other methods of treatment have been exhausted. The Pharmacy and Therapeutic Committee asks the pharmacy to maintain administrative control over the clinical investigation. Duties of the hospital pharmacy include:
  1. Distribution and control of investigational drugs, which includes drug procurement, storage, inventory management, packaging, labeling, distribution, and disposition
  2. Clinical services, such as patient education, staff in-service training, and the monitoring and reporting of adverse drug reactions
  3. Research activities, such as participation in the preparation or review of research proposals and protocols, assisting in data collection and research
  4. Clinical study management, writing reports to drug sponsor
- Physicians initiate the process of prescribing investigational drugs. They must:
  1. Obtain approval for any study of investigational agents from the Institutional Review Board
  2. Complete the Investigational Drug Data Form and return to the pharmacy
  3. Provide the pharmacy with a copy of the signed consent form
  4. Instruct the manufacturer to supply the pharmacy with all pharmacologic and stability data
  5. Make arrangements for the transfer of the drug to the pharmacy
  6. Arrange for the pharmacy to maintain a minimum level of the medication
- In controlled studies, the investigational drugs are received from the sponsoring company. Accurate dispensing records must be kept for the sponsor. These medications need to be kept separately in the pharmacy from other medications. After the study has been completed, the leftover drugs are returned to the sponsor.

RECORD-KEEPING REQUIREMENTS FOR MEDICATION DISPENSING

CONTROLLED SUBSTANCES

All controlled substance prescriptions in System 2, File II should be stamped with a red C 1" in height in the lower right hand corner (Table 2-4). All controlled substance records must be maintained for a minimum of 2 years and are readily retrievable. Readily retrievable refers to being able to provide the records within 48 hr of a request to view the records.

- **Biennial inventory of narcotics:** Must be maintained in the pharmacy.
- **Change of pharmacist-in-charge inventory:** Must be maintained in the pharmacy.
- **Controlled substance invoices:** Must be maintained in the pharmacy. Schedule II invoices should be attached to pharmacy's copy of the DEA Form 222 with the appropriate dating and signature. Schedule III-V need to be stamped with a red C, dated, and signed by the individual checking the invoice. Schedule III-V invoices need to be kept separate from Schedule II invoices.
- **Exempt narcotic log:** Requires name and address of purchaser (must be at least 18 years of age), name of product and date sold, seller's signature, and price of product. The pharmacist must be present in any transaction involving "exempt narcotics".
- **Master formula record:** Work sheets are considered permanent records. Provides directions for compounding and uniform record keeping. Quantities and lot numbers of ingredients used; initials of the preparer and pharmacist who checked the work; and calculations performed to make the compound must be kept.
- **Material Safety Data Sheet (MSDS):** Documentation required by the Occupational Safety and Health Administration (OSHA) that a facility receive this sheet time every time a hazardous chemical is provided to it; hazardous chemicals may be either physical or health hazards.
- **Medication Administration Record (MAR):** Provides documentation that a drug has actually been dispensed in a hospital or long-term facility. MARs are found in hospitals and long-term care facilities.
- **Nonsterile compounded products:** All recipe information is copied and shows step-by-step process. The following information is documented: date prepared, name of ingredients, manufacturer of ingredient, lot number and expiration date of each ingredient, amount or weight of each ingredient, dosage form of each ingredient, pharmacy lot number assigned, technician's initials, pharmacist's initials, date dispensed, patient's name, and medical record number. This information must be maintained for a minimum of 2 years.
- **PoisonLog:** Requires name and address of purchaser (must be at least 18 years of age), name of product and date sold, intended use, seller's signature, and price of product.
- **Prescription hard copy:** On the back of the hard copy of the prescription is a copy label with the initials of the pharmacist or technician who filled the prescription. Prescriptions are filed numerically. Backup copies are made at the end of the day. They must be maintained for a minimum of 2 years.
- **Repackaged medications:** All repackaged medications must be maintained on a log with the following information: date, drug, dosage form, manufacturer, manufacturer's lot number, manufacturer's expiration date, pharmacy lot number, pharmacy expiration date, technician, and pharmacist. The information must be readily retrieved.

AUTOMATIC STOP ORDERS

Used for specific classifications of medications, which can be active for only a limited period after which a new medication order is required to continue. These medications will automatically be stopped after a given period unless other specified by a physician

Examples:
- Analgesics: 30 days
- Antianemia drugs: 30 days

TABLE 2-4   Filing of Prescriptions

SYSTEM	FILE I	FILE II	FILE III
1	CII Separate	CIII-CV	All other prescriptions
2	CII Separate	CIII-CV and all legend drugs	
3	CII-CV	All other prescriptions	

- Antibiotics: 7 days
- Antiemetics: 4 days
- Anticoagulants: 30 days
- Antihistamines: 7 days
- Antineoplastics: 30 days
- Barbiturates: 30 days
- Cardiovascular: 30 days
- Cathartics: 30 days
- Cold preparations: 5 days
- Dermatologic: 30 days
- Diuretics: 30 days

RESTRICTED MEDICATION ORDERS

Restricted drug: A therapeutic agent, admitted to a formulary, which is authorized for a specific doctor or group of doctors by a committee. Guidelines for use include: drugs in the category will be dispensed only if prescribed by a full-time faculty member of the designated group of physicians. Other members of the medical staff may prescribe the drug for an individual patient if they have the drug order authorized by one of the designated doctors.

QUALITY IMPROVEMENT METHODS

- Adequate lighting can prevent errors from occurring
- Bar code scanning for ordering medications to maintain appropriate stock levels
- Be aware of look-alike drug names
- Confirming illegible prescriptions with the physician
- Digital imaging of what the medication should look like and showing manufacturer's container with NDC number
- Double counts of narcotics
- If medications are being counted manually, count in multiples of fives
- Make sure the prescribed agent is appropriate for the clinical situation
- Order should be transcribed and read back to the party giving the order
- Perpetual inventories can reduce possible theft
- Scanning prescriptions can reduce prescription errors
- Tech-check-tech is a method to catch prescription errors
- Verbal orders should only be taken by authorized personnel
- Workflow allows for processing prescriptions in a systematic manner, resulting in speedier processing and fewer prescription errors

PHARMACY CALCULATIONS

ROMAN NUMERALS

Many doctors continue to use Roman numerals when writing for quantities in a prescription or in the directions to the pharmacist. It is imperative that the pharmacy technician be able to correctly interpret these numerals in a prescription. Listed below are the more commonly used Roman numerals.

Ss = ½
I or i = 1
V or v = 5
X or x = 10
L or l = 50
C or c = 100

Rules for interpreting Roman numerals:
1. When a smaller numeral is repeated or follows a larger numeral, the numbers are added. For example:

iii = 1 + 1 + 1 = 3; vii = 5 + 1 + 1 = 7; xvi = 10 + 5 + 1 = 16

2. If a smaller numeral precedes a larger numeral, the smaller numeral is subtracted from the larger numeral. The smaller number in front of the larger number must not be smaller than one tenth of the larger number. For example:

$$\text{iv} = 5 - 1 = 4, \text{ix} = 10 - 1 = 9$$

3. Numerals are never repeated more than three times (i.e., iii = 3, xxx = 30); 4 should be written iv, not iiii; 40 should be written XL instead of XXXX

4. If a smaller numeral is between two larger numerals, the smaller numeral is subtracted from the numeral following it. For example:

$$10 + (5 - 1) = 14, \text{XXIX} = 10 + 10 + (10 - 1) = 29$$

RATIO/PROPORTION

A ratio is a relationship between two parts of a whole or between one part and the whole. A ratio can be written either as 1/2 or 1:2. A proportion is a relationship between two ratios. A proportion may be written as 1/2 = 2/4 or 1:2::2:4. The majority of all pharmaceutical calculations performed in either retail or institutional settings can be accomplished by using proportions.

There are two ways to solve proportion problems. The first involves cross multiplying and dividing, whereas the second method is described as the mean and extremes. Both methods will yield the same answer if set up correctly. Solve the following problem using both methods.

$$\frac{4}{7} = \frac{X}{28}$$

where X is the value we are seeking

Method 1: Cross-multiply and divide

$$\frac{4}{7} = \frac{X}{28}$$

Multiply the numerator on the left hand side of the equation by the denominator on the right hand side (i.e., 4 × 28 = 112).

Multiply the denominator of the left hand side of the equation by the numerator on the right hand side of the equation (i.e., 7 × X = 7X).

Divide both sides of the equation by the side where a number is represented by a number multiplied by X. For example:

$$\frac{112}{7} = \frac{7X}{7}$$
$$16 = X$$

Always make sure that units in the numerator correspond and the units in the denominator are the same. If they are not, the likelihood of an incorrect answer increases.

Method 2: Means and extremes

4:7::X:28, where the first and last number in the series are considered the extremes and the two numbers in the middle are considered the means. In this situation, the 4 and the 28 represent the extremes and the 7 and X represent the means. One multiplies the extremes (4 × 28) and then multiplies the means (7 × X).

$$4 \times 28 = 7 \times X$$
$$12 = 7X$$

Divide both sides of the equation by the side where a number is represented by a number multiplied by X.

$$\frac{112}{7} = \frac{7X}{7}$$
$$16 = X$$

Always make sure the units in the first and third positions are the same and the units in the second and fourth position are the same. If they are not, the likelihood of an incorrect answer increases.

REDUCING AND ENLARGING A FORMULA

When a formula specifies a specific total quantity, one may determine how much of each ingredient is needed to prepare a different total quantity by using this equation:

$$\frac{\text{Total quantity of formula (specified)}}{\text{Total quantity of formula (desired)}} = \frac{\text{quantity of an ingredient (specified) in formula}}{X}$$

METRIC-HOUSEHOLD-APOTHECARY CONVERSION

The practice of pharmacy uses the metric system, the household system, and the apothecary system. A pharmacy technician must be able to calculate doses of medication in any of these systems and to convert them from one system to another system. It is essential that an individual memorize the basic conversions. Using proportions can solve any conversions.

Prefixes

Nano: one billionth of the basic unit
Micro: one millionth of the basic unit
Milli: one thousandth of the basic unit
Centi: one hundredth of the basic unit
Deci: one tenth of the basic unit
Deka: 10 times the basic unit
Hecto: 100 times the basic unit
Kilo: 1,000 times the basic unit

Metric

Length (meter): Commonly used measurements in the practice of pharmacy are millimeter (mm), centimeter (cm), and meter.

$$1,000 \text{ millimeters (mm)} = 100 \text{ centimeters (cm)}$$
$$100 \text{ centimeters (cm)} = 1 \text{ meter (m)}$$

Weight (gram): Commonly used measurements in the practice of pharmacy are microgram, milligram, gram, and kilogram

$$1,000 \text{ micrograms (mcg)} = 1 \text{ milligram (mg)}$$
$$1,000 \text{ milligrams (mg)} = 1 \text{ gram (g)}$$
$$1,000 \text{ grams (g)} = 1 \text{ kilogram (kg)}$$

Volume (liter): Commonly used measurements in the practice of pharmacy are milliliter (mL) and liter (L)

$$1,000 \text{ milliliters (mL)} = 1 \text{ liter (L)}$$

Household

Weight
2.2 lb = 1 kg
Volume
5 mL = 1 teaspoon (tsp)
3 tsp = 1 tablespoon (tbsp)
2 tbsp = 1 fluid ounce (fl oz)
8 fl oz = 1 cup
2 cups = 1 pint (pt)
2 pt = 1 quart (qt)
4 qt = 1 gallon (gal)

Apothecary

Weight:
20 grains (gr) = 1 scruple

3 scruples = 1 dram
8 drams = 1 ounce
12 ounces = 1 pound
Volume:
60 minims = 1 fluid dram
8 fluid drams = 1 fl oz
16 fl oz = 1 pint
2 pints = 1 quart
4 quarts = 1 gallon

Apothecary Metric

16.23 minims = 1 mL
1 fl dram = 5 mL
1 fl oz = 29.57 mL (30 mL)
1 pt = 480 mL
1 gal = 3,840 mL
1 g = 15.432 gr
1 gr = 60 or 65 mg
1 lb (avoirdupois) = 454 g
1 oz (apothecary) = 31.1 g
1 oz (avoirdupois) = 28.35 g

UNITS/MEQ

Several pharmaceutical products made from biologic products are expressed as "units" or International Units. Examples of these products include insulin, heparin, and vitamin E. Units represent an amount of activity within a particular system. Each pharmaceutical product is unique in determining the amount of activity of that product. Units represent a concentration and may be expressed as units/tablet or units/mL.

CALCULATION OF DOSES

There are two methods to determine a dose; the first looks at what one has in stock and what is needed, which can be expressed as **(HAVE) = (NEED)** in the form of a proportion.

The second method uses the desired dose (D), the drug in stock (H), and the quantity in stock (Q) to calculate the amount of medication to give to the patient.

$$D/H \times Q = \text{Amount of medication to give}$$

PERCENTAGES/STRENGTH OF MEDICATION

Percents are another method of showing a relationship between parts and the whole. Percent means "parts per 100." A number less than a one is considered less than 100%, while a number greater than 1 is greater than 100%. A percent can be calculated using ratios, fractions, or decimals.

Rules

1. To convert a decimal to a percent, multiply the number by 100 and add a percent (%) sign (i.e., $0.45 \times 100 = 45\%$; $1.00 \times 100 = 100\%$; $1.25 \times 100 = 125\%$)
2. To convert a percent to a decimal, remove the % sign and divide by 100 (i.e., $95\%/100 = 0.95$; $50\%/100 = 0.50$; $100\%/100 = 1.0$)
3. To convert a fraction to a percent divide the numerator by the denominator and multiply by 100 and add a % sign (i.e., $95/100 = 0.95$ then multiply by $100 = 95\%$)
4. To convert a percent to a fraction, drop the % sign and write the value of the number as the numerator. Place it over a denominator of 100 and reduce it to its lowest terms (i.e., $75\% > 75/100$, reduce to lowest terms where both 75 and 100 are divisible by 25, resulting in an answer of ¾
5. To convert a ratio to a percent, divide the first number by the second number, multiply by 100, and add a % sign (i.e., 1:10 is the same as $1/10 = 0.1$. Next, multiply 0.1 by $100 = 10\%$)

Percents can be calculated by setting up a proportion. The numerator represents parts and the denominators wholes. The left hand side of the equation can be expressed as:

$$\frac{\text{Parts of the whole}}{\text{Whole}}$$

The right hand side of the equation is expressed in a percent form, where the numerator is a percent of the whole; meanwhile, the denominator is considered 100%.

$$\frac{\text{Percent}}{100\%}$$

The equation would look like this:

$$\frac{\text{Parts of the whole}}{\text{Whole}} = \frac{\text{percent}}{100\%}$$

To solve this type of problem, one needs two of the three variables, parts of the whole, the whole, or the percent. Identify the term as a part of the whole, the whole or a percent. After identifying them and placing them in the equation, cross multiply and divide to find the missing term.

CONCENTRATION/DILUTION

A concentration is a strength. It can be expressed as a fraction (i.e., mg/mL, mEq/mL, or units/mL), as a ratio (i.e., 1:100, 1:1,000, or 1:10,000), or as a percent (i.e., 10%, 25%, or 50%). Percents are found in solids (%w/w) and in solutions (% w/v or %v/v). % w/w is the number of grams per 100 g; %w/v is the number of grams per 100 mL; and % v/v is the number of mL/100 mL).

The majority of all problems involving concentrations result in a dilution of a substance. In a daily application, a pharmacist receives an order to prepare a product of a given strength and volume (weight). This is known as the final strength (FS) and final volume (FV). The pharmacist must go to the shelf, choose the product of a given strength (initial strength [IS]) be and determine the amount (initial volume [IV]) needed to prepare the compound. The same process would be done in preparing solids, except an initial weight (IW) and final weight (FW) would substituted for initial and final volumes.

One can use the following equation for this type of situation:

$$\text{Initial volume (IV)} \times \text{initial strength (IS)} = \text{final volume (FV)} \times \text{final strength (FS)}$$

Hints to prevent errors in solving dilution problems:
Initial strength must be larger than final strength.
Initial volume must be less than final volume.
Final volume minus initial volume equals amount of diluent (inert substance) to be added to make the final volume.

POWDER VOLUME

$$\text{Powder volume} = \text{final volume} - \text{diluent volume}$$

Used in the calculation of reconstituting a solution.

ALLIGATION

Alligations are used in pharmacy when a pharmacist or pharmacy technician is compounding either a solution or a solid. The strength being prepared is different from what they have on their shelf. In this situation, they have at least two different concentrations on their shelf—one that is greater than the desired concentration and one that is less than the desired concentration.

For example, a pharmacist receives an order to prepare four ounces of a 10% solution using a 25% and 5% solution. How much of each these should the pharmacist use?

Step 1: Draw a tic-tac-toe table

Step 2: Place the highest concentration in the upper left hand corner, the lowest concentration in the lower left hand corner, and the desired concentration in the middle.

25%		
	10% (4 oz)	
5%		

Step 3: Subtract the desired concentration from the highest concentration and place that number in the lower right hand corner and express the answer as parts. Next subtract the lowest concentration from the desired concentration and place that number in the upper right hand corner and label it as parts.

25%		5 parts
	10% (4 oz)	
5%		15 parts

Step 4: Total the number of parts. 5 + 15 parts = 20 parts

Step 5: Set up a proportion using the parts of the highest and lowest concentration and the total quantity to be prepared.

$$25\%: \frac{5 \text{ parts}}{20 \text{ parts}} \times 4 \text{ ounces} = 1 \text{ oz of } 25\% \text{ needed}$$

$$5\%: \frac{15 \text{ parts}}{20 \text{ parts}} \times 4 \text{ ounces} = 3 \text{ oz of } 5\% \text{ needed}$$

Step 6: Check your work by adding the amounts of each concentration to see if they equal the amount to be compounded.

SPECIFIC GRAVITY

Specific gravity is a ratio expressed as the weight of a substance to the weight of an equal volume of a substance as a standard. Water is the standard that is used and has a specific gravity of 1. Specific gravity can be expressed as

Weight of substance/weight of an equal volume of water

FLOW RATES

Pharmacy technicians must be aware of calculations associated with intravenous fluids. A pharmacy technician must be able to determine the flow rates of intravenous infusions; calculate the volume of fluids administered over a period; and control the total volume of fluids administered to a patient over a period of time.

A variety of IV sets are available to the pharmacist and are identified by the number of drops of a fluid per milliliter. Common IV sets include 10 drops/mL, 15 drops/mL, and 60 drops/mL (minidrip set).

Time of infusion = volume of fluid (or amount of drug)/rate of infusion
Rate of infusion = volume of fluid (or amount of drug)/time of infusion
Infusion rate: Drops/min = (number of mL/hr) × (number of drops/mL)/60 min/hr

CHILDREN'S DOSES

Children will require different amounts of medication than adults. These doses are affected by the individual's age, weight, body surface area, organ development, sex, and disease state. An individual's age is broken down into one of several categories.

Neonates: Birth to 1 month of age
Infant: 1 month to 1 year of age

Early childhood: 1–5 years of age
Late childhood: 6–12 years of age
Adolescence: 13–17 years of age

To calculate the appropriate dosage for children, one of several methods may be used. Young's rule uses age as a guide; Clark's rule uses weight as the determining factor; mg/kg uses weight in terms of kg for a patient, and body surface area uses both height and weight as the basis for choosing a dose.

$$\textbf{Young's rule} = \frac{\text{Age of child (expressed in years)}}{\text{Age of child (in years)} +12} \times \text{adult dose}$$

$$\textbf{Clark's rule} = \frac{\text{Weight of child (expressed in pounds)}}{150} \times \text{adult dose}$$

All four of the these methods require the adult dose and the given parameter to be provided to the practitioner to calculate the appropriate dose. The adult dose may be measured in milligrams, milliliters, units, mEq, or even tablets.

A more accurate method of determining the appropriate dose is based on body surface area (BSA). This method takes into account both the height and weight of the individual (Figure 2-2). If one knows both of these variables, a nomogram (a specialized graph) is referenced. BSA is measured in m^2. The dosage is calculated by:

BSA of child (in m^2)/1.73 m^2 (average adult BSA) × adult dose = approximate dose for child

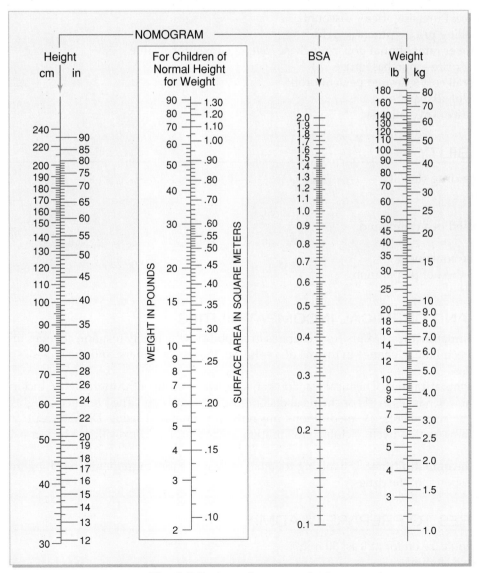

Fig. 2-2 Body surface area chart.

TEMPERATURE CONVERSION

To solve math problems converting Fahrenheit to Celsius or Celsius to Fahrenheit, the following formula can be used:

$$9C = 5F - 160$$

where C represents the temperature in Celsius and F represents the Fahrenheit temperature. Only one of the two variables is required to solve this problem. For example, if an individual were given a temperature of 75°F, they would multiply 75° by 5, subtract 160 from it, and then divide it by 9. The answer would be 23.8°C. On the other hand, if one is told that the temperature was 20°Celsius, multiply the 20 by 9, then add 160 to it, and then divide it by 5, resulting in an answer of 68.

Another way to solve this problem is to use the following equations:

$$F = (C \times 1.8) + 32$$
$$C = \frac{F - 32}{1.8}$$

Either method will yield the same answer.

COMMERCIAL MATH

Cost: Purchase price + cost to dispense
Discount: Purchase price × discount rate
Discounted price: Purchase price − discount
Gross profit: Selling price − purchase price
Inventory turnover rate: Annual dollar purchase/average inventory value
Markup: Selling price − purchase price
Net profit: Overall cost × desired percent profit
Overhead: Sum of all expenses
Profit: Selling price − overall cost

DRUG STABILITY

Factors affecting drug stability:
- Dosage form
- Humidity
- Ingredients used in a compound
- Light
- Material of the container
- Order and method of preparation
- Temperature

PHYSICAL AND CHEMICAL INCOMPATIBILITIES

- **Physical incompatibilities:** Occurs from changes in solubility, which may result in changes in color or the formation of a precipitate. A change in the pH of a solution, the use of buffers, and the type of solvent used may create problems.
- **Chemical incompatibilities:** Chemical reaction between one or more of the ingredients. Incompatibilities may not be noticeable. Changes in pH or chemical decomposition may occur. The presence of light may cause deterioration of the ingredients. IV medications are normally prepared using D5W, except ampicillin, ampicillin/sulbactam, erythromycin lactobionate, imipenem-cilastatin, and oxacillin, which must be mixed with normal saline.
- **Therapeutic incompatibilities:** The mixing together of two or more ingredients, resulting in a change in the therapeutic response of the drugs.

PROCEDURES TO PREPARE IV ADMIXTURES

- Flow hood should be on for at least 30 min
- Wear protective clothing

- Clean laminar flow hood with 70% isopropyl alcohol or other suitable disinfectant pole to hang IV bags, then sides of hood by moving from the back to the front, and finally the bottom of the hood by moving side by side from the back to the front.
- Collect supplies: Check expiration dates and for possible leaks of the bags. Remove dust coverings before placing in the hood. Use presterilized needles, syringes, and filters.
- Position supplies in the hood.
- Sterilize puncture surfaces with an alcohol wipe.
- Prevent coring by placing the vial on a flat surface and insert needle into rubber closure at 45- to 60-degree angle. Use downward pressure on the needle and move needle to a 90-degree angle.
- **Using vials with solutions:** Draw into syringe a volume of air equal to amount of volume being replaced (Figure 2-3). Penetrate vial without coring. Invert vial upside down and pull back on plunger to fill the syringe. Tap air bubbles to come to the top of the syringe. Transfer solution to final container.
- **Vials with lyophilized powder:** Determine the correct volume of diluent and withdraw it. Transfer diluent into vial containing powder. Remove more air from vial than amount of diluent injected. Whirl vial until powder is dissolved. Use new syringe and needle and proceed as if one is using a vial with solution.
- **Using ampules:** If the ampule is not prescored, then score the neck of the ampule with a fine file. Hold ampule upright and tap it. Wipe neck of ampule with alcohol swab. Wrap gauze around the neck and gently snap neck. Inspect and use a filter needle to withdraw. Hold ampule downward at a 20-degree angle and withdraw solution with a filter syringe. Exchange old filter needle with a new filter needle and transfer solution into the final container.

PROCEDURES TO PREPARE CHEMOTHERAPY

- The same aseptic techniques used in preparing IV are used in preparing chemotherapy medications with a few exceptions. Chemotherapy requires a vertical laminar air flow hood, which is smaller than a horizontal laminar flow hood. Special chemotherapy clothing is worn. The hands in a vertical flow hood should not be over the top of any needle, vial, or IV bag.

PREPARING PARENTERAL ANTINEOPLASTICS

- The safety cabinet work surface should be covered with a plastic-backed absorbent paper and disposed of in a biohazard container after use.
- Personnel should be wear surgical gloves and a closed-front surgical gown with knit cuffs. Contaminated gloves or outer gloves should be removed and replaced. If the skin comes in contact with antineoplastics, one should wash the area with soap and water.
- Reconstituted vials should be vented to reduce the possibility of spraying and spillage.
- A sterile alcohol pledget should be wrapped around the needle and vial top during withdraw of solution.
- External surfaces of syringes and IV bags (bottles) should be wiped clean of contamination.
- When using ampules, wrap neck of ampule with sterile alcohol pledget to protect fingers from being cut by the glass.
- Syringes and IV bottles should be properly identified and dated. Cautionary labels should be affixed to the container.
- Safety cabinet should be wiped down with 70% alcohol on completion of compounding.
- Contaminated needles and syringes should be placed in the sharps container. Disposable gowns, gloves, masks, and head and shoe covers should be placed in red biohazard bags.
- Wash hands.
- Dispose of remaining antineoplastic agents according to federal and state regulations.

PROCEDURES TO PREPARE TOTAL PARENTERAL NUTRITION SOLUTIONS

- TPN—total parenteral nutrition—normally contains 50% dextrose, 10% amino acids, and 20% fat. Aseptic technique is required because TPN is infused into the right atrium of the heart. TPN compounders have been developed that include a multichannel pump for the amino acids, dextrose, fats, and other additives that is connected to a personal computer. The computer assists in the calculations and drives the pump. Micro compounding pumps are used for the electrolytes and other additives (Figure 2-4).

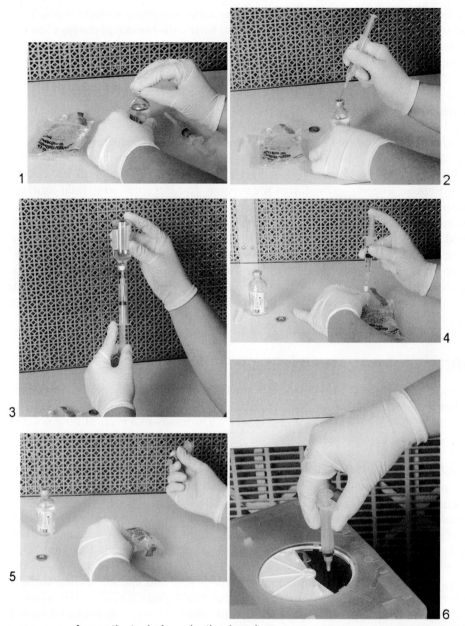

Fig. 2-3 Six-step process of aseptic technique in the hood. (From Hopper T: *Mosby's Pharmacy Technician: Principles & Practice,* Saunders, 2004, St Louis.)

- PPN—Peripheral parenteral nutrition—normally contains 25% dextrose, 10% amino acids, and 10% fat. PPN is a short-term therapy.
- TPN and PPN are premixed from the manufacturer but electrolytes, vitamins, and medications may be added to the nutrients at the pharmacy.

COMPOUNDING TECHNIQUES

Require aseptic technique.

Method 1: Amino acids and dextrose are mixed first. Fats emulsion is added next, followed by the additives.

TPN ORDER SHEET

HOME HEALTH	DATE
PATIENT	ADDRESS

TPN FORMULA:

AMINO ACIDS: ☐ 5.5% ☐ 8.5% ☑ 10%	425	ml
☐ WITH STANDARD ELECTROLYTES		
DEXTROSE: ☐ 10% ☐ 20% ☐ 40% ☐ 50% ☑ 70% (check one)	357	ml
LIPIDS: ☐ 10% ☑ 20% FOR ALL-IN-ONE FORMULA	125	ml

FINAL VOLUME qsad STERILE WATER FOR INJECTION	400mL	1307	ml

Calcium Gluconate	0.465m Eq/ml	5	mEq
Magnesium Sulfate	4m Eq/ml	5	mEq
Potassium Acetate	2m Eq/ml		mEq
Potassium Chloride	2m Eq/ml		mEq
Potassium Phosphate	3m M/ml	22	mM
Sodium Acetate	2m Eq/ml		mEq
Sodium Chloride	4m Eq/ml	35	mEq
Sodium Phosphate	3m M/ml		mM
TRACE ELEMENTS CONCENTRATE	☐ 4 ☐ 5 ☐ 6		ml

Patient Additives:

☐ MVC 9 + 3 10 ml Daily

☐ HUMULIN-R __10__ u Daily

☐ FOLIC ACID_____ mg
_____ times weekly

☐ VITAMIN K_____ mg
_____ times weekly

☐ OTHER: __MVI 12 1.5mL/daily__

☐ OTHER:_____

Directions:

INFUSE: ☑ DAILY
☐ ____ TIMES WEEKLY

OTHER DIRECTIONS:

_____

_____

_____

_____

Rate:	☐ CYCLIC INFUSION:	"	☐ CONTINUOUS INFUSION:	"	☑ STANDARD RATE:
	OVER ____ HOURS	"	AT ____ ml PER HOUR	"	AT __110__ ml PER HOUR
	(TAPER UP AND DOWN)	"		"	FOR __12__ HOURS

LAB ORDERS:

☐ STANDARD LAB ORDERS
SMAC-20, CO2, Mg+2 TWICE WEEKLY
CBC WITH AUTO DIFF WEEKLY
UNTIL STABLE, THEN:
SMAC-20, CO2, Mg+2 WEEKLY
CBC WITH AUTO DIFF MONTHLY

☐ OTHER:_____
_____
_____

VALIDATION:

_____
DOCTOR'S SIGNATURE

Print Name: _____

Office Address: _____

Phone: _____

Fig. 2-4 Example of a total parenteral nutrition (TPN) order. (From Hopper T: *Mosby's Pharmacy Technician: Principles & Practice*, Saunders, 2004, St Louis.)

Method 2: Amino acids are added to the fat emulsion. Dextrose is added next, followed by the additives.
Method 3: Dextrose, amino acids, and fat emulsion are added simultaneously while swirling and mixing. Additives are incorporated last.

PROCEDURES TO PREPARE RECONSTITUTED INJECTABLE AND NONINJECTABLE MEDICATIONS

- **Reconstitution:** Process of mixing a liquid and powder to form a suspension or solution
- **Solvent:** The larger part of the solution
- **Solute:** The agent or ingredient used with solvent
- **Solution:** Solvent + solute
- Measure solute and solvent (distilled water) to be used
- Add solute to solvent in small portions, mix thoroughly
- Check precipitation for solutions or changes in color
- Add new expiration date to product bottle and affix a SHAKE WELL auxiliary label

PROCEDURES TO PREPARE RADIOPHARMACEUTICALS

- Radiopharmaceuticals may be diagnostic or therapeutic; may be oral, IV, or inhaled
- Individual must wear meter indicating the radioactive levels to which the individual is exposed
- Quality control tests are performed to ensure radiopharmaceutical is sterile, pyrogen-free, and pure
- Proper handling of isotopes during preparation and disposal
- Radiopharmaceuticals are to be prepared in vertical flow hood
- Strict packaging requirements for radiopharmaceuticals including the use of special shipping containers
- Safety principles of time, distance, and shielding are observed
- Special training must be completed to work in a nuclear pharmacy

PROCEDURES TO PREPARE ORAL DOSAGE FORMS

- **Unit dose:** Provides medication in the "final unit of use" form. Drug is contained in a small packet. Packet is made of thermal paper and foil laminate; other side is made of poly film material (Figure 2-5).
- Machines may be manual, semiautomatic, or automatic loaded.
- Single drop: 60 packages/min; double drop machine: 120 packages/min.
- Machine drops drug into package, seals package, and, prints medication information in one operation.

PROCEDURES TO COMPOUND STERILE NONINJECTABLE PRODUCTS

Factors to be considered in preparing ophthalmic products include
- **Sterilization:** Can be accomplished by autoclave, filtration, gas, or radiation
- **Clarity:** Free from foreign particles which can be accomplished through filtration
- **Stability:** Affected by chemical nature of the drug substance, pH, method of preparation, solution additives, and packaging.
- **Buffer and pH:** Should be formulated at a pH of 7.4, but rarely occurs. The pH chosen should be optimum for stability.

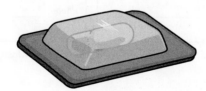

Fig. 2-5 A sample of a blister pack container. (From Hopper T: *Mosby's Pharmacy Technician: Principles & Practice*, Saunders, 2004, St Louis.)

- **Tonicity:** Refers to the osmotic pressure exerted by the salts. An isotonic solution should equal that of sodium chloride 0.9%
- **Viscosity:** Agents are used to prolong contact time in the eye and enhance drug absorption and activity

PROCEDURES TO COMPOUND NONSTERILE PRODUCTS

- **Blending:** An act of combining two substances
- **Comminution:** An act of reducing a substance to small, fine particles
- **Geometric dilution:** A technique used in mixing two ingredients of unequal quantities, where one begins with the smallest quantity and adds an equal quantity of the larger amount. The process continues until all of the quantities are used
- **Emulsifier:** A stabilizing agent in emulsions
- **Flocculating agent:** Electrolytes used in the preparation of suspensions
- **Levigation:** Trituration of a powder drug with a solvent, in which the drug is insoluble with the solvent
- **Mucilage:** A wet, slimy liquid formed as an initial step in the wet gum method
- **Pulverization by intervention:** Reducing the size of a particle in a solid with the aid of an additional material
- **Sifting:** A technique to either blend or combine powders
- **Spatulation:** Mixing powders using a spatula in either a mortar, or an ointment slab, or in a plastic bag. A process used when ingredients may liquefy on mixing. There is no reduction of particle size
- **Thickening agent:** An ingredient used in the preparation of a suspension to increase the viscosity of the suspension
- **Trituration:** A process of rubbing, grinding, or pulverizing a powder to create fine particles
- **Tumbling:** Combining powders in a bag and shaking it

WEIGHING PROCEDURES

- Unlock balance and make sure it is level. Relock balance before placing weights on it
- Placement of weighing papers on pans of scale
- Unlock scale and ensure that it is balanced
- Place weights on right hand pans using forceps
- Place desired material on left hand pans
- Release the beam by unlocking balance
- Lock balance before adding or removing additional powder
- Unlock balance and check for equilibrium
- After the appropriate quantity is on balance, close lid and have pharmacist verify weight
- Remove ingredient and remove weight with forceps

MEASURING USING AN TURISION BALANCE (FIGURE 2-6)

- Leave balance in a draft-free area
- If balance has a level bubble, make sure the bubble is inside the bull's eye and make adjustments using the leveling feet
- Place weighing boat or a single piece of paper on the pan
- When the balance has determined the final weight, press the tare bar to compensate for the weighing boat
- As ingredients are added or removed, the digital display will show the weight

PROCEDURES FOR MEASURING LIQUIDS

- Choose proper size graduate such that quantity to be measured is not less than 20% of the total volume of graduate (Figure 2-7)
- Pour liquid down the center of the graduate slowly and watch the level of liquid rise to desired volume
- Allow time for all liquid to fall in graduate before taking measurement
- Measure level of liquid at eye level and make observation at bottom of meniscus.
- Pour liquid into container and allow for liquid to be completely drained from the graduate.

PROCEDURES TO FILLING CAPSULES

Punch method: Triturate ingredients to the same particle size; mix using geometric dilution. Calculate enough ingredients for several extra capsules. Place powder on ointment slab, where depth of powder is approximately

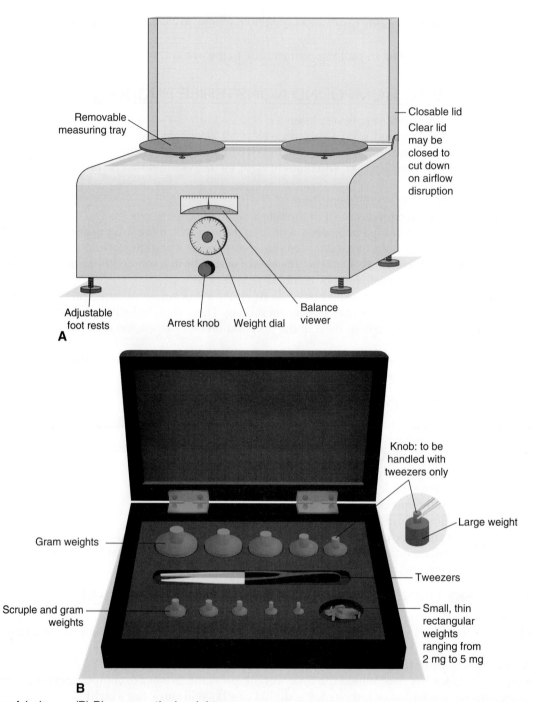

Fig. 2-6 (A) Class A balance. (B) Pharmaceutical weights. (From Hopper T: *Mosby's Pharmacy Technician: Principles & Practice*, Saunders, 2004, St Louis.)

half the length of the capsule body. Hold capsule vertically and punch the open end into the powder until capsule is filled. Place cap on capsule and weigh using an empty capsule as a counterweight. Add or remove ingredient as needed. Hints: Remove exact number of capsules from box; wear finger cots to protect the fingers; roll capsules on a clean towel to remove traces of the drug on the outside; place completed capsules in either a glass or plastic vial; and store in a dry place to prevent them from absorbing moisture or becoming dry (Figure 2-8).
Emulsions: Contains two immiscible liquids, in which one liquid is dispersed throughout another liquid and is aided by a stabilizing agent. May either be oil-in-water (O/W) or water-in-oil (W/O).

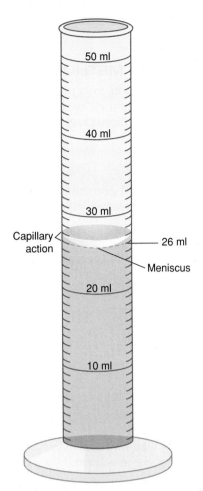

Fig. 2-7 A 50-mL graduate showing the meniscus and proper measurement of solutions. (From Hopper T: *Mosby's Pharmacy Technician: Principles & Practice*, Saunders, 2004, St Louis.)

Number	Approximate amount contained	Example
000	1000 mg	
00	750 mg	
0	500 mg	
1	400 mg	
2	300 mg	
3	200 mg	
4	150 mg	
5	100 mg	

Fig. 2-8 Capsule sizes. (From Hopper T: *Mosby's Pharmacy Technician: Principles & Practice*, Saunders, 2004, St Louis.)

CONTINENTAL METHOD (DRY GUM METHOD)

The primary emulsion is formed from four parts oil, two parts water, and one part gum (emulsifier-acacia). Using a Wedgwood or porcelain mortar, the gum and oil are levigated. Water is added and the trituration continues. After the primary emulsion is formed, additional ingredients may be added and is qs to the initial volume with the external phase.

WET GUM METHOD

Primary emulsion is formed by triturating one part gum and two parts water to form a mucilage. Slowly add four parts oil and triturate slowly. Add additional ingredients.

BEAKER METHOD

Water-soluble and oil-solute ingredients are mixed in separate containers. Both phases are heated to 70°C and are removed from heat. Internal phase is added to the external phase. Final product is cooled to room temperature, but is continually stirred.

POWDERS

Powders are prepared through the use of trituration and geometric dilution.

LIQUID DRUG IN LIQUID VEHICLE

Measure quantities of each liquid in a graduated cylinder. Add drug to vehicle slowly, then shake and stir.

SOLID DRUG IN LIQUID VEHICLE

Weigh solid and measure solvent. One must take into consideration the solubility of the drug and the solvent being used. Triturate drug if needed and dissolve in solvent. May need to heat gently, stir, or shake gently.

NONAQUEOUS SOLUTIONS

Nonaqueous solutions contain solvents other than water, which include elixirs, tinctures, spirits, fluid extracts, glycerates, collodions, liniments, and oleaginous solutions. Prepare by dissolving alcohol-soluble ingredients in alcohol and water-soluble ingredients in water. Add alcohol portion to aqueous portion and stir.

SUPPOSITORIES

Suppository bases may be oleaginous, water soluble, or hydrophilic.

COMPRESSION MOLD

Mix the suppository base and drug ingredients. Force the mixture into a special compression mold.

FUSION MOLD

Active ingredients are dispersed or dissolved in a melted base. Suppository base is melted at a low temperature and the drug is dissolved in it. The base is poured and overfilled into a special suppository mold (metal, plastic, or rubber) and is left to harden. Excess material is removed from the top of the mold.

SUSPENSIONS

The solid drug to be suspended is weighed and is levigated in mortar and pestle with either alcohol or glycerin. A portion of the vehicle is added to mortar and is mixed with the levigated drug until a uniform consistency occurs. This portion of the drug is placed in the final container. The mortar and pestle is rinsed with the balance of the vehicle and the suspension is qs to the final volume with the vehicle being used. A SHAKE WELL label should be affixed to the container. Flocculating and thickening agents may be used in the preparation of a suspension.

SYRUPS

Heat method: Heat needs to be controlled; works fastest, but not all ingredients can be used with heat.
Without heat method: Must use a container that is twice the size of the final volume. The syrup needs to be shaken or stirred.

TABLE **2-5** Property of Ointment Bases

PROPERTY	OLEAGINOUS BASE	ABSORPTION BASE	WATER/OIL EMULSION BASE	OIL/WATER EMULSION BASE	WATER MISCIBLE BASE
Greasiness	Greasy	Greasy	Greasy	Nongreasy	Nongreasy
Occlusiveness	Yes	Yes	Sometimes	No	No
Spreadability	Difficult	Difficult	Moderate to easy	Easy	Moderate to easy
Washability	Nonwashable	Nonwashable	Non or poorly washable	Washable	Washable
Water Content	Anhydrous	Anhydrous	Hydrous	Hydrous	Hydrous
Examples	White petrolatum	Aquaphor	Hydrous lanolin, Eucerin	Hydrophilic ointment	PEG

PROCEDURES TO PREPARE READY-TO-DISPENSE MULTIDOSE PACKAGES

PREPARING OINTMENTS

Ointments can be prepared on an ointment slab. Weigh quantities of each ingredient. Prepare by using geometric dilution and two spatulas to mix the ingredients. Transfer final product into ointment jar by using a spatula. Remove air pockets of ointment by using spatula. Spread evenly in container.

Ointment bases are chosen based on their characteristics to deliver a drug (Table 2-5).

ASEPTIC TECHNIQUES FOR TECHNICIANS

1. No jewelry should be worn in the hood. This includes artificial nails because of microbial growth around or underneath.
2. Long hair should be tied back away from the face.
3. Hands must be washed after entering the IV area and before entering the laminar flow hood (see Figure 2-9).
4. Hands, wrists, and arms to the elbow should be washer with antimicrobial soap and hot water for at least 30 seconds; no more than 90 seconds.
5. Gloves can be worn but should be washed down with 70% isopropyl alcohol after being put on.
6. The surface of the hood should be washed down with 70% isopropyl alcohol using proper method (explained later in this chapter).
7. The hood must run at least 30 minutes before placing medications inside.
8. All vials and ports must be wiped down with alcohol. They should not be sprayed because the alcohol can make contact with the filter in the back of the hood, which breaks down the filter.
9. Hands or any object within the hood cannot block the airflow at any time.
10. Work at least 6 inches into the horizontal hood; keep pens and other objects out of the hood.
11. All needles, syringes, vials and other byproducts must be disposed of improper receptacles.
12. No sneezing talking or coughing can be directed toward the airflow in a laminar flow hood.

INFECTION CONTROL PROCEDURES

UNIVERSAL PRECAUTIONS

1. Applies to all individuals in an institution who may come in contact with blood, other body fluids, or body substances.
2. Latex gloves must be worn when there is a possibility the individual may come in contact with these substances.
3. Hands must be washed after removing the latex gloves.
4. Blood-soaked or contaminated materials must be disposed of in a wastebasket lined with a plastic bag.
5. Specially trained individuals must be notified for cleanup or removal of contaminated waste.
6. Contaminated materials such as syringes, needles, swabs, and catheters must be placed in red plastic containers labeled for disposal of biohazardous materials.
7. A first aid kit must be maintained and adequately stocked if an individual does come in contact with contaminated waste or body fluids. Items to be contained in the first aid kit include adhesive bandages,

alcohol, antiseptic/disinfectant, bleach, disposable latex gloves, disposable towels, medical tape, sterile gauze, and plastic bags for contaminated waste disposal

REQUIREMENTS FOR HANDLING HAZARDOUS PRODUCTS AND DISPOSING OF HAZARDOUS WASTE

- Sharps containers are used for the storage of used syringes, needles, ampules, and vials waiting for disposal. Needles should be clipped or snapped
- Other refuse, such as gloves, gowns, masks, and shoe and head covering should be placed in specially marked biohazard containers. Any clothing or linens that come in contact with body fluids needs to be placed in these receptacles

DOCUMENTATION REQUIREMENTS FOR CONTROLLED SUBSTANCES, INVESTIGATIONAL DRUGS, AND HAZARDOUS WASTES

- **DEA Form 224:** to register a pharmacy with DEA to be able to stock controlled substances
- **DEA Form 222:** to order Schedule II drugs
- **DEA Form 41:** to destroy outdated or unused controlled substances

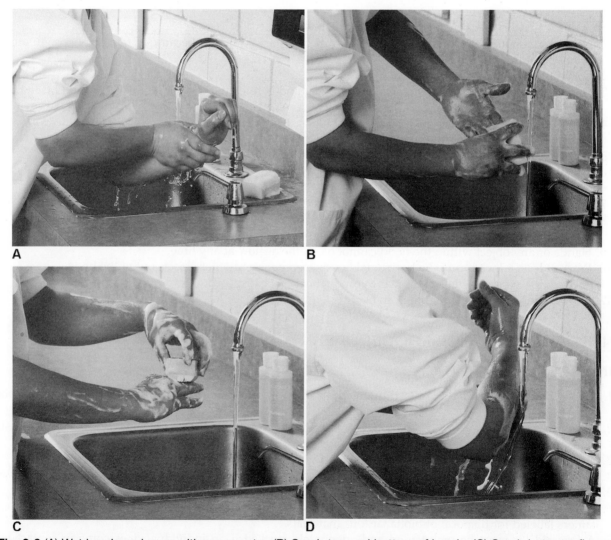

Fig. 2-9 (A) Wet hands and arms with warm water. (B) Scrub top and bottom of hands. (C) Scrub between fingers and up to the elbow. (D) Rinse arms and hands thoroughly. Foot pedals may be used rather than handles. (From Hopper T: *Mosby's Pharmacy Technician: Principles & Practice*, Saunders, 2004, St Louis.)

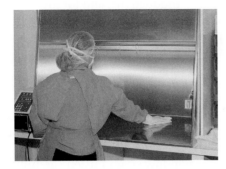

- It is important to be gowned up properly before cleaning the laminar flow hood. All items should be removed from the hood before cleaning.
- Moisten 4 × 4 inch gauze or other disposable cloth or gauze with 70% isopropyl alcohol and wet down the inside of the hood. This includes the sides and tabletop. Make sure you do not spray the HEPA filter at the back or the ceiling inside the hood.
- Then, starting from the top right-hand side of the hood, wipe down, across the surface, and up to the top of the left-hand side of the hood.
- Moving forward a few inches, repeat the motion in the opposite direction.
- The side-to-side, back-to-front motion must be done before using the hood each day. In addition, the hood should be cleaned periodically throughout the course of the day to ensure a sterile environment.

Fig. 2-10 Cleaning the horizontal hood. (From Hopper T: *Mosby's Pharmacy Technician: Principles & Practice*, Saunders, 2004, St Louis.)

- **DEA Form 106:** to report theft of controlled substances
- **Biennial inventory:** Controlled Substance Act of 1970 requires that a pharmacy perform a biennial inventory (every 2 years) of all controlled substances in the pharmacy. An exact count must be performed on all Schedule II drugs and an approximate count performed on Schedules III-V
- **Power of attorney:** Authorizes a pharmacist to order Schedule II drugs
- **Material Safety Data Sheet (MSDS):** Documentation that provides detailed information on the hazards of a particular substance. These hazards may be either physical or health related. Physical hazards may be a chemical that is combustible, flammable, explosive, or corrosive. A health hazard may cause either acute or chronic effects on an individual who has been exposed. Manufacturer is responsible for providing the MSDS to the pharmacy and the pharmacy is responsible to providing the MSDS to the purchaser

INFORMATION FOUND ON AN MSDS FORM

Identification of the substance/preparation: names and alternative names

Composition/information of ingredients: includes uses

Hazards identification: toxicities identified

First aid measures: what to do if inhaled, skin comes in contact with it, eye contact, or ingested

Fire-fighting measures

Accidental release measures

Handling and storage

Exposure controls/personal protection

Physical and chemical properties: includes the form, color, pH, boiling point, melting point, vapor pressure, solubility, partition coefficient, flammable powder class, specific gravity, vapor density, dissociation constant

Stability and reactivity

Toxicologic information: inhalation, skin contact, eye contact, ingestion, long-term exposure

Ecological information: environmental fate and distribution, persistence and degradation, toxicity and effluent treatment

Disposal considerations

Transport information

Regulatory information

Other information

PHARMACY-RELATED COMPUTER SOFTWARE FOR DOCUMENTING THE DISPENSING OF PRESCRIPTIONS OR MEDICATION ORDERS

- Computer software is customized to meet the requirements of the pharmacy.
- Outpatient dispensing software is used to reduce errors, increase productivity, and for inventory management.
- Inpatient sispensing software is used to reduce staff; make accessible to medical staff and to regulate controlled substances. Must interface with various other computer systems in the hospital. Hospitals using robotics possess the capability of scanning unit dose labels and fill patient's orders.

CUSTOMER SERVICE PRINCIPLES

Customer satisfaction is the goal of customer service. Patients coming to a pharmacy do so because they are not feeling well or have a physical ailment. The customer must be treated in a positive manner. The pharmacist should be called to handle any difficult situations.

A technician working on the pharmacy counter or pharmacy window should listen carefully, make eye contact with the patient, repeat what the customer has said, and use positive language to emphasize what can be done rather than what can not be done. If a pharmacy technician is using the telephone, he or she should maintain a pleasant and courteous manner; state the name of the pharmacy and his or her name; adhere to the standard procedures established by the pharmacy, and refer any questions requiring a pharmacist's judgment to the pharmacist.

COMMUNICATION TECHNIQUES

- Appearance
- Empathetic responses to the customer
- Listening
- Nonverbal communication
- Phone skills
- Verbal communication
- Writing skills

PATIENT CONFIDENTIALITY REQUIREMENTS

HIPAA requires that any personally identifiable information be protected as being confidential. Patients will be allowed to access and request copies of their medical records. Health care providers and organizations must provide a written statement that states how medical information will be handled by a provider. Patients are entitled to a complete discussion of health care options from the health care provider. Patients may request that confidential communications is made in a manner that they feel is appropriate. Every organization must have a written privacy procedure. Training must be provided for all employees.

CASH HANDLING PROCEDURES

The technician may be required to ring into the cash register both prescription and other purchases. Many cash registers feature scanners that enter the price into the cash register. If an error occurs, the transaction can be voided and entered manually. The pharmacy technician should accept and count the payment within the sight of the patient. The amount tendered should be entered into the cash register. The amount of change should be counted back to the customer and the customer should be given a cash register receipt. The technician should thank the patient for their purchase.

Checks, debit cards, and credit cards are normally accepted at the pharmacy. Each of these different types of payment may require variations of this process. The pharmacy technician should follow the procedures established by the institution to process these forms of payment.

REIMBURSEMENT POLICIES AND PLANS

- **Average wholesale price applications:** a form of reimbursement that follows the following formula:

$$AWP \pm percentage + dispensing\ fee$$

This form of reimbursement is the most commonly used and encourages a pharmacy to dispense generic medications because the percentage of return is greater for generics than for brand name drugs.

- **AAC:** Actual acquisition cost; the price a pharmacy actually paid for a medication after receiving any discounts from either the manufacturer or the wholesaler. May be used instead of AWP.
- **MAC:** Maximum allowable cost; the maximum price an insurance company will pay for a generic medication.
- **Capitation fee:** A reimbursement system which a pharmacy receives a fixed payment each month per patient, regardless of the number of prescriptions filled or the cost of the prescriptions filled. A practice commonly used by HMOs.
- **Deductible:** A set amount that must be paid by the patient for each benefit period before the insurer will cover additional expenses.
- **Per diem:** A predetermined amount of money, this is paid to an individual or institution for a daily service.

COPAYMENTS
- **Fixed:** The patient pays a fixed or set dollar amount.
- **Percentage:** The patient pays a fixed percentage of the total cost of the prescription.
- **Variable:** Different dollar amount is charged based upon the type of drug dispensed. The variable copay could be for a lifestyle drug, a nonformulary drug, or a medication that has a DAW 2 code.

Third-Party Plans
- **Health maintenance organization (HMO):** The purpose is to keep the patient healthy and is able to control costs by mandating generic usage. It is composed of a network of providers, who are employed by the HMO or have signed contracts with the HMO to adhere to the conditions of the HMO. Expenses are not covered outside of network unless a referral has been made.
- **Preferred provider organization (PPO):** A network of providers contracted by the insurer that offers the most flexibility to the patient. Costs outside the network may be partially reimbursed. They do not require that a physician within the network to make referrals.
- **Point of sale (POS):** A network of providers under contract by the insurer. Patients are required to choose a primary care physician (PCP) and are required to obtain a referral from their PCP for services outside of the network.
- **Medicare:** Federally funded program for individuals over the age of 65, disabled individuals younger than age 65, and patients with kidney failure.
- **Medicaid:** A federally funded program administered by the states. States determine eligibility and services rendered. Prescription drug formularies are used and not all drug products are covered.
- **Patient assistance programs:** Special programs offered by pharmaceutical manufacturers for patients with specific needs, who may be unable to afford their medication.
- **Workman's Compensation:** Federal and state laws require compensation for patients who have been accidentally injured on the job. Prescriptions for medications from the injury are billed either to the state bureau of worker's compensation or to the employer.

LEGAL REQUIREMENTS FOR PHARMACIST COUNSELING OF PATIENT/PATIENT'S REPRESENTATIVE

An offer to counsel must be made to every patient but the patient may refuse. Counseling may include name and description of medication; dosage form; dosage; route of administration; duration of drug therapy; action to take if a dose is missed; common adverse side effects; interactions and contraindications; self-monitoring for drug therapy; prescription refill information; proper storage of medication; and special directions.

CHAPTER 2 REVIEW QUESTIONS

1. What organization establishes standards of practice, addresses the quality of patient care and patient safety; establishes standards and accredits the following health care providers: hospitals, home health care agencies, home infusion providers, long-term care pharmacies, ambulatory infusion pharmacies, and home medical equipment?
    a. DEA
    b. EPA
    c. FDA
    d. JCAHO

2. What is Medicare?
    a. A federal funded program for drug addicts
    b. A federal funded program for elderly and disabled
    c. A federal funded program for the poor
    d. A federal funded program for injured victims of recalled medications

3. What is a deductible?
    a. Special programs offered by pharmaceutical manufacturers for patients with specific needs, who may be unable to afford their medication
    b. A predetermined amount of money that is paid to an individual or institution for a daily service
    c. A set amount that must be paid by the patient for each benefit period before the insurer will cover additional expenses
    d. The patient pays a fixed percentage of the total cost of the prescription

4. What is a Material Safety Data Sheet (MSDS)?
    a. Documentation that indicates the amount of each medication needed and lists the procedures to follow and labeling instructions
    b. Documentation that provides detailed information on the hazards of a particular substance
    c. Medication information sheet provided by the manufacturer that includes side effects, dosage forms, indications, and other important information
    d. A document provided to patients who are taking estrogens and progesterone

5. Where should one place used syringes?
    a. In a biohazard container
    b. In a cardboard box
    c. In a locked cabinet
    d. In a "sharps" container

6. Which of the following is not a universal precaution?
    a. Special handling of chemotherapy agents
    b. Using a sharps container to store used syringes and needles
    c. Wearing jewelry while preparing IV admixtures
    d. Wearing protective clothing while preparing IV admixtures

7. What is the process of mixing a liquid and powder to form a suspension or solution?
    a. Geometric dilution
    b. Levigation
    c. Reconstitution
    d. Trituration

8. Which of the following is not a characteristics of an absorption base?
    a. Anhydrous
    b. Difficult to spread
    c. Nongreasy
    d. Nonwashable

9. What type of order is used for specific classifications or medications that can be active for only a limited period of time after which a new medication order is required to continue?
    a. Automatic stop order
    b. ASAP order
    c. PRN order
    d. STAT order

10. Which reference book provides information on drug prices?
    a. Drug Topics Orange Book
    b. Drug Topics Red Book
    c. National Formulary
    d. US Pharmacopoeia

11. What type of container is impervious to air under normal handling, shipment, storage, and distribution?
    a. Child-resistant
    b. EZ open
    c. Hermetic
    d. Light-resistant

12. What classification of temperature is between 15° and 30°?
    a. Cold
    b. Cool
    c. Excessive heat
    d. Room temperature

13. What number is given by a manufacturer to identify a particular batch of medicine?
    a. Drug schedule
    b. UPC
    c. Lot number
    d. NDC number

14. Which piece of information is not required on a medication order label?
    a. Expiration date of medication
    b. Pharmacist or technician who processed the order
    c. Lot number of medication
    d. Trade or generic name of medication

15. Which of the following medications does not require a patient package insert to be given to the patient?
    a. Accutane
    b. Antidepressants
    c. Estrogens
    d. Oral contraceptives

16. If a pharmacy technician is using the continental (dry gum method), what would he or she be compounding?
    a. Capsules
    b. Emulsions
    c. Suppositories
    d. Syrups

17. What should be used to clean the laminar flow hood?
    a. 70% rubbing alcohol
    b. 70% isopropyl alcohol
    c. 95% isopropyl alcohol
    d. 95% ethyl alcohol

18. What type of substance is composed of 50% dextrose, 20% fat, and 10% amino acid?
    a. Partial parenteral nutrition
    b. Peripheral parenteral nutrition
    c. Total parenteral nutrition
    d. Total peripheral nutrition

19. What technique is used in mixing two ingredients of unequal quantities?
    a. Blending
    b. Geometric dilution
    c. Levigation
    d. Spatulation

20. What type of agent increases the viscosity of a suspension?
    a. Emulsifier
    b. Flocculating agent
    c. Mucilage
    c. Thickening agent

21. What type of ointment base is Aquaphor?
    a. Absorption
    b. Oleaginous
    c. Oil/water emulsion base
    d. Water/oil emulsion base

22. What type of copay is a predetermined amount of money to be paid for each prescription?
    a. Fixed
    b. Maximum allowable
    c. Percentage
    d. Variable

23. Which of the following is not found on an MSDS form?
    a. Accidental release measures
    b. Cost of the product
    c. Exposure controls/personal protection
    d. Handling and storage

24. Which of the following ointment bases is anhydrous?
    a. Absorption
    b. Water/oil emulsion base
    c. Oil/water base
    d. Water-miscible base

25. Who is responsible for providing a pharmacy with the MSDS?
    a. Drug manufacturer
    b. Drug wholesaler
    c. FDA
    d. EPA

26. How many times may a pharmacy transfer a controlled substance prescription of 30 tablets of Tylenol #3 with five refills indicated on the prescription?
    a. 0
    b. 1
    c. 3
    d. 5

27. What does a medication with an FDA therapeutic equivalence code "A" signify?
    a. Drug products that the FDA does not consider at this time to be therapeutically equivalent to other pharmaceutical equivalent products
    b. Drug products that are considered to be therapeutically equivalent to other pharmaceutically equivalent products
    c. Products meeting necessary bioequivalence requirements
    d. Products not presenting bioequivalence problems in conventional dosage forms

28. Which disease is characterized by an imbalance between oxygen supply and demand?
    a. Angina
    b. Hypertension
    c. Myocardial infarction
    d. Stroke

29. What type of a drug interaction occurs when one drug increases or prolongs the effect of another drug?
    a. Addition
    b. Antagonism
    c. Potentiation
    d. Synergism

30. What type of diabetes is caused by taking various medications?
    a. Gestational
    b. Type I
    c. Type II
    d. Secondary

31. What affective disorder is characterized by excessive phases of mania and depression?
    a. Bipolar disease
    b. Epilepsy
    c. Mania
    d. Schizophrenia

32. Which reference book provides monthly updates on FDA-approved medications, orphan drugs, and investigational drugs?
    a. Drug Topics Red Book
    b. Drug Facts and Comparisons
    c. Physicians' Desk reference
    d. Remington's Pharmaceutical Sciences

33. Which of the following DEA numbers is incorrect for Dr. B. Yarhi?
    a. BY1234563
    b. BY5555555
    c. DBY1234563
    d. BY5555517

34. What type of syringe would be used to administer 0.5 mL of amoxicillin pediatric drops?
    a. Low-dose syringe
    b. Oral syringe
    c. Tuberculin syringe
    d. U-100 syringe

35. Which of the following screening/monitoring equipment is used to measure the vital capacity of an individual?
    a. Nebulizer
    b. Peak flow meter
    c. Pneumogram
    d. Sphygmomanmeter

36. Which of the following pumps is used as a PCA?
    a. CADD Prizm PCS pump
    b. CADD-Plus pump
    c. CADD-TPN
    d. Elastometric balloon system

37. Which of the following pieces of equipment would be used by a diabetic?
    a. Glucometer
    b. Echocardiogram
    c. Electrocardiogram
    d. Syringe infusion system

38. Which of the following containers is a single-unit container intended for parenteral administration only?
    a. Tight container
    b. Single-unit container
    c. Single-dose container
    d. Unit-dose container

39. What dosage form can be prepared by the "dry gum method," the "wet gum method," or the "beaker method"?
    a. Capsules
    b. Emulsions
    c. Spirits
    d. Suspensions

40. Which dosage form can be prepared by the "heat method"?
    a. Elixir
    b. Suppository
    c. Syrup
    d. Tincture

41. Which dosage form can be prepared by either the compression mold or the fusion mold?
    a. Pills
    b. Suppositories
    c. Tablets
    d. Timed-released dosage forms

42. What type of an ointment base is white petrolatum?
    a. Absorption base
    b. Oleaginous
    c. Water/oil emulsion base
    d. Water-miscible base

43. Which of the following does not need to be placed in biohazard bag?
    a. Gloves
    b. Gowns
    c. Masks
    d. Needles

44. Which of the following is the price a pharmacy may pay for a medication after receiving a discount?
     a. AAC
     b. AWP
     c. Capitation
     d. MAC

45. Which of the following orders allows for a patient to receive a specific medication at a specific time each day in the hospital?
     a. ASAP orders
     b. Automatic orders
     c. PRN orders
     d. Standing orders

46. What temperature is considered a warm environment?
     a. Between 8 and 15°C
     b. Between 15 and 30°C
     c. Between 30 and 40°C
     d. Above 40°C

47. Which of the following is an automated dispensing device kept on the nursing unit?
     a. Baker Cells
     b. Omni Link Rx
     c. PYXIS Medstation
     c. Safety Pak

48. Which of the following is not required on a medication order label?
     a. Expiration date of medication
     b. Lot number of medication
     c. Medication number
     d. Name and location of patient

49. Which of the following is not found on a patient package insert?
     a. Description of medication
     b. Expiration date and lot number of medication
     c. Indications for medication
     d. Revisions of labeling

50. Which type of pharmacy processes, prepares, and distributes medication from one location?
     a. Centralized dispensing
     b. Decentralized dispensing
     c. Floor stock dispensing
     d. Satellite dispensing

ABBREVIATION QUESTIONS

1. Print the meaning of each abbreviation.
     a. ac =
     b. amp =
     c. bid =
     d. cap =
     e. emuls =
     f. hs =
     g. npo =
     h. oint =
     i. pc =

    j. po =
    k. pr =
    l. q4h =
   m. q6h =
    n. q8h =
    o. qd =
    p. qid =
    q. qod =
    r. stat =
    s. supp =
    t. syr =
    u. tab =
    v. tid =

2. Print the meaning of each abbreviation.
    a. tsp
    b. tbsp
    c. qt
    d. pt
    e. oz
    f. NS
    g. mL
    h. mg
    i. mEq
    j. mcg
    k. lb
    l. kg
   m. gr
    n. g
    o. gal
    p. fl oz
    q. DW
    r. D5W
    s. D5LR
    t. D20W
    u. D10W
    v. cc
   w. ½ NS

3. Print the meaning of each abbreviation.
APhA
ASAP
AWP
CMS
DAW
DEA
EPA
FDA
GERD
GPO
HIPAA
JCAHO
MI
NABP
NF
OSHA
OTC
P & T Committee

PI

U & C

USP

4. Print the meaning of each abbreviation.

3TC

APAP

ASA

AZT

ddi

D4T

$FeSO_4$

HCTZ

INH

KCl

MOM

NTG

Pb

PCN

SMZ-TMP

TCN

PRACTICE LAW QUESTIONS

1. What do the middle four numbers represent in an NDC number?
   a. Drug manufacturer
   b. Drug product
   c. Drug packaging
   d. None of the above

2. The pharmacist fails to place a prescription label on the medication container. Which law is being broken?
   a. Pure Food Drug Act of 1906
   b. Food, Drug and Cosmetic Act of 1938
   c. Durham-Humphrey Act of 1950
   d. Kefauver-Harris Act of 1962

3. An employee injures his back while lifting a carton of medication in the pharmacy. What law allows the employee to collect damages from the employer?
   a. Kefauver-Harris Act
   b. Occupational and Safety Act of 1970
   c. Omnibus Budget Reconciliation Act of 1987
   d. Poison Prevention Act of 1970

4. A patient requests that the pharmacist place their medication in an EZ open container. Which law allows the pharmacist to dispense the prescription in this manner?
   a. Kefauver-Harris Act
   b. Controlled Substance Act of 1970
   c. Occupational and Safety Act of 1970
   d. Poison Prevention Act of 1970

5. A pharmacist prepares a prescription in a mortar and pestle that has been contaminated by antineoplastic agent and dispenses it to a patient. Which law is he or she violating?
   a. Pure Food Drug Act of 1906
   b. Food, Drug and Cosmetic Act of 1938
   c. Durham-Humphrey Act of 1950
   d. Kefauver-Harris Act of 1962

6. Which law allows a pharmacist to accept a telephoned prescription from a physician's office?
   a. Pure Food Drug Act of 1906
   b. Food, Drug and Cosmetic Act of 1938
   c. Durham-Humphrey Act of 1950
   d. Kefauver-Harris Act of 1962

7. Which law allows a pharmacist to dispense nitroglycerin tablets in a child-resistant container?
   a. Durham-Humphrey Act
   b. Kefauver-Harris Act
   c. Controlled Substance Act
   d. Poison Control Act

8. Which law resulted in clearly distinguishing an over-the-counter medication from a prescription medication?
   a. Pure Food Drug Act of 1906
   b. Food, Drug and Cosmetic Act of 1938
   c. Durham-Humphrey Act of 1950
   d. Kefauver-Harris Act of 1962

9. Which law required that the federal legend appear on all prescriptions?
   a. Pure Food Drug Act of 1906
   b. Food, Drug and Cosmetic Act of 1938
   c. Durham-Humphrey Act of 1950
   d. Kefauver-Harris Amendment

10. How long is a DEA Form 222 valid?
    a. 1 week
    b. 1 month
    c. 60 days
    d. 6 months

11. Which law requires that a manufacturer provide Material Safety Data Sheets (MSDS) to a pharmacy for products that are combustible, flammable, or can cause injury to an individual if they come in contact with the substance?
    a. Kefauver-Harris Act
    b. Controlled Substance Act of 1970
    c. Occupational and Safety Act of 1970
    d. Poison Prevention Act of 1970

12. A pharmacist receives a prescription for 40 Percocet tablets, but the pharmacy only has 15 tablets in stock. The patient accepts the 15 tablets: How much time does the pharmacist have to provide the remaining 25 tablets?
    a. 24 hr
    b. 72 hr
    c. 96 hr
    d. 60 months

13. If a patient requests a partial filling of their Tylenol with Codeine #3 prescription, what can the pharmacist do for the patient?
    a. The pharmacist may provide the patient with the requested amount and place the remaining tablets in a bottle for the patient to pick up at a later date.
    b. The pharmacist may provide the patient with the requested amount and inform the patient that the patient must pick the remaining quantity up within 72 hr.
    c. The pharmacist may provide the patient with the requested amount and inform the patient that the patient must pick the remaining quantity up within 6 months of the date of the prescription being filled.
    d. The pharmacist may provide the patient with the requested amount, but can only give the patient the balance if there is a refill indicated on the prescription.

14. Which of the following is a correct DEA number for a Dr. Andrea J. Shedlock, who was Dr. Andrea Costello when she requested her DEA number before she was married?
    a. AC1234563
    b. AS1234563
    c. JC1234563
    d. JS1234563

15. You are working for a chain pharmacy and another member of the chain has run out of DEA Form 222. They ask to borrow one of your DEA Form 222. What would you do?
    a. Because you are members of the same pharmacy chain, you are allowed to let them use of yours because you have the same DEA number.
    b. Give them one of your DEA Form 222 with the agreement that they will replace it after they receive their new ones.
    c. DEA Form 222 are for a specific pharmacy and can only be used by the pharmacy to which it was issued.
    d. Tell them to place an emergency order with the wholesaler and you will provide them with a properly completed DEA Form 222 in 72 hr.

16. You receive a request from another pharmacy for 100 Percocet tablets. What do you do?
    a. You may loan them the requested 100 tablets of Percocet.
    b. You may sell them the 100 tablets of Percocet at the AWP.
    c. You may transfer them the 100 tablets of Percocet through the use of a DEA Form 222.
    d. None of the above can be done.

17. What form is used to report the theft of controlled substances?
    a. DEA Form 41
    b. DEA Form 106
    c. DEA Form 222
    d. DEA Form 224

18. Which of the following is part of HIPAA?
    a. Allows a member of a plan to select any pharmacy for their pharmacy benefit as long as the pharmacy agrees to the terms and conditions of the plan
    b. Allows Rx to appear on a prescription instead of the federal legend
    c. Insurance reform
    d. Prohibits a prescription drug plan from requiring mail order prescription drug coverage without providing a non–mail order coverage

19. Which organization oversees Medicare and Medicaid service?
    a. BOP
    b. CMS
    c. DEA
    d. JCAHO

20. Who reviews INDs?
    a. BOP
    b. DEA
    c. EPA
    d. FDA

21. Which law required opium to have a prescription?
    a. Comprehensive Drug Abuse Prevention and Control Act
    b. Federal Food and Drug Act
    c. Food, Drug and Cosmetic Act
    d. Harrison Narcotic Act

22. Which law required that all narcotics to be labeled "Warning: May be Habit Forming"?
    a. Anabolic Steroids Control Act
    b. Comprehensive Drug Abuse Prevention and Control Act
    c. Harrison Narcotic Act
    d. Prescription Drug Marketing Act

23. Which law requires drug utilization to be performed on all prescriptions?
    a. Dietary Supplement Health and Education Act of 1994
    b. Omnibus Reconciliation Act of 1987
    c. Omnibus Reconciliation Act of 1990
    d. Prescription Drug Equity Law

24. Which law allowed pharmacists to take prescriptions over the telephone from a physician's office?
    a. Durham-Humphrey Amendment
    b. Food, Drug and Cosmetic Act
    c. Kefauver-Harris Amendment
    d. Comprehensive Drug Abuse Prevention and Control Act

25. Which law established tax-free savings accounts?
    a. Freedom of Choice Law
    b. HIPAA
    c. Medicare Drug Improvement and Modernization Act of 2003?
    d. Omnibus Budget Reconciliation Act of 1990

26. Which law stated that a resident's drug regimen must be free of unnecessary medications?
    a. Freedom of Choice Law
    b. HIPAA
    c. Omnibus Reconciliation Act of 1987
    d. Omnibus Reconciliation Act of 1990

27. Which law allows nasal inhalers to be dispensed without a child-resistant container?
    a. Americans with Disabilities Act
    b. Freedom of Choice Law
    c. Occupational Health and Safety Act of 1970
    d. Poison Control Act of 1970

28. Which law lowers the reimbursement rate for durable medical equipment?
    a. Drug Price Competition and Patent Restoration Act
    b. FDA Safe Medical Devices Act of 1990
    c. HIPAA
    d. Medicare Drug Improvement and Modernization Act of 2003

29. Which law prevents reimportation of medication into the United States other than by a manufacturer?
    a. Drug Listing Act of 1972
    b. Drug Price Competition and Patent Restoration Act of 1984
    c. Food, Drug and Cosmetic Act
    d. Prescription Drug Marketing Act

30. Which agency oversees the practice of pharmacy?
    a. APhA
    b. DEA
    c. FDA
    d. State Board of Pharmacy

PHARMACOLOGY REVIEW QUESTIONS

1. Write the generic name for the following brand names.
   a. Premarin
   b. Lipitor
   c. Norvasc
   d. Lanoxin
   e. Zithromax
   f. Zocor
   g. Zestril
   h. Tenormin
   i. Xanax
   j. Cardizem
   k. Glucotrol
   l. Allegra
   m. Procardia
   n. Dilantin
   o. Wellbutrin
   p. Relafen
   q. Risperdal
   r. Serevent
   s. Zantac
   t. Plavix
   u. Azmacort
   v. Amaryl
   w. Phenergan
   x. Nolvadex
   y. Lasix
   z. Vasotec
2. Write the brand names for the following generic names.
   a. cephalexin
   b. fluoxetine
   c. paroxetine
   d. mupirocin
   e. acetaminophen + codeine
   f. propoxyphene N/APAP
   g. triamterene/HCTZ
   h. alendronate
   i. losartan
   j. fluconazole
   k. amitriptyline
   l. rosiglitazone
   m. esomeprazole

     n. olanzapine
     o. montelukast
     p. nefazodone
     q. tolterodine
     r. oxycodone
     s. acyclovir
     t. propranolol
     u. doxycycline
     v. nortriptyline
     w. etodolac
     x. clindamycin
     y. metronidazole
     z. naproxen

3. Which auxiliary labels should be affixed to a prescription container of the following medications?
     a. Vicodin
     b. Glucophage
     c. Coumadin
     d. Cipro
     e. Tetracycline
     f. Deltasone
     g. Biaxin
     h. Ambien
     i. Motrin
     j. Depakote
     k. Xalatan
     l. Antivert
     m. TobraDex
     n. Proventil
     o. Bactrim Suspension
     p. Augmentin
     q. Benzamycin
     r. Minocin
     s. Amoxicillin Suspension
     t. Lotrisone Cream
     u. Feldene
     v. Ritalin
     w. Vicoprofen
     x. Hydrochlorothiazide
     y. Ultram
     z. Humulin N

4. Identify the primary indication for which each brand drug is used.
     a. Premarin
     b. Synthroid
     c. Lipitor
     d. Prilosec
     e. Vicodin
     f. Proventil
     g. Norvasc
     h. Amoxil
     i. Prozac
     j. Zoloft
     k. Glucophage
     l. Lanoxin
     m. Prempro
     n. Paxil

    o. Zithromax
    p. Zestril
    q. Zocor
    r. Prevacid
    s. Augmentin
    t. Celebrex
    u. Coumadin
    v. Vasotec
    w. Lasix
    x. Cipro
    y. Keflex
    z. Deltasone

5. Identify the primary indication for which each generic drug is used.
    a. pravastatin
    b. clarithromycin
    c. norgestimate/ethinyl estradiol
    d. acetaminophen/codeine
    e. atenolol
    f. cetirizine
    g. zolpidem
    h. alprazolam
    i. tramadol
    j. quinapril
    k. diltiazem
    l. glipizide
    m. fexofenadine
    n. triamterene/HCTZ
    o. doxazosin
    p. alendronate
    q. benazepril
    r. nifedipine
    s. sildenafil citrate
    t. ibuprofen
    u. valproate
    v. phenytoin
    w. bupropion
    x. gabapentin
    y. losartan
    z. fluconazole

6. To what drug classification does each drug belong?
    a. sulfasalazine
    b. erythromycin stearate
    c. doxycycline
    d. ranitidine
    e. ampicillin
    f. acyclovir
    g. lamivudine
    h. promethazine
    i. azelastine
    j. codeine
    k. carbamazepine
    l. albuterol
    m. beclomethasone
    n. diphenoxylate + atropine
    o. simethicone

    p. doxazosin
    q. quinidine
    r. amlodipine
    s. verapamil
    t. captopril
    u. hydrochlorothiazide
    v. lovastatin
    w. sumatriptan
    x. estradiol
    y. difluconazole
    z. terbinafine

7. To what drug classification does each drug belong?
    a. fluoxetine
    b. omeprazole
    c. cephalexin
    d. pravastatin
    e. celecoxib
    f. sertraline
    g. atenolol
    h. furosemide
    i. metformin
    j. digoxin
    k. sulfamethoxazole/trimethoprim
    l. ibuprofen
    m. rosiglitazone
    n. salmeterol
    o. cefprozil
    p. quinapril
    q. amitriptyline
    r. lisinopril
    s. imipramine
    t. fluvastatin
    u. ciprofloxacin
    v. indomethacin
    w. hydroxyzine HCl
    x. carbamazepine
    y. diltiazem
    z. triamcinolone

8. To what drug classification does each drug belong?
    a. esomeprazole
    b. prednisone
    c. acetaminophen + codeine
    d. zolpidem
    e. alprazolam
    f. fexofenadine
    g. doxazosin
    h. citalopram
    i. naproxen
    j. oxycodone
    k. carvedilol
    l. etodolac
    m. piroxicam
    n. acetaminophen + hydrocodone
    o. levofloxacin
    p. enalapril

    q. lansoprazole
    r. acetaminophen + oxycodone
    s. tramadol
    t. clotrimazole + nelfinavir
    v. butalbital/codeine/APAP
    w. ketoconazole
    x. clonidine
    y. nadolol
    z. doxycycline

9. Identify one indication for the following herbal agents.
    a. Aloe vera
    b. Cascara sagrada
    c. St. John's wort
    d. Melatonin
    e. Gingko
    f. Glucosamine
    g. Cranberry
    h. Chondroitin
    i. Goldenseal
    j. Echinacea

PRACTICE MATH PROBLEMS

CONVERSIONS

1. How many pounds are equal to 1 kg?
2. How many g are in 5.5 kg?
3. How many g are equal to 2,500 mg?
4. How many mg are equal to 350 mcg?
5. How many cc equal 75 mL?
6. How many tsp equal 120 mL?
7. How many tbsp equal 6 tsp?
8. How many tsp equal 7.5 fl oz?
9. How many fl oz equal 1.5 cups?
10. How many qt equalk 2 gal?
11. How many pt equal 6.5 qt?
12. How many mg equal 7.5 gr?
13. How many gr equal 2 g?
14. How many tsp equal 1 L?
15. How many gr equal 650 mg?
16. How many g equal 125 mg?
17. How many mcg equal 2.4 g?
18. How many tbsp equal 12 tsp?
19. How many fl oz equal 2.5 qt?
20. How many g equal 75 mg?
21. How many ml equal 2 gal?
22. How many gal equal 8 cups?
23. How many g equal 1 lb?
24. How many tbsp equal 6 fl oz?
25. How many tsp equal 2 fl oz?

CALCULATIONS

1. How many colchicine tablets each containing 600 mcg may be prepared from 30 g of colchicine?
2. The prescriber ordered atropine sulfate 0.2 mg sc q6h prn. What is the equivalent dose in micrograms?

3. The physician has ordered Coumadin 5 mg to be taken on Monday, Wednesday, and Friday. On Tuesday, Thursday, Saturday, and Sunday, the patient is to receive 2½ mg. How many mg will the patient take in 1 week?

4. The prescriber ordered 0.05 mg of Sandostatin po, a hormone. How many micrograms are in this dose?

5. You have a 2-mL ampule of caffeine Na benzonatate containing gr viiss. If the physician orders gr v, how many milliliters will you dispense?

6. How many grams of reserpine would be required to make 25,000 tablets, each containing 250 mcg of reserpine?

7. How many mg are in one tablet of Nitrostat 1/150 gr?

8. How many grams of antipyrine should be used in preparing the prescription?
   Rx   Antipyrine 5%
   Glycerin ad   60

9. A pediatric patient is to be given a 70-mg dose of Dilantin by administering an oral suspension containing 50 mg of Dilantin per 5 mL. How many milliliters of the suspension must be administered?

10. A prefilled syringe of furosemide contains 20 mg of drug in 2 mL of solution. How many micrograms of drug would be administered by an injection of 0.5 mL of the solution?

11. The usual dosage range of dimercaprol is 2.5 to 5 mg/kg of body weight. What would be the dosage range in grams for a person weighing 165 lb?

12. How many chloramphenicol capsules each containing 250 mg of chloramphenicol are needed to provide 25 mg/kg of body weight for 1 week for a person weighing 154 lb?

13. Cyclosporine is an immunosuppressive agent administered before and after organ transplantation at a single dose of 15 mg/kg. How many milliliters of a 50-mL bottle containing 100 mg of cyclosporine per milliliter would be administered to a 140-lb kidney transplant patient?

14. How many milliliters of aminophylline injection containing 250 mg in each 10 mL should be used in filling a medication order calling for 15 mg of aminophylline?

15. The dose of a drug is 500 mcg/kg of body weight. How many mg should be given to a child weighing 55 lb?

16. The antiviral ophthalmic drug fomivirsen sodium (Vitravene) has been ordered by the physician, 330 mcg. The vial is labeled 6.6 mg/mL. How many milliliters contain the prescribed dose?

17. The physician ordered 0.725 mg of droperidol (Inapsine) IV stat. The vial reads 2.5 mg in 2 mL. Calculate the amount of drug you will administer to this patient in milliliters.

18. A patient is to receive a 100-mg dose of gentamicin. The medication is available in an 80 mg/mL vial. How many milliliters should the patient receive?

19. A drug has a concentration of 20 mg/mL. How many grams of the drug are in ½ L of the solution?

20. A dose of antacid is 1 tbsp. How many doses can be prepared from a pint bottle?

21. You are to prepare a dose of 300 mg and the tablets are available in 75-mg strength. How many tablets will the pharmacist need to dispense if the patient is to take 300 mg bid for 1 week?

22. What is the percent of a 1:25 (w/v) solution?

23. What is the percent of a 1:200 (w/w) ointment?

24. Convert 25°C to F.

25. Convert 65°F to C.

26. Convert 40°C to F

27. Convert 45°F to C.

28. The drug vial contains 1,000,000 units of penicillin G. The label directions state: Add 2.3 mL of sterile water to the vial, 1.2 mL = 500,000 units. How many milliliters equal 200,000 units?

29. A patient is to receive 25 units of the hormonal drug vasopressin (Pitressin) IM. If the label reads 50 units per 2 mL, how many milliliters will you administer to the patient?

30. The prescriber ordered 175,000 units of urokinase IVPBN. The vial directions read: Add 4.2 mL to vial and each mL will contain 50,000 units. How many milliliters will you prepare?

31. The order is for K-lor 60 mEq po stat. Each packet contains 20 mEq. How many packets of K-L or will you need?

32. A 20% KCL solution has a strength of 40 mEq/tbsp. How many milliliters need to be dispensed for the patient to receive 20 mEq?

33. If the dose of a drug is 150 mcg, how many doses is contained in 0.120 g?

34. If a physician prescribed cephalexin 250 mg qid for 10 days, how many milliliters of cephalexin oral suspension containing 250 mg/tsp should be dispensed?
35. A 25-lb child is to receive 4 mg of phenytoin per kg of body weight as an anticonvulsant. How many milliliters of pediatric phenytoin suspension containing 30 mg/5 mL should the child receive?
36. If a 3-year old child weighing 33 lb accidentally ingested twenty 81-mg aspirin tablets, how much aspirin did the child ingest on a milligram/kilogram basis?
37. The usual pediatric dose of cefazolin sodium is 25 mg/kg/day divided equally into three doses. What would be the single dose in mg for a child weighing 44 lb?
38. If a child is 4 years old and the adult dose of medication is 100 mg, how much medication should the child receive?
39. If a child is 36 months old and the adult dose is 250 mg, how much medication should the child receive?
40. If a child is 2½ years old and the adult dose is 100 mg, how many milligrams should the child receive?
41. If a child weighs 45 lb and the adult dose is 50 mg, how much medication should the child receive?
42. If a child weighs 50 lb and the adult dose is 1 tbsp, how many milligrams should the child receive?
43. If a child weighs 60 lb and the adult dose is 500 mg, how many milligrams should the child receive?
44. If a child weighs 15 kg and the adult dose is 75 mg, how many milligrams should the child receive?
45. If 125 mL of liquid weighs 95 g, what is its specific gravity?
46. A volume of fluid weighs 80 g and has a specific gravity of 1.05. What is its volume?
47. How many grams are in 100 mL of a liquid if its specific gravity is 1.25?
48. What is the specific gravity of a substance that weighs 60 g and occupies a volume 75 mL?
49. How many grams of silver nitrate are needed to make 1 L of a 0.25% solution?
50. A pharmacist has received an order to prepare 1 lb of 5% (w/w) salicylic acid ointment. How much salicylic acid is needed to prepare this ointment?
51. How many grams of NaCl are in 250 mL of ½ NS (0.45%)?
52. How many grams are in 1 L of a 1:200 solution?
53. How many micrograms are in 1.0 mL of a 1:100 solution?
54. If a pharmacist adds 3 g of hydrocortisone to 120 g of a 5% hydrocortisone cream, what is the final percentage strength of hydrocortisone in the product?
55. How many 600-mg ibuprofen tablets will be needed to make 8 oz of a 15% ointment?
56. How many milliliters of a 3% (w/v) solution will be necessary to make 6 oz of a 1:200 solution?
57. A stock bottle of Lugol's solution contains 2 oz from the original pint bottle. The pharmacy technician is able to prepare four 8-oz bottles of a more dilute 4% solution. What was the original percentage strength of the Lugol's solution?
58. You receive an order for 125 mL of 4% acetic acid solution and you have in stock 75% acetic acid solution. How many milliliter of the 75% solution will you need?
59. If 100 mL of 25% (w/v) solution is diluted to 1 L, what will be the percentage strength (w/v)?
60. You are asked to prepare 80 mL of a 72% lidocaine solution and you have in stock a 75% solution. How many milliliters of the 75% solution will you use?
61. The formula for a buffer solution contains 1.24% (w/v) of boric acid. How many milliliters of a 10% (w/v) boric acid solution should be used to obtain the boric acid needed in preparing 1 gallon of buffer solution?
62. How many grams of Eucerin should be added to 4 oz of a 10% ointment to make a 7% ointment?
63. You are asked to prepare 50 mL of a 1:100 rifampin suspension and you have in stock a 1:20 rifampin suspension. How many milliliters of the 1:20 suspension will you need?
64. You are asked to prepare 125 mL of a 1:8 nystatin suspension and you have in stock a 1:6 solution. How many milliliters of the 1:6 nystatin solution will you need?
65. You are asked to prepare 50 mL of a 1:3 folic acid solution and you have in stock a 1:2 solution. How many milliliters of the 1:2 solution will you use?
66. How many milliliters of a 1:50 (w/v) stock solution of a chemical should be used to prepare 2 L of a 1:4000 (w/v) solution?
67. How many milliliters of water should be added to 500 mL of a 1:2000 (w/v) solution to make a 1:5000 (w/v) solution?
68. How much water should be added to 1 quart of 70% isopropyl alcohol to prepare a 20% solution for soaking sponges?

69. How much metoclopramide 5 mg/mL is used to make 10 mL of 0.5 mg/mL solution?
70. Prepare 15 mL of cefazolin dilution 50 mg/mL from a stock of 1 g/5 mL. How many milliliters of the diluent and cefazolin will be needed?
71. Make 30 mL of a vitamin B12 dilution with a concentration of 100 mcg/mL from a stock solution of 1 mg/mL. How much B12 and diluent are needed?
72. You are asked to prepare 36 mL of a 1:4 Bactrim solution and you have in stock 30% solution. How many milliliters of the 30% solution will you use?
73. You are asked to prepare 52 mL of a 28% Flagyl solution and you have in stock 42 g/mL solution. How many milliliters of the 42 g/mL will you use?
74. How many milliliters of a ½% of gentian violet should be used in preparing 500 mL of a 1:100,000 solution?
75. How many milliliters of a 5% stock solution are needed to prepare 1 pint of a solution containing 100 mg of the chemical per liter?
76. How many milliliters of a 95% (v/v) alcohol should be used in preparing a pint of a 75% (v/v) solution?
77. In what proportions should alcohols of 95% and 50% strengths be mixed to prepare 250 mL of a 70% alcohol solution?
78. How many milliliters of a 1:2000 iodine solution and a 7.5% iodine solution are needed to make 120 mL of a 3.5% solution?
79. How many milliliters of a 2.5% (w/v) chlorpromazine hydrochloride injection and how many milliliters of a 0.9% (w/v) sodium chloride injection should be used to prepare 500 mL of a 1.25% (w/v) chlorpromazine hydrochloride injection?
80. How much 10% dextrose solution and 20% dextrose solution should be mixed to prepare 1 L of a 12.5% dextrose solution?
81. In what proportion should 5% and 1% hydrocortisone ointments be mixed to prepare a 2.5% ointment?
82. Prepare 300 mL of 7.5% dextrose using SWFI and D20W. How much of each is needed?
83. Prepare 500 mL of D12.5W. You have on hand D5W, D10W, and D20W. How much of which two solutions will you use?
84. How many grams of a 2.5% hydrocortisone cream should be mixed with 240 g of a 0.25% hydrocortisone cream to make a 1% cream?
85. What is the total volume that will be delivered if a patient receives normal saline solution at 25 mL/hr for 24 hr?
86. Calculate the flow rate to be used to infuse 1,000 mL of NS over 8 hr if the set delivers 10 gtts/mL.
87. 1 L NS is to be administered over 24 hr. The administration set to be used has a DF of 15 gtts/mL. What is the rate of infusion in
    a. mL/hr
    b. gtts/min
88. 1,500 mL TPN solution is given intravenously at 75 mL/hr using an administration set with a drop factor of 20 gtts/mL. If the infusion starts at 0900 hr, when will it end?
89. Medication: Solu-Cortef 250 mg
    Fluid volume: 250 mL
    Time of infusion: 4 hr
    How many mL/hr? How many mg/hr?
90. How many milliliters of IV fluid will a patient receive if infused at the rate of 120 mL/hr over 3½ hr?
91. What will be the rate in gtts/min if a patient receives 1 L of an intravenous fluid over an 8-hr period if the drop factor = 15 gtts/mL?
92. If 1,000 mL at 20 drops/min is administered using a 15 drop set, what is the flow rate in mL/hr?
93. If 500 mL of an intravenous solution contains 0.1 g of a drug, at what flow rate in milliliters per minute should the solution be administered to provide 1 mg/min of the drug?
94. An initial heparin dose of not less than 150 units/kg of body weight has been recommended for open heart surgery. How many milliliters of an injection containing 5,000 heparin units/mL should be administered to a 280-lb patient?
95. An IV piggyback of lincomycin containing 1 g of drug in 100 mL is to be infused over 1½ hours. The IV set is calibrated to deliver 15 gtt/mL. How many drops/minute will the patient receive?

96. An IV piggyback of pentamidine isethionate containing 300 mg of drug in 150 mL of D5W is to be infused over 2 hr. The IV set is calibrated to deliver 20 gtts/mL. How many drops/minute should be administered?

97. An IV piggyback of enalapril maleate containing 10 mg of drug in 50 mL of 0.9% sodium chloride injection is to be infused over 1 hour. The IV set is calibrated to deliver 15 gtts/mL. How many drops/minute should be administered?

98. A physician orders 3 L D5W to be administered over 24 hr. How many drops per minute will be delivered using an administration set calibrated to deliver 30 drops per milliliter?

99. What is the total overhead for a pharmacy that has the following expenses:
    Pharmacist salary (2) $90,000
    Pharmacy technicians (3) $30,000
    Rent $240,000
    Pharmaceutical drugs $2,850,000
    Licenses $545
    Insurance $2,025
    Electricity $3,625
    Gas $8,525
    Water $895
    Supplies $1,255
    Software $995

100. What is the gross profit for a drug that has an AWP of $59.99, a dispensing cost of $3.75, and retails for $67.99?

101. What is the markup for a drug that costs $9.99, a dispensing cost of $2.75, and retails for $13.99?

102. What is the markup rate for a drug that costs $19.99 and retails for $25.99?

103. What is the net profit for a drug that has an AAC of $99.99, a dispensing cost of $4.25, and retails for $112.99?

104. The cost for a bottle of 100 test strips for a glucometer is $67.50. The overhead for the store is $3.50, and the store wants to make a net profit of $23.68. What should the selling price be?

105. How much will a pharmacy pay a wholesaler if the conditions are 2% net 30 if the invoice shows $1,950.00?

106. What will the inventory turnover rate be for a pharmacy if the inventory value is $255,000 and the pharmacy has sales of $3 million?

107. How many inventory turns will a pharmacy experience if they have an initial inventory of $225,000 and a final inventory of $250,000 and have sales totaling $2.6 million during the year?

108. Rx
    | Hydrocodone bitartrate | 0.2 g |
    | Phenacetin | 3.6 g |
    | Aspirin | 6.0 g |
    | Caffeine | 0.6 g |
    | M ft | caps no 24 |
    | Sig | i cap tid prn pain |

    How many milligrams of hydrocodone bitartrate would be contained in each capsule?
    What is the total weight, in milligrams, of the ingredients in each capsule?
    How many milligrams of caffeine would be taken daily?

109.
    | Carafate | 400 mg/5 mL |
    | Cherry syrup | 40 mL |
    | Sorbitol solution | 40 mL |
    | Flavorqs | |
    | Purified water ad | 125 mL |

    Sig: 5 mL tid
    How many 1-g Carafate tablets should be used in preparing the prescription?

110. From the following formula for iodine topical solution, USP, calculate the number of grams of iodine needed to prepare 12 dozen 15-mL containers of the solution.
    | Iodine | 20 g |
    | Sodium iodide | 24 g |
    | Purified water ad | 1,000 mL |

111. From the following formula, calculate the quantities to make 120 mL of benzyl benzoate lotion.
     Benzyl benzoate   125 mL
     Triethanolamine   2.5 mL
     Oleic acid   10 mL
     Purified water, to make 500 mL

112. Each 5 mL of a pediatric cough syrup is to contain the following amounts of medications. Calculate the amount of each ingredient to prepare a gallon of the syrup.
     Dextromethorphan hydrobromide   7.5 mg
     Guaifenesin   100 mg
     Flavored syrup, to make 5.0 mL

113. The following is a formula for psoriasis ointment (*International Journal of Pharmaceutical Compounding* 1998; 2:305). Calculate, in grams, the quantity of each ingredient needed to make a pound of the ointment.
     Coal tar   2.0 g
     Precipitated sulfur   3.0 g
     Salicylic acid   1.0 g
     Lidex ointment   24.0 g
     Aquabase   70.0 g

114. The following is a formula for 100 triple estrogen capsu les (*International Journal of Pharmaceutical Compounding* 1997; 1:187). Calculate the quantities of the first three ingredients in grams and the last two ingredients in kilograms required to prepare 2,500 capsules.
     Estriol   200 mg
     Estrone   25 mg
     Estradiol   25 mg
     Polyethylene glycol   145,020 g
     Polyethylene glycol   335,020 g

Chapter 3

Maintaining Medication and Inventory Control Systems

PHARMACEUTICAL INDUSTRY PROCEDURES FOR OBTAINING PHARMACEUTICALS

- **Group purchasing organization:** Negotiate prices for hospital and institutions; but do not make actual purchase for institution
- **Purchase from drug manufacturers:** Allows pharmacies to purchase in bulk, resulting in a savings for the company. Wholesalers may not always stock specific medications because of storage conditions, expense, or low demand
- **Purchase from wholesalers:** Stocks medications from all manufacturers. Pharmacies are able to purchase when they need a product, rather than far in advance. Wholesalers may provide special services to the pharmacy, such as emergency deliveries, automated ordering systems, or automated purchasing systems
- **Government:** Requires pharmacies to use Drug Enforcement Agency (DEA) Form 222 to purchase Schedule II drugs

PURCHASING POLICIES, PROCEDURES, AND PRACTICES

- **Just-in-time:** Ordering a product before running out and being shipped to pharmacy immediately. The pharmacy will normally receive it the same day or the next business day. A method to keep an inventory low.
- **Point of sale (POS):** Item is deducted from inventory as it is dispensed.
- **Purchase order:** A form that is used to order drugs and supplies from a wholesaler. Information found on a purchase order includes:
  Name and address of the institution
  Shipping address
  Date the order was placed
  Vendor's name and address
  Purchase order number—a tracking number used to identify a purchase order
  Ordering department's name and location
  Expected date of delivery
  Shipping terms
  Account name or billing designation
  Description of items ordered
  Quantity of items ordered
  Unit price
  Extended price

Total price of the order
Buyer's name and phone number

DOSAGE FORMS

Dosage form: A system or device for delivering a drug to a biological system.

SOLIDS

Advantages of Solid Dosage Forms

- Easy to package, transport, store, and dispense
- Convenient for self-medication
- Lacks smell or taste
- Extremely stable for products that are not stable in liquid form
- Predivided dosage form
- Suited for sustained or delayed release medications

Examples of Solid Dosage Forms

- **Tablets:** Prepared either by compressing or by molding. The dosage form is accurate, compact, portable, and easy to administer. May come in various shapes, scored (able to be broken in halves or quarters). The most common types of marketable tablets include standard compressed, enteric-coated, sugar-coated, film-coated, sublingual or buccal, multiple compressed, chewable, or delayed (sustained add action) tablets.
- **Capsules:** A drug is contained in a shell of gelatin (either soft or hard) that dissolves in 10–20 min. Drug may be in either a solid or liquid form. Shape of dosage form may be spherical or ovoid. Capacity of capsule may vary up to 1 g. Can be produced manually by using the punch method.
- **Effervescent salts:** Granules or powders; when dissolved in water, they effervesce and release carbon dioxide.
- **Implants or pellets:** Dosage forms that are placed under the skin through injection and are effective for a long period.
- **Lozenges, troches, or pastilles:** Solid dosage forms with flavoring that dissolve in the mouth.
- **Pellets:** Small cylinders that are implanted subcutaneously for continuous absorption.
- **Plasters:** Medicated or nonmedicated preparations that adhere to the skin by means of a backing material.
- **Powders:** A finely ground substance that can be administered internally or externally. Chief disadvantages are its taste and that it is not stable when exposed to the atmosphere. May be dispensed in a bulk form, a multi-dose form, or as a divided dose such as a powder paper.
- **Suppositories:** A solid dosage form to be inserted in body orifices, such as the rectum, vagina, or urethra. May work either locally or systemically. Mechanism of action is either through melting or dissolving and releases of medication over time. Not all products are available as a suppository; they may be easily expelled from the body and can be erratic in absorption in the body.

Oral Sustained Release Dosage Forms

- Constant release
- Continuous action
- Continuous release
- Controlled action
- Controlled release
- Delayed absorption
- Delayed action
- Depot
- Extended action
- Extended release
- Gradual release
- Long acting
- Long lasting
- Long-term release
- Programmed release

- Prolonged action
- Prolonged release
- Protracted release
- Repeat action
- Repository
- Slow acting
- Sustained action
- Sustained release
- Sustained release depot
- Timed disintegration
- Timed release

LIQUIDS

Advantages of Liquids
- Effective more quickly than a solid dosage form because the drug is already dissolved in a liquid
- Easier to swallow than solid dosage forms for many patients
- Can only be available in liquid form due to convenience of administration
- Uniformity and flexibility of dosage form
- Certain medications may cause gastrointestinal distress if administered in a solid dosage form

Disadvantages of Liquids
- Deterioration and loss of potency occur quicker than in a solid dosage form
- May require special sweetening or flavoring to be palatable
- Incompatibilities of dissolved substances
- May require preservatives to prevent bacteria or mold from developing
- Inaccuracy of measuring a dose may occur
- Bulkier to carry than solid dosage forms
- Interactions may develop from changes in solubility

SOLUTIONS
Contains a solute that is dissolved in a solvent. May be aqueous, alcoholic, or hydroalcoholic.
- **Aromatic waters:** Solutions of water-containing oils, which have a smell and are volatile.
- **Collodions:** Topical dosage form, which contains pyroxylin and is dissolved in alcohol and ether.
- **Elixir:** A clear, sweetened, flavored hydroalcoholic containing water and alcohol, which may be either medicated or not.
- **Enema:** A solution administered rectally for either cleansing or drug administration.
- **Extract:** A process by which active ingredients are removed from their source through the application of solvents.
- **Douche:** An irrigating or bathing solution.
- **Isotonic (iso-osmotic):** Having the same tone or osmolarity of another substance. No loss or gain of water by the cell. Dilution of an isotonic solution may affect the composition of solution. An example is an ophthalmic solution.
- **Liniments:** Either alcoholic or oleaginous solutions or emulsions that are applied through rubbing.
- **Spirits:** Alcoholic or hydroalcoholic solutions containing volatile aromatic ingredients.
- **Syrups:** Aqueous solutions containing sucrose.
- **Tinctures:** Alcoholic or hydroalcoholic solutions of pure chemicals or extracts.

DISPERSIONS
Dispersions: A solute dispersed through a dispersing vehicle.
- **Suspensions:** A two-phase system in which solid particles are dispersed in a liquid vehicle. A suspension may be oral, topical, or injectable. Suspended material should not settle rapidly and pour freely. Topical solutions should be fluid enough to spread over the affected area, but not run off the surface of application; dry quickly; provide a protective film; and have an acceptable color and odor.

- **Emulsions:** One liquid is dispersed in another liquid; may be water in oil (w/o) or oil in water (o/w). Emulsions are stabilized through the use of an emulsifying agent. Oral emulsions are o/w preparations; topical emulsions may be either o/w (washable and nonstaining) or w/o. An o/w will become diluted with water, but a w/o will not.
- **Lotion:** A liquid for topical application that contains insoluble solids or liquids.
- **Gels:** A two-phase system containing an extremely fine solid particle that, when mixed, has a semisolid form. Very difficult to distinguish between the two phases.
- **Ointments:** A semisolid dosage form for topical application. Anhydrous ointments absorb water, but are insoluble in water and are not water washable. Oleaginous ointments are insoluble in water, do not contain or absorb water and are not water washable.
- **Pastes:** Similar to ointments, but contain more solid materials.
- **Creams:** O/W emulsions that are applied topically.

INHALANTS

Inhalants: Gases, vapors, solutions, or suspensions intended to be inhaled either orally or intranasally.
- **Aerosol:** A spray in a pressurized container that contains a propellant, an inert liquid or gas under pressure meant to carry the active ingredient to its location of application. Particles may be either a fine solid or a liquid. Aerosols are used for administration into body cavities. They are convenient and easy to apply.
- **Spray:** A dosage form that consists of a container with a valve assembly that, when activated, will emit a dispersion of liquid, solid, or gaseous material.

TRANSDERMAL

Provides systemic therapy for acute or chronic conditions that do not involve the skin. A transdermal product delivers a controlled dose of medication through the skin and is absorbed directly into the bloodstream. It is a convenient system that results in improved patient compliance, accurate drug dosage, and regulation of drug concentration.

FORMULARY OR APPROVED STOCK LIST

- **Formulary:** A list of drugs that are approved for use in an institution such as a hospital or will be reimbursed by a third-party carrier to a pharmacy. Formulary systems include open formulary (all pharmaceutical products carried), closed formulary (limited number of products of each drug classification covered), or restricted formulary (a hybrid of both open and closed formularies). Formularies may define policies, procedures, and guidelines established by the medical staff regarding a medication's usage. Formularies are revised yearly and a process must be in place for revisions.
- **Pharmacy and Therapeutics Committee:** A committee composed of pharmacists, physicians, nurses, and accountants who develop a formulary for a hospital. The most effective therapeutic agents are chosen for an institution. A formulary may contain a generic and name-brand name index, dosage forms and strengths, formulations, packaging and sizes available, dosage guidelines, approved abbreviations for the institution, policies on investigational medications, electrolyte content of large volume parenterals (LVPs), and lists of available nutritional and sugar-free products.
- **Third-party (managed care) provider:** A provider who may develop a formulary for its members regarding products covered for reimbursement.

PAR AND REORDER LEVELS AND DRUG USAGE

- **PAR value (periodic automatic replacement):** The amount of drug that is automatically reordered. In automatic reordering systems, when a drug falls below a predetermined quantity, it is automatically reordered.
- **Minimum/maximum:** A predetermined number that states the minimum and maximum amount of medication to be kept on a shelf. The smaller the range, the more accurate the quantity to be stocked; eliminates guesswork. The system is based on historical data for an institution and current trends.

INVENTORY RECEIVING PROCESS

1. Verify incoming merchandise (drug, dosage form, strength, package size, number of units, and expiration date) against packing slip or invoice.

2. Any merchandise requiring special storage, such as refrigeration, should promptly be verified and placed in proper conditions to avoid damage or loss of potency.
3. Sign and date invoice.
4. Forward documentation to accounts payable.
5. Place merchandise on shelf and rotate product by placing product with shortest dating in front and longest dating behind it.

BIOAVAILABILITY STANDARDS (I.E., GENERIC SUBSTITUTES)

- **Bioavailability of pharmaceutical products:** A measurement of both the rate of absorption and the total amount of drug that reaches the general circulation from an administered dosage form. Dissolution of the pharmaceutical product affects the absorption of the drug, which is also affected by properties of the drug and the dosage form. All generic drugs must contain the same active ingredients as the original brand indications; meet the same batch requirements for identity, strength, purity, and quality; and yield similar blood absorption and urinary excretion curves as the active ingredient.
- **Therapeutic equivalent:** A drug product that, when administered in the same amount, will provide the same therapeutic effect and pharmacokinetic characteristics as another drug to which it is compared.
- **Therapeutic substitution:** The substitution of a new drug product with another that differs in composition, but is considered to have the same or very similar pharmacologic and therapeutic activity.

REGULATORY REQUIREMENTS REGARDING RECORD-KEEPING FOR REPACKAGED PRODUCTS, RECALLED PRODUCTS, AND REFUNDED PRODUCTS

REPACKAGING

Labeling: Must contain the following information on the label:
- Generic name of the drug
- Strength
- Dosage form
- Manufacturer's name and lot number
- Expiration date after repackaging

Repackaging log: Documentation required for repackaging medication and must be signed by the pharmacist.
- Date of repackaging
- Name of drug
- Manufacturer
- Manufacturer's expiration date and lot number
- Quantity of drug repackaged
- Licensed pharmacist's initials

Expiration date of repackaged drugs: Federal law mandates that the expiration date cannot exceed 6 months and cannot exceed 25% of the remaining time on the manufacturer's original expiration date on the bulk container (Figure 3-1).

RECALLED MEDICATIONS

- Pharmacy notified by manufacturer/wholesaler by mail or fax.
- Pharmacy determines if recalled medication is currently in stock.
- Pharmacy contacts patients who may have received medication. If a customer has the recalled product, the medication should be returned to pharmacy for refund/substitution.
- Recalled medication returned to manufacturer for credit.
- Reorder medication that has been recalled. Notify physician of recalled medication; inquire if the physician wishes to change the medication order especially if product may not be available for a long period.

REFUNDED PRODUCTS

- **Unit dose:** May be redispensed if not tampered with or beyond use date
- **Multidose vial:** Cannot be redispensed

Item	Description
Date	The date that the drug is made, which includes day, month, and year
Drug	Drug name, usually by generic name then brand name if indicated on log sheet
Dosage form	Tablet, capsule, spansule, troche, liquid, etc
Manufacturer	Manufacturer of the drug, usually abbreviated
Manufacturer's lot number	Control number located on the side of the label or on the bottom of the bottle
Manufacturer's expiration date	Located with the lot number; remember that if the date indicates only the month, the drug is good through the end of the month
Pharmacy lot number	Each item repackaged in the pharmacy is given a number consecutive to the previously made batch
Pharmacy expiration date	Calculate the new expiration date, which is 6 months or 1/4 of the time of the manufacturer's expiration date, whichever is less
Technician	Must initial the logbook entry
Pharmacist	Each item made must be checked off by a pharmacist

The information on the label of the unit dose item is much less than what is erequired in the logbook, but it is just as important. The following sample lists the components necessary on a typical unit dose label:

Name of drug
   Generic name
   Trade name (trade name commonly given for the easy identification of the proper medication)

Strength
Dosage form
Pharmacy lot number
Pharmacy expiration date

Fig. 3-1 Example of a record log sheet used for documentation.

POLICIES, PROCEDURES, AND PRACTICES FOR INVENTORY SYSTEMS

Inventory management: Focuses on the procurement; drug storage and inventory control; repackaging and label considerations; distribution systems; and recapture and disposal of used and unused pharmaceutical products.

PURPOSE OF INVENTORY MANAGEMENT
- Provide an adequate stock of pharmaceuticals and supplies
- Reduce unexpected stock-outs and temporary shortages, which may affect patient care
- Reduce carrying cost (financial investment) in drug products
- Minimize costs associated with placing orders to the wholesaler
- Minimize time spent on purchasing functions
- Minimize capital charge on average inventory
- Minimize shrinkage, breakage, and obsolescence of inventory
- Reduce purchasing dollars spent by selecting products with the best price

INVENTORY PRACTICES
- **Cost analysis:** Examining all costs associated in the purchase of a product, which may include acquisition costs, storage costs, costs associated with preparing and packaging a product, and getting the final product to the patient.
- **Formulary:** A basis for the dispensing of medications purchased and prescribed in a hospital or reimbursed under a managed care program. A formulary may be either an open or a closed formulary.

TABLE **3-1** ABC Analysis

ABC ITEM RANK	TOTAL ANNUAL PERCENT OF COSTS	PERCENT OF PRODUCTS
A	80%	20%
B	15%	15%
C	5%	65%
Total	100%	100%

- **Group purchasing organizations:** Organization responsible for negotiating discounted drug prices for hospitals or other institutions with drug manufacturers. They develop contracts with pharmaceutical companies.
- **Just-in-time ordering (JIT):** A strategy of ordering a product before its use. Minimizes tying up funds for long periods and reduces the cost associated with inventory management.
- **Prime vendor agreement:** An agreement between a pharmacy and a wholesaler in which the pharmacy agrees to purchase the majority of its products from that wholesaler return for other considerations.
- **Therapeutic interchange:** A substitution of one medication for another medication that is not generically equivalent but possesses the same therapeutic effect.
- **Want list:** An order of items that are in short supply and need to be reordered from a vendor.

INVENTORY MANAGEMENT STRATEGIES

- **80/20 rule:** 80% of a pharmacy's drug costs are derived from 20% of the pharmaceuticals carried. Focuses on inventory control of the top 20% of the items carried.
- **80/20 report (velocity report):** A detailed summary of purchasing history based on the 80/20 rule.
- **ABC analysis:** A method to identify and define inventory items based on their usage. Products are ranked based on their purchase history and dollar amount of total annual costs. Focuses efforts based on the products that will have the greatest inventory turnover rate (Table 3-1).
- **Compliance reports:** A report summarizing all items that were not purchased on bid.
- **Inventory turnover rate:** A tool to evaluate inventory dollars. Can be calculated using the following formula: Total annual purchases/Inventory value. A greater number of inventory turns improves the financial well being of the institution. Twelve inventory turns per year is considered very good for a pharmacy.
- **Minimum/maximum:** An inventory ordering system that identifies a predetermined order of quantity (par value) and maximum order point of medications. Min/Max ensures that a firm maintains an adequate quantity on its shelves without incurring additional costs from purchasing from a wholesaler or outside vendor.
- **Stock cards:** A card that states how much of a given product the pharmacy should maintain on its shelf based on its purchase history. The level should be a minimum of 1 week and a maximum of 3 weeks. The business will determine the number of days of merchandise it wishes to carry.

PRODUCTS USED IN PACKAGING AND REPACKAGING

- Child-resistant caps required on all prescriptions unless patient or physician requests easy-open containers, patients are being administered medication in institutions, multiple sizes of same product are available and package is marked as not being child resistant, and certain medications are not required to be packaged in child-resistant containers.
- Packaging is light-resistant to prevent ultraviolet rays from breaking the compound down.

RISK MANAGEMENT OPPORTUNITIES

- **Dress code:** Persons involved in the preparation of sterile products should scrub their hands with an appropriate antibacterial agent for a predetermined period of time and dry them with paper towels. Procedure should be repeated if possibility of contamination occurs. Jewelry should not be worn during aseptic technique because of the possibility of contamination. Makeup should not be worn because of the particulate nature of the substance. Clean, particulate-free clothing should be worn.
- **Personal protective equipment (PPE):** Used to place a barrier between the employee and specific substances. PPE includes latex gloves, masks, goggles, face shields, gowns, laboratory coats, shoe coverings, and head coverings.
- **Needle recapping:** Never recap used needles using both hands and any other technique that involves directing the point of the needle toward the body. Use a one-handed "scoop" technique or a mechanical device

designed for holding the needle sheath. Do not remove used needles from disposable syringes by hand and do not bend, break, or manipulate the needles by hand.
- **Use of "sharps" container:** Used disposable syringes are to be placed in the sharp containers (a thick red plastic container) in an area close to where sharps are being used.

THE FOOD AND DRUG ADMINISTRATION'S (FDA) CLASSIFICATIONS OF RECALLS

- **Class I:** Reasonable probability that use of the product will cause or lead to serious adverse health events or death.
- **Class II:** Probability exists that use of the product will cause adverse health events that are temporary or medically reversible.
- **Class III:** Use of product will probably not cause an adverse health event.

SYSTEMS TO IDENTIFY AND RETURN EXPIRED AND UNSALEABLE PRODUCTS

- Policies are established by each pharmacy regarding the process of pulling medications that will expire within a given period.
- A system must be in place in all practices of pharmacy to check for expired medications. Expired medications must be kept away from in-date medications.
- Contracts with wholesalers and manufacturers will determine if products may be returned for partial or full credit. Proper inventory management skills may eliminate the necessity of returns to the manufacturer, if a product is being properly rotated.
- Cytoxic medications are destroyed with biohazardous waste goods.
- The DEA must be notified through the issue of Form 41 for expired controlled substances before destruction may occur. A copy of Form 41 must be maintained for a minimum of 2 years at the pharmacy site.
- Reconstituted or compounded drugs are not returnable to the manufacturer. Other examples of nonreturnable items include partially used bottles of medication.
- Unused unit dose medications may be redispensed after medication has been checked for integrity.

RULES AND REGULATIONS FOR THE REMOVAL AND DISPOSAL OF PRODUCTS

- Medication should never be dispensed to a patient if it has passed its expiration date or will expire before the patient is able to complete the current course of therapy. Multidose containers cannot be redispensed to another patient; unit dose medications can be redispensed to other patients.
- Controlled substances can only be returned to institutions having a DEA number. For example, long-term facilities cannot return controlled substances to pharmacies because long-term care facilities don't have a DEA number.
- Every pharmacy technician in a particular pharmacy should be aware of the pharmacy's disposition procedures. Depending on the vendor or wholesaler, some will accept outdated medication for credit.
- If medication is to be destroyed, the normal means of destruction is either through flushing or rinsing down a sink. The pharmacy technician needs to be familiar with the procedures of the institution regarding outdated products.
- A DEA Form 41 is a triplicate form that needs to be completed before the destruction of controlled substances. The required copies of DEA Form 41 are submitted to the DEA.

LEGAL AND REGULATORY REQUIREMENTS AND PROFESSIONAL STANDARDS GOVERNING OPERATIONS OF PHARMACIES

- **Compounding:** "The preparation, mixing, assembling, packaging, or labeling of a drug or device (1) as the result of a practitioner's prescription drug order or initiative based on the practitioner-patient-pharmacist relationship, or (2) for the purpose of or as an incident to research, teaching, or chemical analysis and not for sale or dispensing. Compounding also includes the preparation of drugs or devices in anticipation of prescription drug orders based on routine, regularly observed prescribing patterns."

- **Manufacturing:** "The production, preparation, propagation, conversion, or processing of a drug or device either directly or indirectly by extraction from substances of natural origin or independently by means of chemical or biological synthesis and includes any packaging or repackaging of the substance(s) or labeling of its container, and the promotion and marketing of such drugs or devices. Manufacturing also includes the preparation and promotion of commercially available products from bulk compounds for resale by pharmacies, practitioners, or other persons."
- **Prepackaging**
  Unit dose system: A system that provides a medication in its final "unit of use." Unit dose packaging machines may be manual, semiautomatic, or automatic. May be a single drop (60 packages/min) or double-drop (120 packages/min).
  Modified unit dose system: A drug distribution system that combines unit dose medications, which are blister-packaged onto a multiple-dose card instead of being placed in a box. Synonymous with "punch cards, bingo cards, or blister cards."
  Blended unit dose system: Combines a unit dose system with a non–unit dose system. May be a multiple-medication package or a modular cassette. Multiple medication package has all the medication, which is administered at the same time. Modular cassette is a combination of cassette or drawer exchange system.

LEGAL AND REGULATORY REQUIREMENTS AND PROFESSIONAL STANDARDS FOR PREPARING, LABELING, DISPENSING, DISTRIBUTING, AND ADMINISTERING MEDICATIONS

- DEA is responsible for enforcing the Controlled Substance Act
- FDA is accountable for ensuring that medications and food are pure, safe, and effective. Can issue drug recalls
- State Board of Pharmacy ensures that specific standards are met for the licensing of pharmacists, permits are issued for a pharmacy, and the requirements are met regarding pharmacy technicians.
- Joint Commission on Accreditation of Healthcare Organizations (JCAHO) requires unit dose dispensing and pharmacy-based intravenous additive programs. Bulk packaging and floor stock have been eliminated due to safety and contamination issues.
- United States Pharmacopoeia sets requirements for labeling of medications, whether they are in multidose vial or unit dose container, an IV admixture or compound.

REQUIRED INFORMATION FOR ALL PRESCRIPTIONS

- Prescriber information:
  Name of physician
  Office address of physician—includes street number, street name (office or suite number if applicable), city, stat, zip code
- Date prescription was written
- Patient information:
Patient's name
Patient's home address—includes number, street, city, state, zip code
- Inscription:
  Name of medication: May be either brand or generic
  Strength of medication
  Quantity of medication to be dispensed
- Subscription: Instructions to the pharmacist
- Physician's signature: Must be in ink; stamped signatures are illegal

REQUIRED INFORMATION ON MEDICATION ORDERS

- Prescriber's information
- Date of order
- Patient information—room number and bed number
- Name, strength, and dosage form of medication
- When to be administered (specific time of day)
- Duration of therapy
- Prescriber's signature

MEDICATION DISTRIBUTION AND CONTROL SYSTEM REQUIREMENTS FOR THE USE OF MEDICATIONS IN VARIOUS PRACTICE SETTINGS

INPATIENT

- Automation is being used to regulate and track controlled substances.
- Bar-coded labels—used as part of automation to reduce errors and to streamline the medication process. Will improve the quality of patient care.
- Computerized dispensing systems are being used because of the need to have medication available 24 hours per day.
- Crash carts or Code Blue carts: A Code Blue in a hospital signifies that a patient is in a life-threatening situation such as the stopping of a patient's heart or a cessation of breathing. Carts are located on the floors of a hospital stocked with the necessary medications for a Code Blue situation and are used to stabilize a patient.
- Robotics is being used to scan unit dose medication and fill a patient's medication cassette.
- Scanning patient identification bracelets—to ensure patient is receiving the proper medication.

OUTPATIENT

- Automated dispensing machines such as Baker cells and PYXIS are being used to improve efficiency.
- Scanning of prescription orders and imaging are being used.

REPACKAGING, STORAGE REQUIREMENTS, AND DOCUMENTATION FOR FINISHED DOSAGE FORMS PREPARED IN ANTICIPATION OF PRESCRIPTIONS OR MEDICATION ORDERS

- Storage of all medications will be based on environmental considerations, security issues, and safety requirements.
- Environmental consideration involves proper temperature, ventilation, humidity, light, and sanitation. Standards for storage will be found in the United States Pharmacopeia and National Formulary under the "General Notices and Requirements" section.
- Faxed prescriptions must not be dispensed until original prescription is presented to the pharmacy. Exceptions exist for emergency prescriptions for Schedule II medications and Schedule II medications in long-term care facilities.
- Master formula must be maintained for any pharmacy engaging in extemporaneous compounding.
- Repackaging log must be maintained in any pharmacy that prepares or repackages medication.

POLICIES, PROCEDURES, AND PRACTICES REGARDING STORAGE AND HANDLING OF HAZARDOUS MATERIALS AND WASTES

The Material Safety Data Sheet (MSDS) provides detailed information on the hazards associated with a particular substance. A hazardous chemical is one that poses a threat to health or safety. A list of hazardous drugs can be found in a patient product insert, in the Physicians' Desk Reference, and in American Hospital Formulary Service Drug Information. These drugs are considered to be hazardous in their final dosage form especially if they are crushed or broken. The manufacturer provides a MSDS to the pharmacy, and the pharmacy must provide it to long-term care facilities.

MEDICATION DISTRIBUTION AND CONTROL SYSTEMS REQUIREMENTS FOR CONTROLLED SUBSTANCES, INVESTIGATIONAL DRUGS, AND HAZARDOUS MATERIALS AND WASTES

CONTROLLED SUBSTANCES

Schedule II medications must be kept in a locked safe in the pharmacy. Schedule III-V medications may be dispersed throughout the pharmacy. Refrigerated Schedule II substances must be kept in a locked refrigerator with no other medications. Controlled substances on a nursing floor must be in a locked cart.

Controlled Substance Administration Record (CSAR): Assists in the accountability of controlled substances in a nursing unit. Controlled substance forms allow a nurse to verify counts of a controlled substance at the change of a shift. Counts must be witnessed by the incoming nurse. A controlled substance usage form monitors receipt, administration, and disposal of individual controlled substances. A separate form is used to account for the amount of controlled substances a patient is taking.

Medication delivery record: Documents receipt of medication on a nursing floor from the pharmacy. Records are checked against records in the pharmacy.

Medication Administration Record (MAR): Documents medication dispensed to a patient.

INVESTIGATIONAL DRUGS

Under the Federal Food, Drug, and Cosmetic Act, a medication must obtain premarketing approval from the government before use. A hospital pharmacy is responsible for the distribution and control of investigational drugs, which includes procurement, storage, inventory management, packaging, labeling, distribution, and disposition of unused drugs. The pharmacy must provide clinical services such as patient education, staff in-service training, monitoring, and reporting of adverse reactions. The pharmacy is involved with research activities, such as participating in the preparation or review of research proposals and protocols, assisting in data collection, and analysis. The pharmacy may undertake clinical study management by providing reports to the sponsor.

HAZARDOUS MATERIALS AND WASTE

The Occupational Health and Safety Act requires that all employees be aware of the hazards of chemicals to which they are exposed. The Hazard Communication Standard is based on the belief that all employees have both a need and a right to be informed of the hazards and identities of the chemicals to which they will be exposed. Every institution handling hazardous chemicals must have a written hazard communication program and they must receive an MSDS from the manufacturer, importer, or distributor for each hazardous chemical in the workplace.

QUALITY ASSURANCE POLICIES, PROCEDURES, AND PRACTICES FOR MEDICATION AND INVENTORY CONTROL SYSTEMS

GUIDE TO PREVENTING PRESCRIPTION ERRORS

The following simple procedures will help avoid errors in the pharmacy.
- Always keep the prescription and the label together during the fill process.
- Know the common look-alike and sound-alike drugs, and keep them stored in different areas of the pharmacy so they will not be easily mistaken (Table 3-2).
- Always question bad handwriting.
- Be aware of insulin mistakes. Insulin brands should be clearly separated from one another. Educate patients to always verify their insulin purchase.
- Clear stock bottles no longer needed away from the work area in a timely fashion. Only keep what is needed for immediate use in the work area.
- Keep dangerous or high-alert medications in a separate storage area of the pharmacy.
- Make sure prescriptions/orders include the correctly spelled drug name, strength, appropriate dosing, quantity or duration of therapy, dosage form, and route. Missing information should be obtained from the prescriber.
- Question ambiguous orders.
- Question the prescription order that uses abbreviations you are not familiar with or that are uncommon. Avoid using abbreviations that have more than one meaning, and verify the meaning of these abbreviations with the prescriber.
- The label should always be compared with the original prescription by at least two people. If an error occurs at this stage, the refills may be filled incorrectly as well (Table 3-3).
- Use the metric system. A leading zero should always be present in decimal values less than one. Remember that an error of this nature will mean a dosage error of at least 10-fold.

What Can the Technician Do to Reduce Errors?
- Do a mental check on dosage appropriateness.
- Keep your work area free of clutter.
- Observe and report pertinent OTC purchases.

TABLE **3-2** Common Look-alike and Sound-alike Medications

Accupril	Accutane	digitoxin	digoxin	Orinase	Ornade
acetazolamide	acetohexamide	diphenhydramine	dimenhydrinate	paroxetine	Paclitaxel
Aciphex	Accupril, Aricept	dopamine	dobutamine	Paxil	Paclitaxel, Taxol
Actos	Actonel	Edecrin	Eulexin	penicillamine	penicillin
albuterol	atenolol	enalapril	Anafranil, Eldepryl	Percocet	Percodan
Aldomet	Aldoril	ERYC	Ery-Tab	pindolol	Parlodel
Alkeran	Leukeran, Myleran	etidronate	etretinate,	Pravachol	Prevacid,
alprazolam	lorazepam		etomidate		propranolol
Amaryl	Reminyl	E-Vista	Evista	prednisolone	prednisone
Ambien	Amen	Femara	femhrt	Prilosec	Prozac
amiloride	amlodipine	Fioricet	Fiorinal	Prinivil	Prilosec, Proventil
amiodarone	amrinone	Flomax	Volmax	Procanbid	Procan SR
amitriptyline	nortriptyline	flurbiprofen	fenoprofen	Provera	Premarin
Apresazide	Apresoline	folinic acid	folic acid	Prozac	Proscar
Arlidin	Aralen	Gantrisin	Gantanol	quinidine	clonidine, Quinamm
Artane	Altace	glipizide	glyburide	quinine	quinidine
asparaginase	pegaspargase	glyburide	Glucotrol	Regroton	Hygroton
Atarax	Ativan	Hycodan	Hycomine	Reminyl	Robinul
atenolol	timolol	hydralazine	hydroxyzine	Retrovir	ritonavir
Atrovent	Alupent	hydrocodone	hydrocortisone	Rifamate	rifampin
Avandia	Coumadin, Prandin	Hydrogesic	hydroxyzine	rimantadine	flutamide
Bacitracin	Bactroban	hydromorphone	morphine	Roxicodone	Roxicet
Benylin	Ventolin	Hydropres	Diupres	Sarafem	Serophene
Brevital	Brevibloc	Hytone	Vytone	Seroquel	Serzone
Bumex	Buprenex	imipramine	Norpramin	Stadol	Haldol
bupropion	buspirone	Inderal	Inderide, Isordil	sulfadiazine	sulfasalazine
Cafergot	Carafate	Indocin	Minocin	Tegretol	Tequin
calciferol	calcitriol	K-Phos	Neutra-Phos-K	terazosin	temazepam
Cardene	Cardizem	Lamictal	Lamisil, Ludiomil	terbinafine	terfenadine
Cataflam	Catapres	Lanoxin	Lasix	terbutaline	tolbutamide
Catapres	Combipres	Lantus	Lente Insulin	Ticlid	Tequin
cefotaxime	cefoxitin	Lioresal	lisinopril	tolazamide	tolbutamide
Cerebryx	Celebrex, Celera	Lithostat	Lithobid, Lithotabs	torsemide	furosemide
Celera	Cerebryx, Celebrex	Lodine	Codeine	trifluoperazine	trihexyphenidyl
chlorpromazine	chlorpromazine,	Lopid	Lorabid	Trimox	Diamox
	prochlorperazine,	lovastatin	Lotensin	Ultram	Ultrase
	promethazine	Ludiomil	Lomotil	Vancenase	Vanceril
Clinoril	Clozaril	Medrol	Haldol	Vasosulf	Velosef
clomipramine	Clomiphene	metolazone	methotrexate,	Versed	Vistaril
clonidine	Klonopin		metoclopramide	Xanax	Zantac
Combivir	Combivent	metoprolol	misoprostol	Xenical	Xeloda
Cozaar	Zocor	metoprolol	metoclopramide	Zantac	Zyrtec
cyclobenzaprine	cyproheptadine	tartrate		Zebeta	Diabeta
cyclophosamide	cyclosporine	Monopril	minoxidil	Zinacef	Zithromax
cyclosporine	cycloserine	nelfinavir	nevirapine	Zocor	Zoloft
Cytovene	Cytosar	nicardipine	nifedipine	Zofran	Zantac
Cytoxan	Cytotec, Cytosar	Norlutate	Norlutin	Zosyn	Zofran
Darvocet-N	Darvon-N	Noroxin	Neurontin	Zovirax	Zyvox
daunorubicin	doxorubicin	Norvasc	Navane	Zyrtec	Zyprexa
desipramine	diphenhydramine	Norvir	Retrovir	Zyvox	Vioxx
Diabeta	Zebeta	Ocufen	Ocuflox		

- Triple check your work.
- Verify your own data entry before processing.

What Can the Pharmacist Do to Reduce Errors?

- Check prescriptions in a timely manner.
- Document all clarifications on orders.

TABLE **3-3** Common Abbreviation Errors

ABBREVIATION	MEANING	MISINTERPRETATION
ac	Before meals	After meals
ad	Right ear	Right eye
ARA-A	Vidarabine	Cytarabine
as	Left ear	Left eye
AU	Both ears	Both eyes
AZT	Zidovudine	Azathioprine
CPZ	Compazine	Chlorpromazine
D/C	Discontinue	Discharge
	Discharge	Discontinue
HCl	Hydrochloride salt	Potassium chloride
HCT	Hydrocortisone	Hydrochlorothiazide
HCTZ 50	Hydrochlorothiazide	Hydrocortisone
IU	International units	Intravenous
MTX	Methotrexate	Mitoxantrone
Nitro Drip	Nitroglycerin infusion	Sodium nitroprusside infusion
od or OD	Right eye	Right ear
os	Left eye	Left ear
ou	Each (both) eye(s)	Each (both) ear(s)
Per os	Orally	Left eye
qd or QD	Each or every day	Four times a day
Qhs	At bedtime	Every hour
qod or QOD	Every other day	Every day or every other day
SC	Subcutaneous	Sublingual
sub q	Subcutaneous	Subcutaneous every
TAC	Triamcinolone	Tetracaine
TIW	Three times a week	Three times a day
x3d	For 3 days	For three doses
%	100%	

- Encourage OTC and herbal remedy documentation.
- Initial checked prescriptions.
- Use the USP-ISMP (Institute for Safe Medication Practices) Medication Error Reporting Form to inform manufacturers of errors caused by commercial packaging and labeling.
- Visually check the product in the bottle.

What Can the Pharmacy Do to Reduce Errors?

- Automate and bar code all fill procedures.
- Encourage physicians to use common terminology and abbreviations.
- Maintain a safe work area.
- Provide adequate computer applications and hardware.
- Provide adequate storage areas.

CHAPTER 3 REVIEW QUESTIONS

1. What is the purpose of a group purchasing organization (GPO) for a hospital pharmacy?
   a. Negotiate prices with drug manufacturers
   b. Negotiate prices with a local drug wholesaler
   c. Purchase drugs from a drug manufacturer for the hospital
   d. Purchase drugs from a local drug wholesaler

2. Which of the following is not an advantage of a solid dosage form?
    a. Convenient for self-medication
    b. Easier to swallow than other dosage forms
    c. Easy to package and dispense
    d. Lacks taste or smell

3. Which dosage form is contained in a gelatin shell?
    a. Capsule
    b. Effervescent salts
    c. Pastilles
    d. Suppositories

4. Which dosage form may be prepared by either compressing or molding?
    a. Capsule
    b. Pellet
    c. Plaster
    d. Tablet

5. Which dosage form releases carbon dioxide when it is dissolved in water?
    a. Effervescent salts
    b. Plasters
    c. Powders
    d. Troches

6. Which of the following is not a disadvantage of liquid?
    a. Deterioration and loss of potency occur quickly
    b. Easier to swallow than solid dosage forms
    c. Interactions develop due to changes in solubility
    d. Requires sweetening and flavoring to be palatable

7. Which type of solution is a clear, sweetened, flavored hydroalcoholic containing water and alcohol?
    a. An aromatic water
    b. An elixir
    c. A suspension
    d. A syrup

8. What type of dispersion is either water in oil or oil in water?
    a. An emulsion
    b. A gel
    c. A lotion
    d. An ointment

9. Which of the following is not required on the label of a repackaged medication?
    a. Date of repackaging
    b. Generic name of the medication
    c. Manufacturer's name and lot number
    d. Expiration date after repackaging

10. Which of the following information is not required on a repackaging log?
    a. Date of repackaging
    b. Expiration date after repackaging
    c. Pharmacist's initials
    d. Quantity of drug repackaged

11. Which regulatory agency may issue a drug recall?
    a. BOA
    b. DEA
    c. FDA
    d. JCAHO

12. What type of unit dose system may be referred to as a "punch card" or "bingo card"?
    a. Blended unit dose system
    b. Modified unit dose system
    c. Modular cassette unit dose system
    d. Multiple medications package unit dose system

13. What type of agreement is between a pharmacy and a wholesaler, in which the pharmacy agrees to purchase the majority of its product from that wholesaler?
    a. Prime purchaser agreement
    b. Prime vendor agreement
    c. Purchase order
    d. Velocity agreement

14. Which of the following dosage forms is an aqueous solution containing sucrose?
    a. Elixir
    b. Spirit
    c. Syrup
    d. Tincture

15. Which of the following dosage forms is not an example of dispersion?
    a. Gel
    b. Liniment
    c. Lotion
    d. Suspension

16. Which of the following dosage forms is not an example of a solution?
    a. Elixir
    b. Emulsion
    c. Enema
    d. Syrup

17. Which of the following dosage forms is not an example of a sustained release dosage?
    a. Controlled action
    b. Depot
    c. Pastille
    d. Repository

18. Which type of solution is a topical dosage form containing pyrotoxin and is dissolved in alcohol and ether?
    a. Collodion
    b. Extract
    c. Liniment
    d. Spirit

19. How many phases are in a suspension?
    a. 2
    b. 3
    c. 4
    d. 5

20. Which type of dispersion is similar to an ointment but contains more solid materials?
    a. Cream
    b. Gel
    c. Lotion
    d. Paste

21. Which committee develops a formulary for an institution?
    a. BOP
    b. FDA
    c. JCAHO
    d. P&T

22. What is the maximum amount of time that can be assigned to a repackaged drug?
    a. 3 months
    b. 6 months
    c. 9 months
    d. 12 months

23. What is the subscription on a prescription?
    a. Any special instructions or directions to the pharmacist
    b. Directions to be typed on the prescription label
    c. Name, strength, and quantity of medication
    d. The Rx symbol

24. What types of substances require a Material Safety Data Sheet?
    a. Hazardous drugs and chemicals
    b. Investigational drugs
    c. IV admixtures
    d. OTCs

25. What type of products must be isotonic?
    a. External medications
    b. Ophthalmic products
    c. Oral inhalation products
    d. Otic preparations

Participating in the Administration and Management of Pharmacy Practice

THE PRACTICE SETTING'S MISSION, GOALS AND OBJECTIVES, ORGANIZATIONAL STRUCTURE, AND POLICIES AND PROCEDURES

- **Mission statement:** states the purpose and goals of an organization
- **Organizational structure:** shows the chain of command in an organization. Examples of organizational structure include matrix and product line. Matrix emphasizes overlapping of responsibility among departments and common areas of decision making. Product line is organized along a common product or service being offered
- **Policy:** a definite course or method of action; a plan establishing goals and objectives
- **Procedure:** process of accomplishing a task to ensure efficiency and consistency; a step-by-step method to accomplish a policy

Policy and procedure are found in all types of pharmacy practice. They are required by professional and regulatory agencies, such as ASHP, APhA, and JCAHO. Policy and procedures provides standards for the operation of a pharmacy. The policy and procedure manual can be used a reference book and can be used to promote safety in the workplace.

LINES OF COMMUNICATION THROUGHOUT THE ORGANIZATION

- Face-to-face meetings
- Telephone
- Voicemail
- E-mail
- Memorandums (written letters)

PRINCIPLES OF RESOURCE ALLOCATION

- **Cross-training (cross-functional):** Bringing together persons from different functions to work on a common task; designed to help improve lateral communication. They have the ability solve problems based on "total systems thinking." They have the ability to work well based on better information and speed of transmitting the information.
- **Multiskilling:** Team members are trained in skills to perform more than one job.

- **Scheduling:** Productivity reports can be used to show the peak times of the day when prescription processing is heaviest and when prescriptions are being picked up by customers. The staff should be scheduled based on these times.
- **Self-managing teams:** Teams that are empowered to make decisions about planning, doing, and evaluating their daily work.
- **Virtual groups:** Convene and operate with members linked together electronically via computers.
- **Workflow:** An organized way of performing a task. It is efficient in nature and it is a repeatable, defined set of activities.

PRODUCTIVITY, EFFICIENCY, AND CUSTOMER SATISFACTION MEASURES

- Customer service—follow up survey with customers. Use of focus groups to gauge opinions of customers comparing customer service of one location or organization to another
- Efficiency—inventory turnover rates, reduction in prescription errors per shift
- Productivity—prescriptions filled per pharmacist per hour

WRITTEN, ORAL, AND ELECTRONIC COMMUNICATION SYSTEMS

Organizational communication: process by which information is exchanged in an organizational setting
Channel richness: the capacity of a channel to convey information effectively. Listed below, the channels are shown in decreasing order of channel richness.
- Face-to-face: most effective
- Telephone
- E-mail
- Written memos
- Letters
- Posted notices
- Bulletins: least effective
Formal channels: follow the chain of command or hierarchy in an organization
Informal channels: do not follow chain of command; allow for the transfer of information through networks and acquaintances

REQUIRED OPERATIONAL LICENSES AND CERTIFICATES

- All pharmacists must have licenses on site (which may include continuing education documentation)
- Business license
- Drug Enforcement Agency (DEA) Form 222 to order Schedule II medications
- DEA Form 224 to order controlled substances
- DEA Form 41 to destroy controlled substance
- JCAHO accreditation is highly recommended for hospitals and long-term care facilities, such as nursing homes
- Permits to collect taxes if any products are sold and tax is to be collected
- Pharmacist-in-charge must have appropriate documentation to order Schedule II medications, such as the "power of attorney"

ROLES AND RESPONSIBILITIES OF PHARMACISTS, PHARMACY TECHNICIANS, AND OTHER PHARMACY EMPLOYEES

The primary duty of a pharmacy technician is to assist the pharmacist. Pharmacy technicians provide technical assistance in the pharmacy, but are not involved in judgmental duties. Listed below are duties associated with community, institutional (i.e., hospital), and managed care pharmacy technicians.

RESPONSIBILITIES OF COMMUNITY TECHNICIANS

- Help patients who are dropping off or picking up prescription orders
- Enter prescription orders into the computer
- Create a profile of the patient's health and insurance information in the computer or update the patient's profile

- Assist the pharmacist, under direct supervision, in the practice of pharmacy, in accordance with local, state, federal, and company regulations
- Communicate with insurance carriers to obtain payment for prescription claims
- At point of sale, verify that customer receives correct prescription(s)
- Complete weekly distribution center medication orders, place orders on shelves, and verify all associated paperwork
- Assist the pharmacist with filling and labeling prescriptions
- Prepare the pharmacy inventory
- Screen telephone calls for the pharmacist
- Communicate with prescribers and their agents to obtain refill authorization
- Compound oral solutions, ointments, and creams
- Prepackage bulk medications
- Maintain an awareness of developments in the community and pharmaceutical fields that relate to job responsibilities and integrate them into own practices
- Assist in training new employees
- Assist other pharmacy technicians
- Assist pharmacist in scheduling and maintaining workflow
- Maintain knowledge of loss prevention techniques

RESPONSIBILITIES OF INSTITUTIONAL TECHNICIANS

- Rotate through all work areas of the pharmacy
- Transport medications, drug-delivery devices, and other pharmacy equipment from the pharmacy to nursing units and clinics
- Pick up copies of physician orders, automated medication administration records, and unused medications from the nursing units and return them to the pharmacy
- Fill patient medication cassettes
- Prepare medications and supplies for dispensing, including:
  1. prepacking bulk medications, compounding ointments, creams, oral solutions, and other medications
  2. preparing chemotherapeutic agents
  3. compounding total parenteral nutrition solutions
  4. compounding large-volume intravenous mixtures
  5. packaging and preparing drugs being used in clinical investigations
  6. preparing prescriptions for outpatients
  7. checking continuous unit dose medications
  8. controlling and auditing narcotics/stock substance
- Assist pharmacists in entering medication orders into the computer system
- Prepare inventories, order drugs and supplies from the storeroom, receive drugs, and stock shelves in various pharmacy locations
- Screen telephone calls
- Perform monthly nursing unit inspections, maintain workload records, and collect quality assurance data
- Assist in training new employees
- Assist other pharmacy technicians
- Coordinate insurance billing including third party prescriptions
- Deliver unit dose to automated dispensing technology
- Triage telephone/window inquiries

RESPONSIBILITIES OF MANAGED CARE TECHNICIANS

- Under the supervision of a pharmacist: daily handling of ongoing pharmacy benefit telephone calls from members, pharmacy providers, and physicians
- Troubleshoot third-party prescription claims questions with an understanding of online rejections and plan parameters
- Develop and maintain an electronic service log on all telephone calls with complete follow-up history
- Develop a trending report on the aforementioned service calls with an eye toward forecasting possible trends in pharmacy service
- Provide as-needed telephone and administrative support for the department

LEGAL AND REGULATORY REQUIREMENTS FOR PERSONNEL, FACILITIES, EQUIPMENT, AND SUPPLIES

- Drug storage—all Schedule II forms must be stored in a locked safe (either combination or key lock); Schedule III-V's may be dispersed throughout the pharmacy with the other medications; refrigerated medication must be stored in a refrigerator.
- Equipment—required equipment in all pharmacies includes a Class A balance, pharmacy weights; equipment for reconstitution such as graduate cylinders, various mortars and pestles for mixing; spatulas, and stirring rods. Laminar air flow hoods are required for preparing intravenous preparations and chemotherapy agents.
- Facilities—State Boards of Pharmacy require a minimum amount of counter space in a pharmacy, an alarm system to be activated when the pharmacy is not open, separate refrigerators for refrigerated medications and controlled substances (must be lockable), a safe for Schedule II medications, and a sink with hot and cold water. The pharmacy must be kept clean and uncluttered.
- Personnel—pharmacists must be licensed by the State Board of Pharmacy in which they practice. Pharmacists must maintain their licensure by meeting specific requirements established by the Board of Pharmacy, which include continuing education. Pharmacy technicians must follow state regulations set by the Board, which may include registering with the Board of Pharmacy, becoming certified either by the PTCB or the state, and maintaining their certification, which may include continuing education.
- Prescription storage—prescriptions, biennial inventories, invoices, and Forms 222 and 41 must be readily retrievable (able to be produced within 72 hours of the request). Prescriptions may be filed either by separating the Schedule II, Schedule III-V, and non-controlled prescriptions; or filing the Schedule II-V separate from the nonscheduled drugs.

PROFESSIONAL LIBRARY

All pharmacies must have a professional library. Required books include the Federal Control Substance Act, USP and NF, and other texts (statute) required by the State Board of Pharmacy. Examples of reference books that may be found in a pharmacy library include the following.

American Drug Index 2002. St. Louis, MO: Facts and Comparisons, 2002.

This standard reference work contains more than 20,000 entries on drugs and drug products, including alphabetically listed drug names, cross-indexing, phonetic pronunciations, brand names, manufacturers, generic or chemical names, composition and strength, pharmaceutical forms available, package size, use, and common abbreviations. It also contains a listing of orphan drugs. The work is available in hardbound and CD-ROM editions. *http://www.factsandcomparisons.com*

American Hospital Formulary Service Drug Information 2002 (AHFS). Bethesda, MD: American Society of Health-System Pharmacists, 2002.

The complete text of roughly 1,400 monographs covering about 50,000 commercially available and experimental drugs, including information on uses, interactions, pharmacokinetics, dosage, and administration. *http://www.ashp.org*

Ansel, H.C., et al. *Pharmaceutical Dosage Forms and Drug Delivery Systems.* 7th ed. Baltimore: Williams & Wilkins, 1999.

A superb survey of contemporary dosage forms and delivery systems. *http://www.lww.com*

Drug Facts and Comparisons. St. Louis, MO: Facts and Comparisons, 2002.

This comprehensive source of information about 16,000 prescription and 6,000 over-the-counter drugs contains monographs about individual drugs and groups of related drugs; product listings in table format providing information on dosage forms and strength, distributor names, costs, package sizes, product identification codes, flavors, colors, and distribution status; and information on therapeutic uses, interactions, and adverse reactions. The publication includes an index of manufacturers and distributors and controlled substance regulations. This reference work is available in hardbound form, on CD-ROM, or in a loose-leaf form that is updated monthly. *http://www.factsandcomparisons.com*

Drug Information Fulltext (DIF). Norwood, MA: Silverplatter.

A searchable computer database combining two publications: the *American Hospital Formulary Service Drug Information* and the *Handbook on Injectable Drugs.* This database is available on a hard disk, on CD-ROM, or via the Internet. *http://www.silverplatter.com*

Drug Interaction Facts. St Louis, MO: Facts and Comparisons, 2002.

This reference, available as a hardbound book, CD-ROM, or loose-leaf book that is updated quarterly, provides comprehensive information on potential interactions that can be reviewed by drug class, generic drug name, or trade name. Provides information on drug–drug and drug–food interactions. *http://www.factsandcomparisons.com*

Food and Drug Administration. *Approved Drug Products with Therapeutic Equivalence Evaluations.* Washington, DC: US Government Printing Office.

Revised annually, with monthly updates, this source lists drug products approved for use in the United States. Also known as the *Orange Book* because of its orange-colored cover, it is available online at *http://www.fda.gov/cder/ob/default.htm.* The URL of the FDA is *http://www.fda.gov*

Fudyuma, J. *What Do I Take? A Consumer's Guide to Nonprescription Drugs.* New York: HarperCollins, 1997.

A simple-to-read guide to over-the-counter drugs.

Goodman & Gilman's The Pharmacological Basis of Therapeutics. 10th ed. New York: McGraw-Hill, 2002.

An authoritative text on pharmacology and therapeutics containing 67 articles by leading experts in the field. This text provides information for pharmacists to help them answer clinical questions about how drugs work under different conditions in the body. *http://www.pbg.mcgraw-hill.com*

Index Nominum. Geneva: Swiss Pharmaceutical Society, 1995.

A compilation of synonyms, formulas, and therapeutic classes of more than 7,000 drugs and 28,000 proprietary preparations from 27 countries. Available in text and CD-ROM formats.

The International Pharmacopoeia. 3rd ed. New York: World Health Organization, 1994.

Recommended production methods and specifications for drugs, in four volumes. *http://www.who.ch*

Koda-Kimble, M., and Young, L.Y. *Applied Therapeutics: The Clinical Use of Drugs.* 6th ed. Vancouver, WA: Applied Therapeutics Inc., 1995.

MedCoach CD-ROM (Windows, NT, and Macintosh). Rockville, MD: United States Pharmacopeia Convention, 1997.

A database of information for patients on more than 6,000 generic and brand-name drug products, over-the-counter drugs, nutritional and home infusion items, test devices, and infant formulas. Provides information for patients on proper drug use and preparation, drug and food interactions, side effects/adverse effects, therapeutic contraindications, and product storage. Information is tailored to particular patients' needs (e.g., pediatric, male or female, geriatric). Subscription includes quarterly updates. *http://www.usp.org*

Orange Book. See Food and Drug Administration.

Patient Drug Facts, 1996: Professionals Guide to Patient Drug Facts. St. Louis, MO: Facts and Comparisons, 1996.

This is a comprehensive guide to patient counseling about drugs, available in loose-leaf format for verbal patient counseling and in PC format (on disk) for creation of patient handouts. *http://www.factsand comparisons.com*

Physicians' Desk Reference (PDR). 58th ed. Oradell, NJ: Medical Economics, 2004.

Available in hardbound and CD-ROM form, with two supplements published twice a year, this standard reference work contains information from package inserts for more than 4,000 prescription drugs, as well as information on 250 drug manufacturers. *http://www.medec.com*

Stringer, J.L. *Basic Concepts in Pharmacology: A Student's Survival Guide.* 2nd ed. New York: McGraw-Hill, 2001.

Survey of basic pharmacological concepts for students. *http://www.pbg.mcgraw-hill.com*

United States Pharmacopeia, 23rd Rev.—National Formulary. 20th ed. Rockville, MD: United States Pharmacopeial Convention, 2001.

Combined compendium of monographs setting official national standards for drug substances and dosage forms (*United States Pharmacopeia*) and standards for pharmaceutical ingredients (*National Formulary*). Available in book or CD-ROM form and in English- and Spanish-language editions. *http://www.usp.org*

USP Dictionary of USAN and International Drug Names. Rockville, MD: United States Pharmacopeial Convention, 2001.

An authoritative guide to drug names, including chemical names, brand names, manufacturers, molecular formulas, therapeutic uses, and chemical structures. *http://www.usp.org*

USP Drug Information (USP DI). Vol. I. *Drug Information for the Health Care Professional.* Rockville, MD: United States Pharmacopeial Convention, 2002.

A comprehensive source of in-depth drug information, available in book or CD-ROM form and in English- and Spanish-language editions. Describes medically accepted uses of more than 11,000 generic and brand-name products. *http://www.usp.org*

USP Drug Information (USP DI). Vol. II. *Advice for the Patient.* Rockville, MD: United States Pharmacopeial Convention, 2002.

Contains monographs corresponding to those in the USP DI, Vol. I, but simplified for the purpose of patient education and counseling. Available in English- and Spanish-language editions. *http://www.usp.org*

USP Drug Information (USP DI). Vol. III. *Approved Drug Products and Legal Requirements.* Rockville, MD: United States Pharmacopeial Convention, 2002.

Therapeutic equivalence information and selected federal requirements that affect the prescribing and dispensing of prescription drugs and controlled substances. Includes the FDA *Orange Book*; USP-NF requirements for labeling, storage, packaging, and quality; federal Food, Drug, and Cosmetic Act provisions relating to drugs for human use; portions of the Controlled Substance Act Regulations; and the FDA's Good Manufacturing Practice regulations for finished pharmaceuticals. *http://www.usp.org*

Benitz, W.E., and Tatro, D.S. *The Pediatric Drug Handbook*. 3rd ed. St. Louis, MO: Mosby-Year Book, 1995.

Information on drugs, dosage forms, and administration for pediatric patients. *http://www.mosby.com*

Davies, D.M. *Textbook of Adverse Drug Reactions*. 5th ed. New York: Oxford University Press, 1999.

A standard textbook on the subject. *http://www.oup-usa.org*

Goldfrank's Toxicologic Emergencies. 6th ed. New York: Appleton & Lange, 1998.

Information on treating toxicological emergencies. The medical titles of Appleton & Lange are distributed by McGraw-Hill and may be found at that Web site: *http://www.pbg.mcgraw-hill.com*

Handbook of Nonprescription Drugs. 2 vols. 11th ed. Washington, DC: American Pharmaceutical Association, 1996-1997.

A reference work on over-the-counter medications. *http://www.aphanet.org*

Hunt, Max L., Jr. *Training Manual for Intravenous Admixture Personnel*. 5th ed. Chicago: Bonus Books, 1995.

A manual for training people to create parenteral preparations. *http://www.bonus-books.com*

The King Guide to Parenteral Admixtures, 2001 Edition. Napa, CA: King Guide Publications, 2001.

Available in four loose-leaf volumes, on microfiche, and on CD-ROM, the *King Guide* provides 350 monographs on compatibility and stability information critical to determining the advisability of preparing admixtures of drugs for parenteral administration. The guide is updated quarterly. *http://www.kingguide.com*

Nahata, M.C., and Hipple, T.F. *Pediatric Drug Formulations*. 3rd ed. Cincinnati, OH: Harvey Whitney, 1997.

Information on formulation and compounding of drugs for pediatric patients. *hwb@eos.net*

Poisindex System. Englewood, CO: Micromedex.

A computerized poison information system. *http://www.mdx.com*

Remington. *The Science and Practice of Pharmacology*. 20th ed. Lippincott, 2000.

The compounding "bible" of the pharmacy profession.

Stoklosa, Mitchell J., and Ansel, H.C. *Pharmaceutical Calculations*. 11th ed. Baltimore, MD: Williams & Wilkins, 2001.

A clear, concise, thorough introduction to pharmaceutical mathematics. *http://www.lww.com*

Trissel, L.A. *Handbook on Injectable Drugs, with Supplement*. 11th ed. Bethesda, MD: American Society of Health-System Pharmacists, 2000.

Provides information on stability and compatibility of injectable drug products, including formulations, concentrations, and pH values. *http://www.ashp.org*

Understanding and Preventing Errors in Medication Orders and Prescription Writing. Bethesda, MD: United States Pharmacopeial Convention, 1998.

An education resource, consisting of lecture materials, videotapes, and 35-mm slides describing medication errors that arise from poorly written orders and prescriptions, using examples of actual reports received through the USP Medication Errors Reporting Program. Contains recommendations for preventing errors. *http://www.usp.org* (search within USP Educational Programs)

PROFESSIONAL STANDARDS

The Joint Commision on the Accreditation of Healthcare Organizations (JCAHO) requires the following:
- Unit dose systems are preferred over floor stock inventories in hospitals and long-term care facilities.
- Internal and external products must be kept in separate locations in a pharmacy to prevent an error from occurring.
- Discourages the use of professional samples to be dispensed to patients because of the potential to be out of date before being administered to patients and they may cause a bias toward the purchase of a medication.
- Intravenous admixtures are prepared in a pharmacy using aseptic technique and a laminar flow hood.

Both state JCAHO and the State Boards of Pharmacy require that the pharmacy receive the physician's prescription or a copy of the original prescription when filling medication orders.

QUALITY IMPROVEMENT STANDARDS AND GUIDELINES

- Encouraging pharmacies to report errors and find causes for the error without fear of punishment
- Establish the maximum number of prescriptions a pharmacist may fill during a shift

- Improving lighting in a pharmacy
- Improving workflow in a pharmacy
- Limiting the number of hours a pharmacist or technician may work in a given pay period
- Limiting the number of pharmacy technicians a pharmacist may supervise during a shift
- Requiring certification of technicians (25 states have required that technicians be certified and register with the Board of Pharmacy to assist a pharmacist)

STATE BOARD OF PHARMACY REGULATIONS

Every pharmacy technician must be familiar with regulations governing the practice of pharmacy in their respective state by the State Board of Pharmacy. These regulations may include registering with the State Board of Pharmacy, maintaining their certification status and continuous education requirements. All pharmacy technicians must obey all state statutes in addition to federal statutes.

STORAGE REQUIREMENTS AND EXPIRATION DATES FOR EQUIPMENT AND SUPPLIES

- Cardiopulmonary resuscitation training and certification may be required of all employees. Each employee is responsible for maintaining his or her certification.
- Employees should know location and usage of the automated external defibrillator kit.
- Fires extinguishers must be certified on a yearly basis. Personnel should know the location of fire extinguishers in a facility.
- First aid kits need to be periodically checked to ensure contents have not expired.
- Pharmacy balances require certification by the Department of Taxation on a yearly basis.
- Laminar flow hoods need to be certified every 6 months unless the HEPA filter becomes damaged, which will require certification.

STORAGE AND HANDLING REQUIREMENTS FOR HAZARDOUS SUBSTANCES

- **Chemotherapeutics** and cytoxic materials must be prepared in a biological safety cabinet or vertical flow hood and placed in bags identifying them as such. The preparer should wear a gown, goggles, and two pairs of gloves to protect him or her from possible contamination. A 4 × 4 piece of gauze should be kept inside the hood in case of a spill. A preparer should know the location of the clean-up kit.
- **Hazardous substances** include syringes, needles, and toxic medications. Used needles and syringes should be placed in a red plastic "sharps" container to be autoclaved and disposed. Toxic substances (i.e., chemotherapeutic agents) should be placed in a red biohazard bag to be picked up by the appropriate authorities for destruction.
- **Radiopharmaceuticals:** A pharmacy must be designed to protect employees from radiation exposure; prevent radioactive contamination of pharmacy work areas and equipment; ensure proper ventilation of the pharmacy; provide for the safe disposal of radioactive waste; limit access into the pharmacy; and ensure security of the pharmacy.

A nuclear pharmacy has designated rooms to perform specific functions

- **Breakdown room:** area where empty or used radiopharmaceuticals are returned and dismantled for reuse
- **Order entry area:** prescription orders for radiopharmaceuticals are entered
- **Compounding area:** compounding or dispensing areas
- **Quality control area:** quality assurance tests are performed before delivery
- **Packaging area:** finished product is packaged for delivery
- **Storage and disposal area:** storage area for radioactive waste
- **Requires special equipment:** fume box, glove box, dose calibrator, Geiger-Muller counter, dosimeter, lead-lined refrigerator and freezer, lead-lined storage boxes, autoclave, heating equipment, testing equipment, centrifuge, lead barrier shield, stainless steel sink, shower, and respirator.

US Department of Transportation (DOT) regulates the shipment of hazardous materials under the Hazardous Materials Transportation Act of 1994. Radioactive materials are considered hazardous materials. The DOT has set regulations regarding packaging, labeling, and transporting of radioactive materials.

The shipping container (metal) for transporting radioactive material must be able to maintain the integrity of the product during shipping. The container must be specifically labeled based on the activity of the radioactive material; Radioactive White I, Radioactive Yellow II, and Radioactive Yellow III, which contains the highest concentration of radiation. The container must have a "Caution: Radioactive Label" with the name of the nucleotide, the quantity, date, and time.

Shipping papers must be inside the shipping container and include the following information: name of nucleotide, quantity, form, label category, emergency response telephone number, information regarding emergency personnel, and pharmacy name. The driver carries a copy of the shipping papers. A placard must be on the vehicle if it is carrying Radioactive Yellow III material. Shipped material must be braced inside the transportation vehicle.

PROCEDURES FOR THE TREATMENT OF EXPOSURE TO HAZARDOUS SUBSTANCES

- Chemotherapy spill kits should be used for the cleanup of accidental spills of antineoplastic agents. These kits include waste disposal bags, respirator, latex gloves, heavy utility gloves, eyeglasses, gowns, shoe covers, toweling, and sealable bags.
- The technician should know the location of Material Safety Data Sheets (MSDS) and follow the directions on them for a particular item. After completion of the cleanup, an incident report should be filed with the supervisor.
- If a hazardous substance comes in contact with the skin, it must be washed immediately with soap and water for at least 5 minutes. If a substance comes in contact with the eyes, they should be rinsed for 15 minutes. This can be done at the eyewash station.

SECURITY SYSTEMS FOR THE PROTECTION OF EMPLOYEES, CUSTOMERS, AND PROPERTY

- All pharmacies are required to have a workable alarm service when the pharmacy is closed
- Closed-circuit televisions and hold-up alarm buttons may be installed in pharmacies, but it is at the discretion of the institution
- Each facility (organization) will have established policies and procedures to ensure the safety of staff, customers, and property
- Facilities may provide lockers for employees' belongings in a secure area
- Keys may be required to be signed out from a security location to gain access to a pharmacy
- Motion detectors must be installed and in working condition
- Only licensed pharmacists may dispense a prescription and supervise a pharmacy technician
- Only pharmacists or designated employees will have access to keys to open or close the pharmacy
- Security requirements that restrict access to medications to "authorized personnel only" occur because of legal, institutional, and standards of practice
- Volatile substances must be stored in an area that is properly ventilated and has been designed to prevent explosion
- Touch pads and scannable identifications may be used for an employee to gain access to a particular area

LAMINAR FLOW HOOD MAINTENANCE REQUIREMENTS

1. The blower of the laminar air flow hood should be kept on at all times. If it is shut down, then it must be in operation for at least 30 min before use.
2. The hood is wiped down with 70% isopropyl alcohol beginning with the bar, followed by the sides, and continuing from the area closest to the filter, working outward and wiping from the top edge of the side to the bottom.
3. The bench is cleaned last by beginning from the back of the bench and wiping from side to side and moving outward.
4. The laminar flow hood should be cleaned at the beginning of every shift and whenever a spill occurs. Sanitizing agent should not be sprayed because the HEPA filter may become damp and develop a hole in it.
5. The flow hood needs to be certified every 6 months or whenever the HEPA filter becomes wet.

SANITATION REQUIREMENTS

- Counting trays should be cleaned with alcohol after every use to prevent cross-contamination from occurring, which might result in an allergic reaction in another patient. A separate counting tray should be used for chemotherapeutic agents only.
- Proper hand-washing techniques include washing the hands and arms with hot water and Betadine; scrubbing both the top and bottom of the hands; scrubbing between the fingers up to the elbow; and rinsing arms and hands thoroughly.
- Every pharmacy must have running hot and cold water. A mild detergent may be used to clean instruments used in extemporaneous compounding; 70% isopropyl alcohol should be used to clean all countertops in the pharmacy. All pharmacy equipment should be kept clean and in good condition.
- Microorganisms can be introduced into the laminar flow hood by jewelry, cosmetics, coughing or sneezing (if a mask is not worn), or loose facial hair.
- The laminar flow hood should provide a Class 100 clean environment and the work surface should be cleaned with 70% isopropyl alcohol. The prefilter and the HEPA filter need to be maintained such that particles greater than 3 microns cannot enter the sterile area.
- Radiation may be used in hospitals to sterilize supplies, vitamins, antibiotics, syringes, and needles.

EQUIPMENT CALIBRATION AND MAINTENANCE PROCEDURES

- Automated compounding and repackaging equipment must be calibrated before each use.
- A buffer room must be at least a Class 100,000 clean room but may be a Class 10,000 clean room.
  Class 100 Area: an area in which there are no more than 100 particles 0.5 micron and larger per cubic foot of air
  Class 10,000 Area: an area in which there are no more than 10,000 particles 0.5 micron and larger per cubic foot of air
  Class 100,000 Area: an area in which there are no more than 100,000 particles 0.5 micron and larger per cubic foot of air
- **Class A balance:** can accurately weigh 120 mg to 15 g.
- **Class B balance:** can weigh 650 mg to 120 g. Prescription balances should be placed on a level counter away from customer traffic. Before weighing, place equal size glassine papers on the pans of the balance and "zero out" or level until indicator on the balance shows both pans are of even weight. This procedure needs to be done before each weighing.
- **Graduates**
  TC (to contain): volume measured on the scale is equal to the volume of liquid inside the graduate
  TD (to deliver): allows one to measure the amount of liquid needed by considering the residual amount of liquid that is left inside the graduate once the liquid is poured out
- A HEPA filter is monitored by introducing aerosolized Emery 3004 into the plenum of the laminar flow hood while monitoring the penetration of the Emery 3004 on the downstream side of the HEPA filter. No more than 0.01% of the upstream concentration may be detected downstream from the HEPA filter.
- Laminar flow hoods must be turned on for a minimum of 30 min before being used. The velocity of air from the HEPA filter is measured using a volumeter. Average air velocity is 90 linear feet per minute ± 20 percent.
- Pharmacy balances (scales) need to be evaluated on a yearly basis by the Department of Taxation for accuracy.
- Pharmacy weights need to be calibrated once per year.

SUPPLY PROCUREMENT PROCEDURES

- Procurement includes drug selection, source selection, cost analysis, group purchasing, prime vendor relationships, purchasing procedures, record keeping, and receiving control.
- Drug selection includes a cost analysis (cost per dose, cost per day, or cost per treatment). Cost-benefit examines the perceived benefit versus the cost of the medication.
- Source selection is deciding whether a generic or brand-name drug is to be purchased. It examines the therapeutic equivalency of the products. Examination of the reputation of the drug manufacturer and knowledge of drug analysis data is taken into consideration. Consideration of product is affected by the *ASHP Guidelines for Selecting Pharmaceutical Manufacturers and Suppliers.*

- Cost analysis is an examination of acquisition and storage costs; costs associated with the time required preparing or packaging a drug.
- Group Purchasing Organizations (GPO) allow hospitals to purchase medications at a lower cost based on volume. Group purchasing organizations negotiate prices, but do not make the purchase for an institution. The ability to purchase contract items is known as a "bid or contract compliance."
- Prime vendor means purchasing as many products as possible from one source, a wholesaler. When choosing a "primary vendor," one should consider the following: delivery rate of items, 24-hour emergency service, computer system for ordering drugs from the vendor, electronic order entry devices, bar-coded shelf labels, competitive pricing, purchasing history reports (80/20 and compliance reports), pricing updates, and drug recalls.
- Purchasing procedures include negotiating discounts, payment schedules, terms of payment, prepayment, nonperformance penalties, and returned and damaged goods policy.
- Keeping records must be maintained to meet government regulations, standards of practice requirements, accreditation standards, policies, and management information. Records may include purchase orders that authorize the purchase of a product.
- Receiving procedures include shipments, invoices, and purchase orders that must be reconciled by item; quantity and strength of each item must be checked; prices on invoice should correspond to price that had been negotiated; and discrepancies must be addressed promptly to pharmacist and the vendor.

TECHNOLOGY USED IN THE PREPARATION, DELIVERY, AND ADMINISTRATION OF MEDICATION

- Accusource monitoring system—automated TPN compounder with total nutrient admixture
- Baker cells—an example of an automated counting/filling device. Each cell contains a particular medication. The desired quantity is entered and the Baker cell counts the desired quantity for the pharmacist
- Bar scanners—the FDA has proposed that bar codes be placed on all human drugs and biologicals, which will result in an improvement in both patient and medication safety. The potential for errors will be greatly reduced because the right patient will be receiving the right drug and dose at the right time through the right route.
- Enteral pump—a special pump to infuse enteral substances into the stomach
- Gravity infusion system—a stationary infusion system using a minibag that is regulated by the patient
- Homerus—centralized robotic unit-dose dispensing device. Has ability to individually package medications from bulk and deliver bar-coded medications to 24-hour patient-specific bins and return medication to bins on discharge of patient
- Infusion control devices
  Nonmechanical rate controller (dial calibrated gravity flow regulator, such as Dial-a-Flow or Rate Regulator)
  Nonmechanical external pump (elastometric balloon system—a stationary infusion system controlled by the use of a special tube. Examples include Intermate, ReadyMed, MedFlo II, Eclipse, and Homepump).
  Spring-controlled pump such as the SideKick
  Mechanical peristaltic pumps deliver a controlled amount of medication at a controlled rate, such as the CADD line of products. CADD-Plus—an ambulatory-specific therapy pump used to infuse antibiotics. CADD-Prizm PCS Pump—an ambulatory-specific therapy infusion pump. Patient-controlled analgesia (PCA) used to infuse analgesics. CADD-TPN—an ambulatory-specific infusion pump, used in the infusion of total parenteral nutrition. Other examples includes Verifuse, Alm-Plus, Provider 6000, and WalkMed PIC
  Mechanical piston pump—similar to mechanical peristaltic pump, except that it is controlled by a piston that is electromagnetically operated by a battery; the advantage of the system is miniaturization. An example is the Lifecare Omni-Flow 4000
  Implantable pumps—implanted under the skin with a catheter entering a vein. Examples include the Syncromed and Infusaid
- Physician order entry system results in a reduction of medical errors by having complete and accurate information, accurate dose calculation, and appropriate clinical decision support
- Mobile robots that travel through a hospital to the various nursing units delivering medication
- PYXIS is an automated point-of-use storage system for making floor stock items available to nursing staff
  Servers are connected to a PYXIS server and link hospital billing and information systems together
- Syringe infusion system is a stationary infusion system requiring the use of a special syringe

PURPOSE AND FUNCTION OF PHARMACY EQUIPMENT

EXTEMPORANEOUS COMPOUNDING EQUIPMENT

- **Beakers**—may be either glass or plastic and are used to estimate and mix solutions
- **Class A (III) balance**—required in all pharmacies. Used to weigh small quantities of weight. Has a sensitivity requirement of 6 mg
- **Counter balance (bulk balance)**—two-pan balance used to weigh quantities up to 5 kg. Sensitivity of 100 mg
- **Digital balances**—are sensitive to a tenth of a mg and are used to replace Class A balances
- **Compounding slab (ointment slab)**—used for mixing compounds
- **Filter paper**—can be used to weigh or filter a solution
- **Forceps**—used to pick up prescription weights. Forceps are used to ensure that oil is not deposited on the weight and affect it
- **Funnels**—used to filter or pour liquids
- **Glass stirring rods**—used to stir solutions and suspensions
- **Glycine paper**—used under substances to be weighed
- **Graduates**—used to measure liquids. There are two types of graduates: conical and cylindrical (most accurate method to measure a volume). Graduates will either be "TD" or "TC." "TD" means the volume delivered is the exact amount desired and the residual remaining solution is in addition to the volume measured. "TC" will hold the desired volume but, when transferred, a residual remains, making the amount measured inaccurate
- **Master formula sheet (pharmacy compounding log)**—lists the ingredients and their quantities and the procedures to follow in the preparation
- **Mortar and pestle**—used to mix ingredients. Glass is used for mixing liquids and semisolid dosage forms. Wedgwood is used in the trituration of crystals, granules, and powders. Porcelain is similar to Wedgwood and is more commonly used in the blending of powders
- **Pharmaceutical weights**—brass weights measured in both metric and apothecary systems. They should never be touched by the hand; should be stored in a clean state; and should be calibrated once per year
- **Pipettes**—used to measure volumes less than 1.5 mL
- **Sink**—used to wash and clean equipment and hands
- **Spatulas**—used to transfer solid ingredients to weighing pans and compounding activities. May be either hard rubber (used for corrosive ingredients), plastic, or steel. Hard rubber is used in the compounding of ingredients that react with metal. Stainless steel is most commonly used for its flexibility and ability to remove materials from a mortar

IV ADMIXTURES

- **70% isopropyl alcohol**—used to clean laminar air hood surfaces
- **Administration sets**—disposable, sterile tubing that connects the IV solution to the injection site
- **Alcohol pads**—used to clean the ports on an IV bag, the rubber stopper of a vial, or the area of the skin before an injection
- **Ambulatory pumps**—a small, lightweight and portable pump worn by a patient. May either be therapy-specific or for multiple therapies
- **Ampule breaker**—a device used to break the neck of an ampule. May range from 1 to 50 mL
- **Ampules**—elongated glass container in which the neck is broken off
- **Catheters**—devices that are inserted into veins for direct access to the vascular system. May either be peripheral venous catheters or a central venous catheter
- **Clamps**—adjust the rate and shutting down of the flow. Types of clamps include slide clamps, screw clamps, and roller clamps
- **Depth filter**—a filter that works by trapping particles as solution moves through channels
- **Drip chamber**—a hollow chamber where drops of the IV solution accumulate. The purpose of the drip chamber is to prevent air bubbles from entering the tubing
- **Filters**—used to remove particulate material and microorganisms from solution. Can be attached to the end of a syringe, the end of the administration kit, or the end of the needle
- **Filter needles**—needles that include a filter that prevents glass from entering the final solution when drawing from an ampule
- **Filter straws**—used for pulling medication from ampules
- **Final filters**—a filter used before the solution enters the patient's body

- **Flexible bag**—plastic container that may hold volumes ranging from 50 to 3,000 mL
- **Heparin lock**—a short piece of tubing attached to a needle or catheter when the tubing is filled with heparin to prevent potential clotting
- **Infusion pumps**—regulate the flow of medication into a patient. May either be stationary or ambulatory
- **Laminar Flow Hoods:**

Type A hoods—recirculate a portion of the air (after first passing through a HEPA filter) within the hood and exhaust a portion of this air back into the parenteral room

Type B1 hoods—exhaust most of the contaminated air through a duct to the outside atmosphere. This air passes through a HEPA filter

Type B2 hoods—exhaust all of the contaminated air to the outside atmosphere after passing through a HEPA filter. Air is not recirculated within the hood or returned to the parenteral room atmosphere

Type B3 hoods—use recycled air within the hood. All exhaust air is discharged to the outside atmosphere. A Type A hood may be converted to a Type B3 hood

- **Large-volume parenterals (LVP)**—parenterals with a volume greater than 100 mL
- **Male/female adapters**—available in a universal size. Fit a syringe on each end and are used in the mixing of the two contents
- **Membrane filters**—consist of small pores that retain particles that are larger than the pores. Membrane filters may be placed between syringe and needle before a medication is introduced into an LVP or SVP
- **Minibags**—contain volumes between 50 and 100 mL
- **Multidose vial**—contains a preservative to prevent bacterial contamination and allows for multiple doses of variable amounts. Rubber closure reseals after syringe is withdrawn from it
- **Needles**—composed of a hub and a shaft and are designated by two numbers (gauge and length). The gauge measures the diameter of the needle bore; the larger the gauge the smaller the bore. The length of the needle is measured in inches
- **Needle adapter**—a needle or catheter may be attached to it
- **Piggy backs**—a small volume solution added to an LVP
- **Roll clamp**—allows for variable flow rates
- **Single-dose vial**—does not contain a preservative and must be discarded after one use
- **Small-volume parenterals (SVP)**—packaged products that are either directly administered to the patient or added to another parenteral. Contain a volume of 100 mL or less
- **Spike**—a rigid, sharpened plastic piece that is inserted into the IV bag
- **Syringe**—components of a syringe include plunger, plunger flange, barrel, and tip (Figure 4-1)
- **Syringe caps**—a sterile cap used to prevent contamination of syringes during the transportation out of the pharmacy
- **Syringes needles**—components include hub, shaft, bevel, lumen, and point (Figure 4-2)
- **Transfer needles**—specially designed needles that look like two needles attached together at the hub. Are used to transfer sterile solutions from one vial directly into another without the use of a syringe
- **Tubing for pumps**—tubing is specific for manufacturer's machine
- **Tubing transfer sets**—blood transfer sets; used to transfer large containers into empty containers
- **Vials**—glass or plastic containers with rubber stoppers. Single-dose vials do not contain a preservative, whereas multidose vials do.
- **Solutions used**

  ¼ NS—one fourth normal saline (0.225% sodium chloride)

  ½ NS—one half normal saline (0.45% sodium chloride)

  D10W—10% dextrose in water

  D5NS—5% dextrose in normal saline (0.9% solution)

  D5W—5% dextrose in water

  LR—Lactated Ringer's solution

  NS—normal saline solution (0.9%)

  SW—sterile water

TYPES OF WATER

- **Purified water USP**—not intended for parenteral administration; used in the reconstitution of oral products
- **Water for injection USP**—is not sterile and cannot be used in aseptic compounding of sterile products
- **Sterile water for injection USP**—has been sterilized, but has no antimicrobial agents; can be used in parenteral solutions

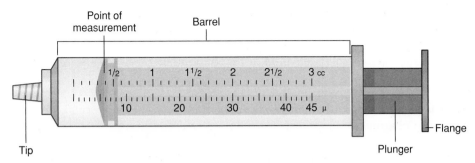

Figure 4-1 Parts of a syringe.

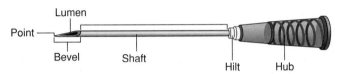

Figure 4-2 Parts of a needle.

- **Bacteriostatic water for injection USP**—sterile water with antimicrobial agents that can be used for injection
- **Water for injection USP**—not sterile; has no antimicrobial agents and cannot be used for aseptic compounding
- **Sterile water for irrigation USP**—has been sterilized but contains no antimicrobial agents, used as an irrigating solution

DOCUMENTATION REQUIREMENTS FOR ROUTINE SANITATION, MAINTENANCE, AND EQUIPMENT CALIBRATION

- Balances—-must be certified yearly by the state Department of Taxation
- Laminar hoods and HEPA filters—need to be certified a minimum of every 6 months or when the HEPA filter is wetted or the laminar flow hood is moved. Validation is documented evidence that provides a high degree of assurance that the process will produce a product with predetermined specifications.

THE AMERICANS WITH DISABILITIES ACT REQUIREMENTS

Americans with Disabilities Act—a federal civil rights law that prohibits discrimination against people with disabilities in everyday activities, such as buying an item at the store, going to the movies, enjoying a meal at a local restaurant, exercising at the health club, or having a car serviced at a local garage.

To meet the goals of the ADA, the law established requirements for businesses of all sizes. These requirements went into effect on January 26, 1992. Businesses that serve the public must modify policies and practices that discriminate against people with disabilities; comply with accessible design standards when constructing or altering facilities; remove barriers in existing facilities where readily achievable; and provide auxiliary aids and services when needed to ensure effective communication with people who have hearing, vision, or speech impairments. All businesses, even those that do not serve the public, must comply with accessible design standards when constructing or altering facilities.

MANUAL AND COMPUTER-BASED SYSTEMS FOR STORING, RETRIEVING, AND USING PHARMACY-RELATED PHARMACY INFORMATION

MANUAL PROCESSING OF MEDICATION ORDERS

- Medication order is written in patient chart
- Copy of medication order is removed from chart
- Order is picked up at nursing station, faxed, or tubed to the pharmacy

- Medication order is entered into the pharmacy computer system
- Pharmacist reviews and verifies medication order
- Medication order is filled by technician and checked by pharmacist
- Patient-specific medication is manually delivered or tubed to nursing unit

AUTOMATIC PROCESSING OF MEDICATION ORDERS

- Physician or physician's representative enters medication order directly into hospital computer service, which communicates order to pharmacy
- Pharmacist reviews and verifies order
- RN retrieves medication from point-of-use automated medication station
- Pharmacy technician fills inventory as medication supplies fall below par

Drug interactions—OBRA 90 requires that all pharmacists perform a Drug Utilization Review (DUR) during the processing of prescriptions. The DUR will alert the pharmacist of any potential drug interactions or contraindication a patient may experience while taking a prescribed medication.

Patient profiles—patient profiles are required to be maintained by a pharmacy as a result of OBRA 90. Information to be collected includes personal information such as name, home address, home telephone number, and patient's birthday; billing information such as insurance carrier (plan and group number); disease states of the patient; and drug allergies of the patient.

Label generation—labels are generated on successful adjudication of an insurance claim or if the patient is a cash customer.

SECURITY PROCEDURES RELATED TO DATA INTEGRITY, SECURITY, AND CONFIDENTIALITY

The second part of HIPAA was enacted in April 2005 and requires that pharmacies have established appropriate safeguards to prevent a patient's information from becoming compromised by an outside source.

KNOWLEDGE OF DOWNTIME EMERGENCY POLICIES AND PROCEDURES

A pharmacy technician should be familiar with procedures to be followed when a system is down. These procedures may include manual filling of prescriptions and reentering the information into the computer system when the system returns to normal. The pharmacy technician should know how to bill prescriptions during an emergency.

BACK UP AND ARCHIVING PROCEDURES FOR STORED DATA AND DOCUMENTATION

Computer systems need to be backed up at regularly scheduled times (possibly daily) to prevent loss of data if the system goes down for whatever reason.

Defragmentation of computer files reorganizes files that have been stored on a computer.

LEGAL REQUIREMENTS REGARDING ARCHIVING

Federal law requires the following documents be maintained for a minimum of 2 years and be readily retrievable (able to be produced within 72 hr of inquiry):

DEA Forms 41, 106, 222, and 224
All prescriptions containing controlled substances
All controlled substance invoices
All initial narcotic inventories, biennial inventories, and change of pharmacist inventories
All exempt narcotic and poison sales records
If a particular state requires retention of greater than 2 years for these records, a pharmacy must adhere to the regulations, whichever is the more stringent of the two

HEALTH CARE REIMBURSEMENT SYSTEMS

Acute care: Does not allow pharmacy to make a profit. Pharmacy-related expenses are incorporated into the per diem hospital charge.

Ambulatory care parenteral therapy: Centers for Medicare and Medicaid services has created a list of health insurance continuation program (HICP) codes for drugs in this setting. Reimbursable costs are also included. Other fees include a professional fee component and a facility fee.

Cognitive services: These services include prescriptive authority by the pharmacist, administration of medications by the pharmacist, patient assessment and treatment, pharmacist intervention with prescribers and other health care providers, patient education, and patient reassessment and monitoring. Reimbursement is based on prior years' data.

Community care: Cost of medication + Dispensing fee for dispensing, monitoring, and record keeping.

Disease state management services: HCFA 1500 form may be used for billing of these services.

Long-term care: Per diem reimbursement (predetermined daily rate) that is based on prior medication costs of the facility. Formulary control is important. Regulatory agencies have developed lists of medication that they have deemed unnecessary based on excessive adverse effects and poor outcomes obtained.

BILLING AND ACCOUNTING POLICIES AND PROCEDURES

Allowances: a deduction is given from the purchase price by the seller to the purchaser

Average cost method: an inventory costing method that uses the weighted average unit cost to allocate the costs of goods available for sale to inventory and cost of goods sold

Cosigned goods: goods held for sale by one party (the consignee) although ownership of the goods is retained by another party

Cost of goods available for sale: the sum of the beginning merchandise inventory and the cost of goods purchased

Cost of goods purchased: the sum of the net purchases and freight charges associated with a product

Cost of goods sold: the total cost of merchandise sold during the period, determined by subtracting ending inventory from the cost of goods available for sale

Credit terms: specify the amount of cash discount and time period during which it is offered. They indicate the length of time in which the purchaser is expected to pay the full invoice price. An example includes 2/10, where a 2% discount can be taken off of the invoice price less any returns or allowances, if the invoice is paid within 10 days of the invoice date

Current replacement cost: the current cost to replace an inventory item

Days in inventory: measure of the average number of days the inventory is held; calculated as 365 divided by inventory turnover rate

Depreciation: a process of allocating to expense the cost of a plant asset over its useful life in a rational and systematic manner. It is not a process of asset valuation. Depreciation takes into account the cost (all expenditures necessary to acquire the asset and make it ready for intended use); the useful life (estimate of the expected life based on need for repair, service life, and vulnerability to obsolescence); and the salvage value (an estimate of the asset's value at the end of its useful life). Can be computed by either the straight-line, declining-balance, or units of activity method

First in, first out (FIFO): an inventory costing method that assumes the cost at the earliest goods purchased is the first to be recognized as the cost of the goods sold

FOB destination: freight terms indicating that the goods are placed free on board at the buyer's place of business and the seller pays the freight cost; goods belong to the seller while in transit

FOB shipping point: freight terms indicating that the goods are placed free on board the carrier by the seller; the buyer pays the freight cost; goods belong to the buyer while in transit

Gross profit (gross margin): excess of net sales over the cost of goods sold

Gross profit rate: gross profit expressed as a percentage by dividing the amount of gross profit by net sales

Inventory turnover rate: a ratio that measures the number of times on average the inventory sold during the period; computed by dividing cost of goods sold by the average inventory during the period

Last in, first out (LIFO): an inventory costing method that assumes that the costs of the latest units purchased are the first to be allocated to cost of goods sold

Lower of cost or market (LCM) basis: a basis whereby inventory is slated at the lower of cost or market (current replacement cost)

Net profit: Sales − Cost of goods − Expenses

Net purchases: purchases less purchase returns and allowances and purchase discounts

Net sales: sales less sales returns and allowances and sales discounts

Periodic inventory system: an inventory system in which costs are allocated to ending inventories and cost of goods sold at the end of the period. Cost of goods is computed at the end of the period by subtracting the ending inventory (costs are assigned to a physical count of items on hand) from the cost of goods available for sale

Purchase discount: a cash discount claimed by a buyer for prompt payment of a balance due

Purchase invoice: a document that supports each credit purchase

Sales discounts: a reduction given by a seller for prompt payment of a credit sale

Specific identification method: an actual physical flow costing method in which items still in inventory are specifically costed to arrive at the total cost of the ending inventory

Weighted average unit cost: average cost that is weighted by the number of units purchased at each unit cost

INFORMATION SOURCES USED TO OBTAIN DATA IN A QUALITY IMPROVEMENT SYSTEM

Controlled substance form—Allows a nursing staff to verify controlled substances at each change of shift of nurses. Monitors receipt, administration, and disposal of a controlled substance.

Medication administration record (MAR)—Documents medication administered to a patient. It includes the drug, dose, route of administration, frequency of administration, and administration times. The MAR lists the patient's allergies and diagnoses. It is used every time a medication is administered.

Medication delivery record—Provides accountability for medication distribution between the pharmacy and hospital or long-term care facility. It lists the medication found in a particular delivery.

Patient profile—A patient profile may be either a hard or a computerized list of a patient's prescriptions (medications) and other information A patient profile will identify the patient by name, social security number, birth date, and gender. It provides billing information, such as insurance (group number, patient's identification, patient's relationship to the cardholder [spouse, dependent]). A patient profile contains a patient's medical history that includes current conditions, known allergies, and adverse reactions. It provides a listing of medications, whether legend or OTC, that have been filled for the patient, including dates, quantities, directions for use, and physician's name. It may list whether the patient requests EZ open containers or use of generic medications if authorized by the physician.

Physician order sheet (POS)—List of all of the physician's orders for a patient, which includes both drug and nondrug orders. Nondrug orders may include allergies, diagnoses, diet orders, directives, laboratory orders, and orders for ancillary services such as physical therapy, occupational therapy, respiratory therapy, or speech therapy.

Resident monitoring form—Documents behavior of a patient and any precipitating factors, drug and nondrug intervention, outcomes, and adverse reactions.

Treatment administration record (TAR)—Documents external treatments given to a patient in a hospital or long-term care facility.

PROCEDURES TO DOCUMENT OCCURRENCES SUCH AS MEDICATION ERRORS, ADVERSE EFFECTS, AND PRODUCT INTEGRITY

The following agencies track medication errors.
- AHRQ—Agency for Healthcare Research and Quality
- AMA—American Medical Association
- ASHP—American Society of Health System Pharmacists
- CDER—Center for Drug Evaluation and Research
- FDA—Food and Drug Administration Med Watch: a voluntary program reporting adverse health events and problems with medical problems
- JCAHO—Joint Commission on Accreditation of Healthcare Organizations

STAFF TRAINING TECHNIQUES

Training—a set of activities that provides the opportunity to acquire and improve job related skills. Should include both technical (i.e., computer and systems technology) and soft skills (i.e., diversity and sexual harassment)

On-the-job training—involves job instruction while performing the job in the actual workplace
Apprenticeships—learning a trade from an experienced worker
Internship—a form of on-the-job training for which the intern may or may not be paid
Job rotation—provides a wide range of experience in different kinds of jobs in a firm. May include mentoring
Off-the-job training—involves lectures, videos, and simulations

EMPLOYEE PERFORMANCE EVALUATION TECHNIQUES

Performance appraisal—a process of systematically evaluating performance and providing feedback on which performance adjustments can be made. Performance appraisals define specific job criteria against which performance will be measured, measure past job performance accurately, justify rewards given to individuals/groups, and define the development experiences the rate needs to enhance performance in the current job and to prepare for future responsibilities.
Output measures—performance dimension of interest is a quantitative.
Activity measures—a rating system based on an evaluator's observation and rating.
Ranking—a comparative technique of performance appraisal that involves rank ordering of each individual from best to worst on each performance dimension.
Paired comparison—a comparative method of performance appraisal whereby each person is directly compared with every other person.
Forced distribution—a method of performance appraisal that uses a small number of performance categories, such as "very good," "good," "adequate," and "very poor" and forces a certain proportion of people into each.
Graphic rating scales—a scale that lists a variety of dimensions thought to be related to high performance outcomes in a given job and that the individual is expected to exhibit.
Critical incident diary—a method of performance appraisal that records incidents of unusual success or failure in a given performance aspect.
Behaviorally anchored rating scales—a performance appraisal approach that describes observable job behaviors, each which is evaluated to determine good versus bad performance.
Management by objective—a process of joint goal setting between a supervisor and a subordinate.
360 evaluations—a comprehensive approach that uses self-ratings, customer ratings, and others outside the work force.

EMPLOYEE PERFORMANCE FEEDBACK TECHNIQUES

Feedback—the process through which the receiver communicates with the sender by returning another message. Examples of giving constructive feedback:
1. Give directly and in a spirit of mutual trust
2. Be specific
3. Give when receiver is most ready to accept
4. Be accurate, check validity with others
5. Focus on things the receiver can control
6. Limit how much the receiver gets at one time

CHAPTER 4 REVIEW QUESTIONS

1. Which type of mortar and pestle is used to mix liquids?
   a. Glass
   b. Porcelain
   c. Wedgwood
   d. None of the above

2. Who is responsible for the transportation of hazardous materials?
   a. Department of Transportation (DOT)
   b. Environmental Protection Agency (EPA)
   c. Food and Drug Administration (FDA)
   d. Joint Commission on Accreditation of Healthcare Organizations (JCAHO)

3. How often must HEPA filters be certified?
    a. Every 3 months
    b. Every 6 months
    c. Every year
    d. Every 2 years

4. Which of the following symbols indicates the highest level of radiation?
    a. Radioactive White I
    b. Radioactive Yellow II
    c. Radioactive Yellow III
    d. Radioactive Orange IV

5. How often must laminar flow hoods be certified?
    a. Every 3 months
    b. Every 6 months
    c. Every year
    d. Every 2 years

6. Which reference book is a compendium of monograph-setting official national standards for drug substances, dosage forms, and standards for pharmaceutical ingredients?
    a. Approved Drug Products with therapeutic Equivalence Evaluations
    b. Drug Facts and Comparisons
    c. PDR
    d. USP-NF

7. What is the sensitivity of a Class A Balance?
    a. 5 mg
    b. 6 mg
    c. 10 mg
    d. 20 mg

8. What type of spatula should be used in measuring corrosive ingredients?
    a. Plastic
    b. Rubber
    c. Steel
    d. All of the above

9. What type of alcohol should be used to clean a laminar flow hood?
    a. 70% Isopropyl alcohol
    b. 70% Methyl alcohol
    c. 70% Rubbing alcohol
    d. All of the above

10. What is the name of the opening of a needle?
    a. Bevel
    b. Hilt
    c. Lumen
    d. Shaft

11. What type of environment should a laminar flow hood provide?
    a. Class 100 area
    b. Class 1,000 area
    c. Class 10,000 area
    d. Class 100,000 area

12. What is used to measure volumes less than 1.5 mL?
    a. 5-mL conical graduate
    b. 5-mL cylindrical graduate
    c. Pipette
    d. Syringe

13. How are disease management services reimbursed?
    a. Capitation
    b. Cost of service + cost to monitor + cost for record keeping
    c. Fee-cost spread
    d. HCFS 1500 form

14. Who is responsible for pharmaceuticals in transit if they are designated as "FOB destination"?
    a. Buyer
    b. Drug manufacturer
    c. Drug wholesaler
    d. Seller

15. Which of the following is not a duty of an institutional pharmacy technician?
    a. Compound parenteral medications
    b. Enter prescription orders into the computer
    c. Fill patient medication cassettes
    d. Transport medications throughout the institution

16. Which of the following is not true regarding the JCAHO's policies toward the pharmacy in an institution?
    a. External and internal products should not be stocked next to each as to avoid errors
    b. IV admixtures are prepared in a pharmacy using aseptic technique and a laminar flow hood
    c. Professional samples should be dispensed as soon as the pharmacy receives them to prevent them from going out of date
    d. Unit doses are preferred over a traditional vial system

17. What type of balance can weigh objects between 650 mg and 120 g?
    a. Class A
    b. Class B
    c. Electronic balance
    d. Triple beam

18. How long should the blower be on for a laminar air flow hood?
    a. 10 min
    b. 15 min
    c. 20 min
    d. 30 min

19. What type of laminar flow hood can be converted to a Type B3 hood?
    a. Type A hood
    b. Type A1 hood
    c. Type B1 hood
    d. Type B2 hood

20. How often does a pharmacy balance need to be certified?
    a. Every 3 months
    b. Every 6 months
    c. Every 9 months
    d. Every 12 months

21. Where is a finished radiopharmaceutical product stored?
    a. Breakdown room
    b. Compounding area
    c. Packaging area
    d. Storage and disposal area

22. Which is the most effective method of communication?
    a. E-mail
    b. Face to face
    c. Memos
    d. Telephone

23. Which of the following does the JCAHO not certify?
    a. Hospitals
    b. Long-term care facilities
    c. Nursing homes
    d. Retail pharmacies

24. What type of balance must a pharmacy have?
    a. Class A
    b. Class B
    c. Electronic
    d. Triple beam

25. What is the air velocity of a laminar flow hood?
    a. 70 linear feet/min (±20%)
    b. 80 linear feet/min (±20%)
    c. 90 linear feet/min (±20%)
    d. 100 linear feet/min (±20%)

Chapter 5

Practice Examinations

PRACTICE EXAMINATION I

Select the response that best answers the question.

1. Which drug classification should not be taken with potassium-sparing diuretics?
    a. ACE inhibitors
    b. Beta-blockers
    c. Calcium channel blockers
    d. Nitrates

2. Which of the following would be a correct DEA number for Dr. A. Shedlock?
    a. AB135426
    b. BS2456879
    c. FS1578926
    d. MS2254235

3. A pharmacy technician receives a prescription to make 4 oz of a 10% solution and has a 25% stock solution on hand. How much diluent will be added to fill this prescription?
    a. 7.2 mL
    b. 48 mL
    c. 72 mL
    d. 300 mL

4. How many refills may a physician order for a Schedule II drug?
    a. 0
    b. 1
    c. 5
    d. Unlimited refills in a 1-year time frame

5. Which of the following dosage forms is not a solid dosage form?
    a. Capsule
    b. Elixir
    c. Plaster
    d. Powder

6. What do the three sets of numbers in an NDC number reflect?
    a. Drug manufacturer, drug product, and the year an NDA was filed
    b. Drug manufacturer, drug product, and package size
    c. Drug manufacturer, drug name, and drug strength
    d. None of the above

7. Which of the following drugs is not a beta-blocker?
   a. Atenolol
   b. Metoprolol
   c. Nifedipine
   d. Propranolol

8. What is the meaning of the following signa: "i gtt ou tid ud?"
   a. Instill 1 drop in each ear three times a day as directed.
   b. Instill 1 drop in each eye two times a day as directed.
   c. Instill 1 drop in each eye three times a day as needed.
   d. Instill 1 drop in each eye three times a day as directed.

9. If a patient is hypokalemic, the patient has
   a. Low sodium.
   b. High sodium.
   c. Low potassium.
   d. High potassium.

10. Which of the following solutions is the most diluted?
    a. 25%
    b. 20%
    c. 2.5%
    d. 0.25%

11. What does the following abbreviation "UTI" stand for?
    a. Undiagnosed treatment inconclusive
    b. Upper respiratory infection
    c. Urethral tract infection
    d. Urinary tract infection

12. Which of the following drugs is not used as a prophylactic product?
    a. Amoxicillin
    b. Imitrex
    c. Norgestimate/ethinyl estradiol
    d. Propranolol

13. How many teaspoon doses are in a pint of elixir?
    a. 24
    b. 48
    c. 72
    d. 96

14. What does the term "overhead" refer to in business?
    a. All of the costs associated with a business
    b. Ceilings
    c. Inventory
    d. Payroll

15. What does the abbreviation "FDA" refer to?
    a. Food and Drug Abuse
    b. Food and Drug Administration
    c. Food and Drug Association
    d. Free Drug Assistance

16. In which schedule would you find the combination product oxycodone + acetaminophen?
    a. Schedule II
    b. Schedule III
    c. Schedule IV
    d. Schedule V

17. Which vitamin will increase the blood coagulation of a patient taking Coumadin?
    a. Vitamin B1
    b. Vitamin B6
    c. Vitamin C
    d. Vitamin K

18. How many days does a pharmacy have to fill a prescription of Accutane?
    a. 1 day
    b. 7 days
    c. 30 days
    d. 180 days

19. How many day(s) will 40 tablets last if the patient is taking the medication "ii bid?"
    a. 1 day
    b. 5 days
    c. 10 days
    d. 20 days

20. How many drops per milliliter does a "mini-drip" system provide?
    a. 10
    b. 15
    c. 30
    d. 60

21. What is the maximum number of refills allowed for a Schedule IV drug?
    a. 0
    b. 1
    c. 5
    d. Unlimited

22. Which of the following would not be a correct auxiliary label for a patient taking doxycycline?
    a. Avoid dairy products
    b. Avoid sunlight
    c. Not to be taken by pregnant women or children younger than age 9
    d. Take on an empty stomach

23. How many times a day would a patient take a medication if it was "q6h?"
    a. 3
    b. 4
    c. 6
    d. 8

24. The cost of 100 tablets of a particular medication is $2.00. What would the retail price be if there were a 30% gross profit?
    a. $0.60
    b. $2.00
    c. $2.30
    d. $2.60

25. Which organ would be affected if the root word "nephro" was indicated?
    a. Ear
    b. Heart
    c. Kidney
    d. Liver

26. How many grams of 20% zinc oxide ointment would contain 10 g of zinc oxide?
    a. 5 g
    b. 10 g
    c. 20 g
    d. 50 g

27. Which of the following drugs would be administered to a patient if he or she had received an overdose of heparin?
    a. Aspirin
    b. Phytonadione
    c. Protamine sulfate
    d. Warfarin

28. Which vitamin deficiency may result in scurvy?
    a. Vitamin A
    b. Vitamin B1
    c. Vitamin C
    d. Vitamin D

29. What does the term "od" mean?
    a. Right ear
    b. Right eye
    c. Left ear
    d. Left eye

30. Which of the following products can be used as a smoking-cessation product and as an antidepressant?
    a. Bupropion
    b. Nicotine
    c. Trazodone
    d. Zolpidem

31. What is the generic name for Lodine?
    a. Diclofenac
    b. Etodolac
    c. Naproxen
    d. Oxaprozin

32. What is the percentage strength of a solution that is made by adding 100 mL of purified water to 600 mL of a 25% solution?
    a. 4.2%
    b. 12.5%
    c. 21.4%
    d. 30.00%

33. An intravenous solution containing 20,000 units of heparin in 500 mL of a 0.45% sodium chloride solution is to be infused at a rate of 1,000 units per hour. How many drops per minute should be infused to deliver the desired dose if the intravenous set is calibrated at a rate of 15 gtt/mL?
    a. 0.42 gtt
    b. 6 gtt
    c. 16 gtt
    d. 32 gtt

34. The adult dose of a drug is 200 mg. What is the dose for a 5-month-old infant?
    a. 0.267 mg
    b. 0.667 mg
    c. 6.67 mg
    d. 66.7 mg

35. How much medication should a 70-lb child receive if the adult dose is 250 mg?
    a. 70 mg
    b. 79 mg
    c. 116 mg
    d. 1458 mg

36. If a patient is suffering from a hepatic disorder, which organ is involved?
    a. Heart
    b. Kidney
    c. Liver
    d. Stomach

37. Which of the following ratings indicates that the drug is contraindicated in pregnancy?
    a. A
    b. B
    c. C
    d. X

38. Which of the following drugs should be taken with food?
    a. Amoxicillin
    b. Minocycline
    c. Nitrofurantoin
    d. Tetracycline

39. What term refers to the amount of money a patient must pay in a given time period before the third-party insurer will make a payment?
    a. AWP + dispensing fee
    b. Capitation
    c. Copayment
    d. Deductible

40. Which of the following drugs does not need to be packaged in a child-resistant package?
    a. Digoxin
    b. Ibuprofen
    c. Nitroglycerin
    d. Simvastatin

41. The following prescription is presented to the pharmacy:
    Hctz 50 mg #30
    i tab po qod c OJ

    How many days will the prescription last the patient?
    a. 15
    b. 30
    c. 45
    d. 60

42. What system does tuberculosis affect?
    a. Cardiovascular
    b. Digestive
    c. Endocrine
    d. Respiratory

43. Which of the following is not an input device for a computer?
    a. Bar Code Technology
    b. Keyboard
    c. Printer
    d. Touch screen applications

44. Where would meperidine be stored in the pharmacy?
    a. In the refrigerator
    b. In the pharmacy safe
    c. With the "fast movers"
    d. With the pills and tablets

45. What is the maximum number of refills allowed on Accutane prescriptions?
    a. 0
    b. 1
    c. 6
    d. 12

46. What type of label is placed on medications to warn patients or provide additional information?
    a. Auxiliary label
    b. Patient Product Insert
    c. Patient profile
    d. Prescription label

47. Where should an otic product be placed?
    a. In the ear
    b. In the eye
    c. In the rectum
    d. Under the tongue

48. If a patient is experiencing a dry, nonproductive cough, what classification of drug should the patient take?
    a. Antihistamine
    b. Antitussive
    c. Decongestant
    d. Expectorant

49. Which of the following drugs is not available as an OTC product?
    a. Ibuprofen
    b. Naproxen sodium
    c. Ranitidine
    d. Tramadol

50. How many grams of boric acid are required to make 4 fl oz of the following boric acid solution?
    Boric acid 50 g
    Purified water qs to make 1,000 mL
    a. 0.006 g
    b. 0.06 g
    c. 0.6 g
    d. 6 g

51. Which of the following is the strongest dose?
    a. NTG 1/100 gr
    b. NTG 1/150 gr
    c. NTG 1/200 gr
    d. NTG 1/400 gr

52. What is the generic name for Micronase?
    a. Glimepiride
    b. Glipizide
    c. Glyburide
    d. Pioglitazone

53. Which of the following antidepressants may be used to treat bedwetting in small children?
    a. Amitriptyline
    b. Desipramine
    c. Doxepin
    d. Imipramine

54. Which of the following products is not indicated as a smoking-cessation product?
    a. Habitrol
    b. NicoDerm
    c. Wellbutrin
    d. Zyban

55. Which of the following antifungal agents is not available as an OTC product?
    a. Clotrimazole
    b. Itraconazole
    c. Miconazole
    d. Terbinafine

56. Which of the following is not a brand of verapamil?
    a. Calan
    b. Coreg
    c. Isoptin
    d. Verelan

57. Which of the following is not a task completed by pharmacy technicians?
    a. Counseling patients
    b. Inventory management tasks
    c. Ordering medications
    d. Refilling prescriptions

58. Which drug law stated that all drugs must be pure, safe, and effective?
    a. FDCA 1938
    b. Durham-Humphrey Amendment
    c. Kefauver-Harris Amendment
    d. Poison Prevention Act of 1970

59. Which insulin has the longest duration of action?
    a. NPH insulin
    b. Lente insulin
    c. Regular insulin
    d. Ultralente insulin

60. What is the correct interpretation of the following signa: 1 tsp PCN 250 mg po qid for 10 days?
    a. Take one tablespoonful of penicillin 250 mg by mouth four times a day for 10 days.
    b. Take one teaspoonful of penicillin 250 mg by mouth every other day for 10 days.
    c. Take one teaspoonful of penicillin G 250 mg by mouth four times a day for 10 days.
    d. Take one teaspoonful of penicillin 250 mg by mouth four times a day for 10 days.

61. What does the root word "cardio" mean?
    a. Heart
    b. Lungs
    c. Skin
    d. Stomach

62. Which of the following would not be a reason for a prescription to be rejected by an insurance provider?
    a. Compounded drugs with one ingredient being a legend drug
    b. Incorrect NDC number
    c. Invalid ID number
    d. Prescription coverage has expired

63. How much 1% boric acid solution and 5% boric acid solution are needed to make 30 mL of 3% boric acid solution?
    a. 5%-20 mL; 1%-10 mL
    b. 5%-5 mL; 1%-5 mL
    c. 5%-10 mL; 1%-20 mL
    d. 5%-5 mL; 1%-25 mL

64. Which of the following does not increase the level of cholesterol in the body?
    a. Corticosteroids
    b. Loop diuretics
    c. Nitroglycerin
    d. Thiazide diuretics

65. Which of the following drugs is not a proton pump inhibitor?
    a. Esomeprazole
    b. Itraconazole
    c. Lansoprazole
    d. Pantoprazole

66. Which reference book is a compilation of package inserts?
    a. Drug Topics Red Book
    b. Facts and Comparisons
    c. Physicians' Desk Reference
    d. USP-DI

67. Which of the following migraine preparations is a controlled substance?
    a. Butorphanol
    b. Sumatriptan
    c. Tramadol
    d. Zolmitriptan

68. How old must a person be to purchase an exempt narcotic?
    a. 12 years
    b. 16 years
    c. 18 years
    d. 21 years

69. Which of the following drugs is not an antifungal agent?
    a. Fluconazole
    b. Miconazole
    c. Nystatin
    d. Sulfisoxazole

70. Which of the therapeutic equivalence codes states that the product meets the necessary bioequivalence requirements?
    a. AA
    b. AB
    c. B
    d. BC

71. Which of the following would not be used in the preparation of intravenous medications?
    a. Ampules
    b. Class A prescription balance
    c. Laminar flow hood
    d. Syringes

72. Which of the following drugs is safe to take for an HA if the patient experiences peptic ulcer disease?
    a. Acetaminophen
    b. Acetylsalicylic acid
    c. Ibuprofen
    d. Naproxen sodium

73. A pharmacy technician receives a medication order that requires them to add 40 units of insulin to an intravenous solution. How many mL will they need?
    a. 0.3 mL
    b. 0.4 mL
    c. 0.5 mL
    d. 0.6 mL

74. Which of the following factors does not affect the route of administration?
    a. Disease state
    b. Ease of administration
    c. Rate of action
    d. Shape of the dosage form

75. Which instrument should be used to measure a volume less than 1.0 mL?
    a. Beaker
    b. Conical graduate
    c. Cylindrical graduate
    d. Pipette

76. What standards must be followed during extemporaneous compounding?
    a. DEA
    b. FDA
    c. GMP
    d. OBRA 90

77. Which of the following might be used to treat arthritis?
    a. Feverfew
    b. Ginger
    c. Ginkgo
    d. Glucosamine

78. What is the generic name for Glucophage?
    a. glipizide
    b. glyburide
    c. metformin
    d. pioglitazone

79. What is the generic name for Zithromax?
    a. azithromycin
    b. clarithromycin
    c. minocycline
    d. ofloxacin

80. What does AWP represent?
    a. Actual warehouse price
    b. Actual wholesale price
    c. Average wholesale price
    d. Average wholesale promotion

81. Which dosage form is described as "solid particles dispersed in liquid vehicle?"
    a. Emulsions
    b. Gel
    c. Lotion
    d. Suspensions

82. If a patient is to receive 5 mg/kg of a drug, how much should a 176-lb patient receive?
    a. 40 mg
    b. 193.6 mg
    c. 1936 mg
    d. 0.4 g

83. Which law is being violated if a prescription is dispensed without a valid prescription?
    a. Controlled Substance Act of 1970
    b. Durham-Humphrey Amendment
    c. FDCA 1938
    d. OBRA 90

84. Which of the following is not an effect of narcotics?
    a. Analgesia
    b. CNS stimulation
    c. Euphoria
    d. Sedation

85. How many 150-mg clindamycin capsules are required to compound a prescription reading "clindamycin 2%, propylene glycol 5%, isopropyl alcohol qs ad 480 mL"?
    a. 10
    b. 64
    c. 96
    d. 112

86. Which dosage form features a gelatin shell?
    a. A caplet
    b. A capsule
    c. An enema
    d. A suppository

87. A pharmacy is reimbursed by an insurance company for AWP + $3.25 per prescription. If the AWP for 100 tablets is $120.00, how much will the pharmacy be reimbursed for a prescription of 30 tablets?
    a. $36.00
    b. $39.25
    c. $120.00
    d. $123.25

88. How many milliliters of water should be mixed with 1200 mL of 65% (v/v) to make a 45% (v/v) solution?
    a. 533 mL
    b. 667 mL
    c. 830 mL
    d. 1733 mL

89. How many 500-mg doses can be prepared from a 10-g vial of cefazolin?
    a. 15
    b. 20
    c. 25
    d. 50

90. How much time does a pharmacist have to complete the partial filling of a Schedule II prescription?
    a. 24 hr
    b. 48 hr
    c. 72 hr
    d. 96 hr

91. Which of the following could be used to prepare an ointment if another technician is using the ointment slab?
    a. A graduate
    b. A mortar
    c. Parchment paper
    d. Weighing paper

92. Which drug classification of antibiotics should not be taken if the patient is allergic to penicillin?
    a. Aminoglycosides
    b. Cephalosporins
    c. Macrolides
    d. Quinolones

93. What is the most common route of administration?
    a. Inhalation
    b. Inunction
    c. Oral
    d. Rectal

94. How many inches inside a laminar airflow hood should one prepare a sterile product?
    a. 4
    b. 6
    c. 10
    d. 12

95. Which of the following is not true when ordering Schedule II drugs?
    a. Form 222 is a triplicate form
    b. Form 222 must be kept in a secure location
    c. If an error is made on a Form 222, one can cross it out and initial it
    d. A maximum of 10 different drugs can be ordered on one form

96. Which process brings a drug from the administration site into the bloodstream?
    a. Absorption
    b. Distribution
    c. Metabolism
    d. Elimination

97. How much dextrose does 1 L of D10W contain?
    a. 10 mg
    b. 100 mg
    c. 1 g
    d. 100 g

98. Which of the following is not a side effect of decongestants?
    a. Decreased blood pressure
    b. Elevated blood pressure
    c. Increased heart stimulation
    d. Increased CNS stimulation

99. A pharmacy bases its retail prices on AWP plus a professional fee as follows:

Fee	AWP
$2.25	Less than $25.00
$3.25	$25.01–$50.00
$10.00	$50.01–$75.00
$20.00	More than $75.01

    A prescription is presented that reads "Sig: 2 tabs bid × 25 days." If the AWP of this drug is $321.66 for 500 tablets, what will be the retail price of the prescription?
    a. $66.53
    b. $70.20
    c. $74.33
    d. $85.25

100. How many milliliters of water must be added to 250 mL of a 0.9% (w/v) stock solution of sodium chloride to prepare a ½ NS solution?
    a. 125
    b. 250
    c. 375
    d. 500

101. A patient has been ordered PB ¼ gr; how many 15 mg tablets should the patient receive?
    a. 1
    b. 2
    c. 3
    d. 4

102. A pharmacy technician is preparing heparin 25,000 units in 500 mL of D5W. The appropriate concentration on the label should read:
    a. 50 units/mL.
    b. 75 units/mL.
    c. 100 units/mL.
    d. 125 units/mL.

103. How many 2-teaspoon doses can be prepared from 1 L of a solution?
    a. 50
    b. 100
    c. 500
    d. 1000

104. Which method of administration is used to provide medication to an unconscious patient?
    a. Inunction
    b. Inhalation
    c. Parenteral
    d. Peroral

105. What is the purpose of the DEA?
    a. Accepting NDAs from manufacturers
    b. Enforcing the Controlled Substance Act of 1970
    c. Licensing pharmacists
    d. Overseeing the MedWatch program

106. Which liquid form is a dispersion in which one liquid is dispersed in another immiscible liquid?
    a. Emulsion
    b. Lotion
    c. Ointment
    d. Suspension

107. Who may accept new prescriptions phoned in from a physician's office according to federal law?
    a. Pharmacists
    b. Pharmacy aides
    c. Pharmacy clerks
    d. Pharmacy technicians

108. Which term on a prescription is an instruction to the pharmacist?
    a. Inscription
    b. Rx
    c. Signa
    d. Subscription

109. Why are amber vials used to package medications?
    a. To clearly identify oral products from topical products
    b. To prevent an individual from identifying a medication
    c. To prevent moisture from getting inside the container
    d. To protect the medication from ultraviolet light and possible degradation

110. What components would be found in total nutrient admixture?
     a. Amino acids-dextrose-lipids
     b. Amino acids-dextrose-proteins
     c. Amino acids-dextrose-vitamins
     d. Amino acids-dextrose-minerals-vitamins

111. Which law is being violated if an employer discriminates against a potential employee because of medical reasons that would not prevent him or her from properly performing the job?
     a. ADA
     b. Any Willing Provider
     c. OSHA
     d. Prescription Drug Equity Act

112. Which of the following drugs is not a macrolide?
     a. Azithromycin
     b. Clarithromycin
     c. Doxycycline
     d. Erythromycin-sulfisoxazole

113. What does IV mean?
     a. Intravenous
     b. Intravenous piggyback
     c. Intravenous push
     d. Involuntary

114. Who is the primary source of medication for community pharmacies?
     a. Chain pharmacy warehouses
     b. GPOs
     c. Manufacturers and wholesalers
     d. Store-to-store vendors

115. Who develops the formulary for a hospital?
     a. Board of directors of the hospital
     b. FDA
     c. GPO
     d. P&T committee

116. Which medication should be dispensed to a pregnant woman with hypertension?
     a. Lisinopril
     b. Methyldopa
     c. Nifedipine
     d. Verapamil

117. What does "qsad" mean on a prescription?
     a. A sufficient quantity
     b. A sufficient quantity for the right ear
     c. A sufficient quantity to make
     d. To make for the right ear

118. Which reference book is the official compendium of pharmaceutical products in the United States?
     a. Facts and Comparisons
     b. Physicians' Desk Reference
     c. Remington's Pharmaceutical Sciences
     d. USP-NF

119. What is the purpose of a Group Purchasing Organization?
    a. Negotiates prices for hospital pharmacies
    b. Purchases medications for hospital pharmacies
    c. Purchases medications for community pharmacies
    d. Purchases medications for managed care pharmacies

120. How long must controlled substance records be retained according to federal law?
    a. 6 months
    b. 1 year
    c. 2 years
    d. 7 years

121. Which gland influences water balance, body temperature, appetite, and emotions?
    a. Hypothalamus
    b. Pancreas
    c. Thymus
    d. Thyroid

122. Which of the following drug classifications would use pulse dosing?
    a. Antibiotics
    b. Anticonvulsants
    c. Antidepressants
    d. Antifungal

123. Which pharmacy law clearly defined adulteration and misbranding?
    a. Pure Drug Act of 1906
    b. Food, Drug and Cosmetic Act of 1938
    c. Durham-Humphrey Amendment
    d. Poison Control Act of 1970

124. Which drug classification ends in "-pril?"
    a. ACE inhibitors
    b. Benzodiazepines
    c. Corticosteroids
    d. H2 antagonists

125. What advice should not be given to a patient taking penicillin products?
    a. Do not take with juices or colas
    b. May cause drowsiness
    c. Take on an empty stomach
    d. Take with water

126. How much gentian violet is in 100 mL of a 1:10,000 solution?
    a. 0.01 mg
    b. 10 mg
    c. 0.01 g
    d. 10 g

127. A drug is available in the following strengths and dosage forms: 125-mg tablets, 250-mg capsules, 125-mg/5 mL liquid. A child weighs 55 lb and the recommended dose is 10 mg/kg/24 hr and is to be given in either 6- or 12-hr intervals. Which of the following would not be an appropriate regimen?
    a. One 125-mg tablet every 12 hr
    b. One 250-mg capsule every 12 hr
    c. One teaspoon of 125 mg/5 mL liquid every 12 hr
    d. 1/2 of a 125-mg tablet every 6 hr

128. A dermatologist prescribes 2 oz of the following compound:

LCD	2%
Salicylic acid	5%
Yellow petrolatum	qs ad

    The pharmacy prepares a 500-g bulk container and repackages it in 2-oz containers. How much salicylic acid is needed to compound 500 g?
    a. 0.5 g
    b. 2.5 g
    c. 5 g
    d. 25 g

129. A manufacturer's invoice totals $500.00 with the terms 3% net. How much should be remitted to the manufacturer if it is paid in 30 days?
    a. $15.00
    b. $150.00
    c. $485.00
    d. $500.00

130. A patient is to receive 1 L of D5/0.45 NS with 20 mEq solution over 24 hr. What is the flow rate?
    a. 21 mL/hr
    b. 24 mL/hr
    c. 41 mL/hr
    d. 84 mL/hr

131. What color C should be stamped on controlled substance prescriptions?
    a. Black
    b. Blue
    c. Green
    d. Red

132. What type of mortar and pestle should be used in mixing liquid compounds?
    a. Glass
    b. Latex
    c. Porcelain
    d. Wedgwood

133. What is the markup rate for a prescription that costs $35.00 and retails for $50.00?
    a. 30%
    b. 43%
    c. 57%
    d. 70%

134. The infusion rate of an IV is over a-12 hr period. The total exact volume is 800 mL. What would be the infusion rate in mL/min?
    a. 0.56 mL/min
    b. 1.11 mL/min
    c. 2.7 mL/min
    d. None of the above

135. You have a 10% solution of dextrose. How many grams of dextrose are in 500 mL of this solution?
    a. 50 mg
    b. 500 mg
    c. 5000 mg
    d. 50 g

136. How many 5-gr tablets are required to make 650 mL of a 1:200 solution?
    a. 5
    b. 10
    c. 15
    d. 20

137. On the state board exam, a label shows that the medication is dispensed in a 4-oz bottle and is a 5% solution. How much medication is present in the bottle?
    a. 6 mg
    b. 24 mg
    c. 6 g
    d. 24 g

138. What is the flow rate to be used to infuse 1000 mL of NS over 4 hr if the set delivers 10 gtt/mL?
    a. 25 gtt/min
    b. 35 gtt/min
    c. 41 gtt/min
    d. 82 gtt/min

139. Two tablespoonfuls of 85% boric acid solution are diluted to 10%. How many 3-oz bottles will the technician be able to fill with the diluted solution?
    a. 1
    b. 2
    c. 4
    d. 8

140. What does Syrup USP contain?
    a. Alcohol in water
    b. Oleaginous in water
    c. PEG in water
    d. Sucrose in water

PRACTICE EXAMINATION II

Select the response that best answers the question.

1. Which of the following interpretations of the following signa is correct: 30 mL MOM po ac and hs prn
    a. Take one teaspoonful of Milk of Magnesia by mouth before meals and at bedtime as needed
    b. Take one tablespoonful of Milk of Magnesia by mouth after meals and at bedtime as needed
    c. Take 1 oz of Milk of Magnesia by mouth after meals and at bedtime as needed
    d. Take 1 oz of Milk of Magnesia by mouth before meals and at bedtime as needed.

2. Five pints of diluted hydrochloric acid weigh 2.79 kg. What is its specific gravity?
    a. 0.56
    b. 0.86
    c. 1.16
    d. 1.79

3. Which of the following is not a side effect of steroidal medications?
    a. Bruising
    b. Inflammation
    c. Moon face
    d. Weight gain

4. What is the generic name for the brand name drug, Bactrim DS?
   a. Amoxicillin/clavulanate
   b. Cephalexin
   c. Sulfamethoxazole/trimethoprim
   d. Sulfamethoxazole/trimethoprim DS

5. What does the suffix "-ectomy" mean?
   a. Disease
   b. Hardening
   c. Removal
   d. Vomiting

6. How many grams of 2.5% hydrocortisone cream should be mixed with 240 g of 0.25% hydrocortisone cream to make a 1% hydrocortisone cream?
   a. 120
   b. 180
   c. 240
   d. 360

7. What is the maximum number of refills allowed for a Schedule III drug?
   a. 0
   b. 1
   c. 5
   d. 6

8. How many days would 40 capsules of a medication last if the directions were "i cap qid"?
   a. 4
   b. 6
   c. 8
   d. 10

9. Which of the following interpretations of the following signa is correct: "ii gtt os bid?"
   a. Instill 2 drops in right ear twice a day
   b. Instill 2 drops in right eye twice a day
   c. Instill 2 drops in left ear twice a day
   d. Instill 2 drops in left eye twice a day

10. Which of the following is not a duty performed by a pharmacy technician?
    a. Answering telephones
    b. Counseling patients
    c. Preparing prescription labels
    d. Pricing prescriptions

11. Which of the following drugs is not a form of estradiol?
    a. Climara
    b. Estrace
    c. Estraderm
    d. Premarin

12. Which of the following would not be used in extemporaneous compounding?
    a. Class A balance
    b. Compounding slab
    c. Graduate cylinder
    d. Laminar flow hood

13. What does the term "gram" measure?
    a. Distance
    b. Vision
    c. Volume
    d. Weight

14. Which of the following side effects may result from taking thiazide diuretics?
    a. Hypocalcemia
    b. Hypoglycemia
    c. Hypokalemia
    d. Hypourticaria

15. What does DUR mean?
    a. Directions Under Review
    b. Doctor Under Review
    c. Drug Used Rectally
    d. Drug Utilization Review

16. Approximately how many liters are in 1 qt?
    a. 1
    b. 2
    c. 3
    d. 4

17. What is the maximum number of different items that may be ordered on a Form 222?
    a. 5
    b. 10
    c. 15
    d. 20

18. Which of the following drugs is a Schedule II drug?
    a. Acetaminophen with codeine
    b. Alprazolam
    c. Cocaine
    d. Flurazepam

19. What does hypoglycemia mean?
    a. High blood pressure
    b. High blood sugar
    c. Low blood pressure
    d. Low blood sugar

20. How many days would 40 capsules of a medication last if the directions were "i cap qid ac and hs?"
    a. 4
    b. 8
    c. 10
    d. None of the above

21. How many 4-oz bottles of an exempt narcotic may be purchased every 48 hr by an individual?
    a. 0
    b. 1
    c. 2
    d. None of the above

22. In what proportion should 20% zinc oxide be mixed with white petrolatum (diluent) to produce a 3% zinc oxide ointment?
    a. 1 part ZnO and 1 part white petrolatum
    b. 3 parts ZnO and 17 parts white petrolatum
    c. 3 parts ZnO and 14 parts white petrolatum
    d. 17 parts ZnO and 3 parts white petrolatum

23. If 120 mL of a 2% (w/v) are diluted with water to 1 pint, what will be the strength of the dilution?
    a. 0.25%
    b. 0.5%
    c. 1.0%
    d. 8.0%

24. Gentamicin 120 mg in 100 mL D5W is administered over 30 minutes every 8 hours with a 10 drop kit. What will the gtt/min be?
    a. 2
    b. 4
    c. 16
    d. 33

25. Where would one place a medication if the directions said "au"?
    a. Each ear
    b. Each eye
    c. Left ear
    d. Left eye

26. If a child weighs 8 kg and the adult dose is 10 mL, how much medication should the child receive?
    a. 0.5 mL
    b. 1.2 mL
    c. 4.0 mL
    d. 6.7 mL

27. What is the correct dosage for a 25-lb child if the adult dose is 100 mg?
    a. 7.6 mg
    b. 17 mg
    c. 68 mg
    d. 113 mg

28. What is the generic for Lipitor?
    a. Atorvastatin
    b. Fluvastatin
    c. Pravastatin
    d. Simvastatin

29. Which of the following drugs would not be used to treat COPD?
    a. Albuterol
    b. Guaifenesin
    c. Ipratropium bromide
    d. Salmeterol

30. When is trazodone contraindicated?
    a. Children suffering from enuresis
    b. Elderly females suffering from Alzheimer disease
    c. Elderly males suffering from erectile dysfunction
    d. Young males

31. What is the flow rate of 1 L of NS to be infused over 8 hr?
    a. 8 mL/hr
    b. 12.5 mL/hr
    c. 125 mL/hr
    d. 1,000 mL/hr

32. What term describes the response when two or more drugs combine to provide a response that is greater than the sum of the two individual drugs?
    a. Additive effect
    b. Potentiation
    c. Synergistic effect
    d. None of the above

33. What is the proper dosage for a 6-year-old child if the adult dose is 10 mg?
    a. 33 mcg
    b. 3.3 mg
    c. 33 mg
    d. 333 mg

34. Which of the following herbal products would be used as a laxative?
    a. American ginseng
    b. Cascara sagrada
    c. Goldenseal
    d. Melatonin

35. What is inventory?
    a. Expired merchandise
    b. Merchandise available for sale
    c. Merchandise to be ordered
    d. Overstock merchandise

36. What size syringe should be used to measure 0.6 mL of fluid?
    a. 1 mL
    b. 5 mL
    c. 10 mL
    d. 20 mL

37. If 150 mL of a substance weighs 170 g, what is its specific gravity?
    a. 0.88
    b. 1.0
    c. 1.13
    d. 1.25

38. In multiples of what number should tablets or capsules be counted at a time using a spatula and a pill tray?
    a. 1
    b. 2
    c. 5
    d. 10

39. How many milligrams are equal to 2 grains?
    a. 1 mg
    b. 13 mg
    c. 130 mg
    d. 1,300 mg

40. How many days will the following prescription last?
    Amoxicillin 125 mg/5 mL   75 cc
    i tsp po tid
    a. 1
    b. 5
    c. 10
    d. 15

41. Which of the following drugs will produce an adverse effect if alcohol is consumed during the course of therapy?
    a. Disulfiram
    b. Guaifenesin
    c. Hydrochlorothiazide
    d. Triamcinolone

42. What does the suffix "-osis" mean?
    a. Abnormal condition
    b. Inflammation
    c. Study of
    d. Treatment

43. Which dosage form may either be oil-in-water or water-in-oil?
    a. Capsule
    b. Emulsion
    c. Suspension
    d. Suppository

44. How many kilograms are in 4.4 lb?
    a. 0.2
    b. 2.0
    c. 20
    d. 200

45. What is the direction for airflow in a horizontal laminar airflow hood?
    a. From the back of the hood to the front
    b. From the bottom of the hood to the top
    c. From the front of the hood to the back
    d. From the top of the hood to the bottom

46. How many milliliters of a 1:50 (w/v) stock solution can be prepared from 1 pint of a 5% stock solution?
    a. 96
    b. 192
    c. 720
    d. 1,200

47. Which organization is responsible for drug recalls?
    a. Boards of Pharmacy
    b. DEA
    c. FDA
    d. NABP

48. Which DAW code should be used if the physician authorizes the use of a generic drug, but the patient requests the brand name drug?
    a. 0
    b. 1
    c. 2
    d. 3

49. At what standard time would a patient receive medication if it was 0800 hr military time?
    a. 7 AM
    b. 8 AM
    c. 7 PM
    d. 8 PM

50. By what route should Phenergan 25 mg suppository be taken?
    a. PO
    b. PR
    c. SL
    d. TOP

51. Which of the following drugs is not a quinolone?
    a. Ciprofloxacin
    b. Norflex
    c. Norfloxacin
    d. Floxin

52. If a medication has an expiration date of 3/06, when will it expire?
    a. The first day of June 2003
    b. The last day of June 2003
    c. The first day of March 2006
    d. The last day of March 2006

53. Which of the following medications could be used as a prophylactic for migraines?
    a. Imitrex
    b. Inderal
    c. Midrin
    d. Stadol

54. Which of the following is not an antiviral agent?
    a. Acyclovir
    b. Clotrimazole
    c. Didanosine
    d. Zidovudine

55. Which term refers to the name of the medication, its strength, and the quantity to be dispensed?
    a. Inscription
    b. Rx
    c. Signa
    d. Subscription

56. What is the cost for 24 mg of an active ingredient used in a compound if the bulk bottle of the active ingredient costs $250.00/g?
    a. $1.50
    b. $3.00
    c. $6.00
    d. $9.00

57. A 1,000-mL IV bag was hung at 0800 and is to run at 100 mL/hr. What time would the next bag be needed?
    a. 1200 hr
    b. 1400 hr
    c. 1600 hr
    d. 1800 hr

58. How often should a fentanyl patch be changed?
    a. Once per day
    b. Every 3 days
    c. Once per week
    d. Once per month

59. Which of the following professional licenses is not allowed to prescribe medications?
    a. DDS
    b. LCSW
    c. MD
    d. PA

60. What does the term "PCA" represent?
    a. Patient-calibrated analysis
    b. Patient-controlled analgesia
    c. Partially collapsed artery
    d. Perennial circumvented arteriosclerosis

61. What is MedWatch?
    a. A device that signals that an another IV bag needs to be hung in an institution
    b. A reporting program available to pharmacies indicating physicians who may be overprescribing narcotics
    c. A reporting program available to healthcare providers to report adverse events that pose a serious health threat
    d. A service established by the AARP to monitor polypharmacy in the elderly

62. What is the name of the opening of a needle?
    a. Bevel
    b. Hilt
    c. Lumen
    d. Point

63. Which of the following would not be found on a CSAR?
    a. Amount of medication administered
    b. Amount of medication wasted
    c. Date and time of the administration of a drug
    d. Expiration date of the drug administered

64. Which form is required to dispense controlled substances?
    a. Form 222
    b. Form 224
    c. Form 225
    d. Form 363

65. Which of the following is not an abbreviation for extended-release forms of medication?
    a. CD
    b. CR
    c. ERF
    d. SR

66. Which of the following capsule sizes contains the smallest quantity?
    a. 0
    b. 1
    c. 2
    d. 4

67. What is the generic name for Tenormin?
    a. Atenolol
    b. Carisoprodol
    c. Nadolol
    d. Propranolol

68. Which of the following is not a manner for a new prescription to be presented for filling at a pharmacy?
    a. Called by the physician
    b. Called by the patient
    c. Fax
    d. Presented by the patient

69. Which of the following medications is not measured in International Units?
    a. Heparin
    b. Insulin
    c. Vitamin B
    d. Vitamin E

70. What term can be described as "the rules of a facility or institution"?
    a. Policy
    b. Procedure
    c. Protocol
    d. Standard

71. What type of alcohol is used to clean a laminar airflow hood?
    a. Ethyl alcohol
    b. Isopropyl alcohol
    c. Methyl alcohol
    d. Rubbing alcohol

72. What is the meaning of the abbreviation "BS"?
    a. Blood sugar
    b. Blood-in-stools
    c. Body surface
    d. Bowel syndrome

73. What is the brand name for enalapril?
    a. Accupril
    b. Monopril
    c. Vasotec
    d. Zestril

74. What should a patient take for a headache if he or she is taking warfarin?
    a. APAP
    b. ASA
    c. Narcotic analgesics
    d. NSAIDs

75. Which of the following drugs may be used to counteract the side effects of antipsychotic medications?
    a. Benztropine
    b. Citalopram
    c. Propranolol
    d. Zolpidem

76. Dissolve 40 g of urea in enough liquid to make a 20% solution. What is the total volume?
    a. 2 mL
    b. 8 mL
    c. 20 mL
    d. 200 mL

77. Which of the following drugs should be avoided in the treatment of asthmatics?
    a. Antihistamines
    b. Beta-blockers
    c. NSAIDs
    d. All of the above

78. To what classification does Tessalon Perles belong?
    a. Antitussive
    b. Antihistamine
    c. Decongestant
    d. Expectorant

79. Which of the following drugs is not available as an OTC?
    a. Aluminum hydroxide-magnesium hydroxide
    b. Lansoprazole
    c. Omeprazole
    d. Ranitidine

80. Which of the following is the generic name for Pepcid?
    a. Cimetidine
    b. Famotidine
    c. Nizatidine
    d. Ranitidine

81. Which of the following is not a task a pharmacy technician would perform?
    a. Counting medication
    b. Extemporaneous compounding
    c. Reconstituting medications
    d. Signing a Form 222

82. What is the flow rate of 1,000 mL of Ringer's lactate to be infused over 8 hr?
    a. 6.25 mL/hr
    b. 12.5 mL/hr
    c. 62.5 mL/hr
    d. 125 mL/hr

83. How many grams of fluorouracil will a 154-lb patient receive in 5 successive days at a dosage rate of 12 mg/kg/day?
    a. 0.84
    b. 1.848
    c. 4.2
    d. 9.24

84. Interpret the following signa "ii caps stat, then i cap q hr, max 5 caps/12 hr."
    a. Take 2 capsules by mouth immediately, then 1 capsule at bedtime, maximum of 5 capsules in 5 hours
    b. Take 2 capsules by mouth immediately, then 1 capsule each hour, maximum of 5 capsules in 12 hours
    c. Take 11 capsules by mouth immediately, then 1 capsule at bedtime, maximum of 5 capsules within the next 12 hours
    d. Take 11 capsules by mouth immediately, then 1 capsule each hour, maximum of 5 additional capsules in 12 hours

85. Which part of the body would be affected by the root word "arthro"?
    a. Arm
    b. Artery
    c. Joint
    d. Membrane

86. What type of drug is affected by MAC?
    a. Discontinued drugs
    b. Investigational drugs
    c. Nonproprietary drugs
    d. Proprietary drugs

87. Which of the following classifications of antidepressants needs to be washed out of the body before switching to another antidepressant?
    a. Lithium
    b. MAOIs
    c. SSRIs
    d. TCAs

88. Which of the following is not required on a prescription label?
    a. Directions for usage
    b. Drug name with strength and quantity
    c. Physician's DEA number
    d. Prescription or serial number

89. Prepare 2.5 L of a 1:20 solution from a 30% solution. How much water was added?
    a. 417 mL
    b. 2,083 mL
    c. 2,500 mL
    d. 15,000 mL

90. How many pairs of latex gloves should be worn when preparing IV admixtures?
    a. 0
    b. 1
    c. 2
    d. 3

91. Which of the following drugs could be used prophylactically for dental procedures?
    a. Ampicillin
    b. Amoxicillin
    c. Ibuprofen
    d. Naproxen sodium

92. A pharmacy technician is preparing an IV admixture and notices on the medication order the abbreviation "NS." What does NS mean?
    a. Nasal solution
    b. Normal saline
    c. Normal solution
    d. No smoking while the patient is receiving the IV

93. Which medication should not be prescribed for young males?
    a. Desyrel
    b. Paxil
    c. Prozac
    d. Zoloft

94. Which of the following drugs is not a Schedule II drug?
    a. Codeine
    b. Fentanyl
    c. Lorazepam
    d. Methylphenidate

95. Which of the following drugs needs to placed in a child-resistant container?
    a. Inhalation products
    b. Mebendazole tablets
    c. Ranitidine
    d. Sublingual nitroglycerin tablets

96. Which of the following dosage forms bypasses the digestive system?
    a. Capsule
    b. Enteric coated table
    c. Oral tablet
    d. Sublingual tablet

97. Which pharmacy reference book contains drug costs?
    a. Blue Book
    b. Orange Book
    c. Red Book
    d. White Book

98. A patient weighs 60 lb and has been given a prescription in which he or she is to receive 3 mg/lb each day. How many mg will he or she receive each day?
    a. 170
    b. 175
    c. 180
    d. 185

99. Why would a pharmacy receive a noncompliance report?
    a. The pharmacy failed to maintain adequate controlled substance records and has been cited by the DEA on an audit
    b. The pharmacy failed to properly fill out a Form 222
    c. The pharmacy failed to purchase medications from a specific vendor, which had been negotiated by the GPO
    d. The pharmacy purchased more drugs than it is permitted based on its budget

100. What is another name for a nonproprietary drug?
     a. Brand name drug
     b. Generic drug
     c. Investigational drug
     d. OTC

101. How old must one be to purchase an exempt narcotic?
     a. 16 yr
     b. 18 yr
     c. 21 yr
     d. 65 yr

102. What type of interaction occurs when a patient takes tetracycline with milk?
     a. Adverse effect
     b. Drug-drug
     c. Drug-food
     d. Synergistic

103. At what standard time would a patient receive a medication if the military time was 1800 hr?
     a. Midnight
     b. 8 AM
     c. 6 PM
     d. 8 PM

104. When does a "Code Blue" occur?
     a. When a patient is experiencing a heart attack
     b. When a patient quits breathing
     c. A and B
     d. None of the above

105. Which of the following is not used to treat gastrointestinal problems?
     a. Antacids
     b. Histamine 2 receptor agonists
     c. Histamine 2 receptor antagonists
     d. Proton pump inhibitors

106. Which of the following products should not be chewed?
     a. Azatadine
     b. Azelastine
     c. Benzonatate
     d. Fexofenadine

107. What is the generic name for Retrovir?
     a. Didanosine
     b. Lamivudine
     c. Stavudine
     d. Zidovudine

108. How many minutes should a pharmacy be allowed to deliver a "stat" order?
     a. 5–15 min
     b. 5–30 min
     c. 30–45 min
     d. 45–60 min

109. Which formula for calculating a child's dosage is the most accurate?
    a. Body surface area
    b. Clark's rule
    c. Fried's rule
    d. Young's rule

110. Convert 10 degrees Celsius to Fahrenheit.
    a. −12
    b. 32
    c. 42
    d. 50

111. An IV order calls for the addition of 45 mEq of $CaCO_3$ (calcium carbonate). You have a 25-mL vial of calcium carbonate 4.4 mEq/mL. How many milligrams of this concentration do you need to add to this IV?
    a. 5.6
    b. 8.4
    c. 10.2
    d. 12.8

112. What vitamin deficiency may result in beriberi?
    a. Vitamin A
    b. Vitamin B1
    c. Vitamin C
    d. Vitamin D

113. Who is the person in whose name an insurance policy is held?
    a. Beneficiary
    b. Dependent
    c. Subscriber
    d. Patient

114. What classification of drugs may yield side effects such as dry mouth, difficult urination, or constipation?
    a. Alpha-blockers
    b. Anticholinergics
    c. Beta-blockers
    d. Cholinergics

115. It is recommended that 25 mg/kg of a drug be given every 6 hr to a child weighing 13.2 lb. How many milligrams of a drug would be used for each dose?
    a. 75
    b. 150
    c. 330
    d. 600

116. In this formula, how much talc is needed to fill 120 g of the compound?
    Nupercainal ointment   4%
    Zinc oxide   20%
    Talc   2%

    a. 1,200 mg
    b. 1,500 mg
    c. 2,400 mg
    d. 120 g

117. Which of the following is not a method to reduce hypertension?
    a. Increase physical inactivity to regular aerobic physical activity
    b. Increase the amount of sleep an individual receives at night
    c. Reduce high sodium intake to moderate sodium intake
    d. Reduce excess alcohol consumption to moderate alcohol consumption

118. The following medications—Diovan HCT, Dyazide, Hyzaar, and Zestoretic—are combination products used in the treatment of cardiovascular disease. Which medication is found in all of them?
    a. Hydrochlorothiazide
    b. Lisinopril
    c. Triamterene
    d. Valsartan

119. Which of the following is an antidote for an excess of warfarin?
    a. Heparin
    b. Enoxaparin
    c. Phytonadione
    d. Protamine sulfate

120. What is the percent equivalent of a 1:10 ratio?
    a. 0.01%
    b. 0.1%
    c. 1.0%
    d. 10.0%

121. To what does an NDC number on a prescription bottle refer?
    a. Drug product
    b. Drug manufacturer
    c. Quantity package
    d. All of the above

122. What does MDI mean?
    a. Medical diagnosis included
    b. Medical doctor under investigation
    c. Metered dose inhaler
    d. Multidose inhaler

123. Which term refers to the vehicle that contains the dissolved drug?
    a. Solute
    b. Solution
    c. Solvent
    d. Syrup

124. What term refers to an abnormal heartbeat?
    a. Arrhythmia
    b. Bradycardia
    c. Flutter
    d. Tachycardia

125. How much hydrocortisone is found in a 1-oz tube of hydrocortisone 1% cream?
    a. 0.3 mg
    b. 3.0 mg
    c. 0.3 g
    d. 3.0 g

126. Who licenses pharmacists in each state?
    a. DEA
    b. FDA
    c. Federal government
    d. State Boards of Pharmacy

127. What is the meaning of fibromyalgia?
    a. Brittle hair and nails
    b. Chronic pain in the muscles
    c. Inflammation of tendon
    d. Lymph node disease

128. What is the minimum weighable quantity for a Class A balance?
    a. 120 mg
    b. 150 mg
    c. 250 mg
    d. 500 mg

129. What type of dosage form is prepared using the "punch method"?
    a. Capsules
    b. Emulsions
    c. Suppositories
    d. Tablets

130. What type of documentation does OSHA require for pharmacies that handle hazardous chemicals?
    a. Manufacturer Safety Documentation Sheets
    b. Manufacturer Sheets for Documentation of Safety
    c. Material Safety Data Sheets (MSDS)
    d. Mixture Safety Documentation Sheets

131. Where should a patient store a prescription of liquid amoxicillin suspension?
    a. In a bathroom vanity
    b. In a kitchen cupboard
    c. In the refrigerator
    d. Does not matter where it is stored

132. A pharmacy wants to mark up a product by 30%. How much would an item cost with this mark up if its original cost was $4.50?
    a. $5.85
    b. $6.23
    c. $6.40
    d. $7.10

133. What is the generic name for Depakote?
    a. Divalproex
    b. Gabapentin
    c. Primidone
    d. Valproic acid

134. Which of the following is not found on a Master Formula Sheet used in compounding?
    a. Amount of ingredient needed
    b. Color of ingredient
    c. Manufacturer's lot number and expiration date
    d. Name of individual who weighed or measured ingredient

135. What is the meaning of "ou" on a prescription?
   a. Each ear
   b. Each eye
   c. Left eye
   d. Right ear

136. What piece of equipment reduces the risk of contamination when preparing IV admixtures?
   a. Foot pedal sinks
   b. Humidifiers
   c. Laminar flow hoods
   d. Ultraviolet lighting

137. What type of formulary is a limited list of drugs?
   a. Closed formulary
   b. Open formulary
   c. Restricted formulary
   d. None of the above

138. What type of copayment is a different dollar amount based upon the type of drug being dispensed?
   a. Fixed copayment
   b. Percentage copayment
   c. Variable copayment
   d. None of the above

139. How often is the Physicians' Desk Reference published?
   a. Biannually
   b. Biennially
   c. Every 6 months
   d. Yearly

140. What is the route of administration for a prescription to be taken "po?"
   a. Buccally
   b. Orally
   c. Rectally
   d. Sublingually

PRACTICE EXAMINATION III

Select the response that best answers the question.

1. How long must a laminar airflow hood be on before being used?
   a. 15 min
   b. 30 min
   c. 1 hr
   d. 2 hr

2. What does the abbreviation "hs" mean on a prescription?
   a. At bedtime
   b. Hours
   c. House
   d. None of the above

3. Which of the following drugs is not a cephalosporin?
   a. Keflex
   b. Lorabid
   c. Suprax
   d. Vantin

4. Which of the following drugs is not an NSAID?
   a. Colchicine
   b. Celecoxib
   c. Ibuprofen
   d. Oxaprozin

5. Which of the following is true concerning nitrofurantoin?
   a. It should be taken as a loading dose
   b. It should be taken at breakfast only
   c. It should be taken with alcohol
   d. It should be taken with food

6. What auxiliary label should be included on a container of medication that has the following signa: "i gtt os bid"?
   a. For external use
   b. For the ear
   c. For the eye
   d. Use rectally

7. Where would a buccal tablet be placed?
   a. Between the cheeks
   b. Orally
   c. Rectally
   d. Under the tongue

8. Which of the following would be found on a hospital medication order but not on a retail prescription?
   a. Dosage schedule
   b. Drug name
   c. Drug strength
   d. Patient name

9. Which of the following drugs would be contraindicated with vitamin K therapy?
   a. Glyburide
   b. Heparin
   c. Pentoxifylline
   d. Warfarin

10. What does the suffix "-ectomy" mean?
    a. Disease
    b. Hardening
    c. Removal
    d. Vomiting

11. What is the maximum number of refills allowed for a Schedule III drug?
    a. 0
    b. 1
    c. 5
    d. 10

12. A technician is given 120 mL of a 50% (w/v) potassium chloride solution and is told to add 6 oz of sterile water to it. What will be the final (w/v) percentage concentration of the solution?
    a. 10
    b. 20
    c. 33
    d. 47

13. What is the purpose of post-marketing monitoring of new drugs?
    a. Ensure GMP
    b. Monitor the quality of new drugs
    c. Removal of unsafe drugs
    d. Testing for purity and effectiveness of new drugs

14. What disease may result in the formation of a goiter?
    a. Cancer
    b. Hypertension
    c. Hypoglycemia
    d. Hyperthyroidism

15. Which type of insulin can be added to an IV solution?
    a. Extended insulin zinc
    b. Isophane insulin
    c. NPH insulin
    d. Regular insulin

16. What is a drug monograph?
    a. A picture of the drug from the manufacturer
    b. A price list for the drug from the manufacturer
    c. Literature on the drug
    d. Literature on the drug manufacturer

17. What may a pharmacy technician do as a result of OBRA 90?
    a. Call a physician and recommend a different drug dosage
    b. Counsel a patient with regard to their drug therapy
    c. Offer to counsel a patient, if allowed by state law
    d. Screen patient profiles for drug-disease contraindications

18. How many milliliters are in 1 cubic centimeter?
    a. 1
    b. 2
    c. 5
    d. 10

19. Which of the following drugs will produce an adverse effect if alcohol is consumed during the course of therapy?
    a. Amoxicillin
    b. Azithromycin
    c. Metronidazole
    d. Nitrofurantoin

20. How much guaifenesin with codeine would you dispense for a 5-day supply if the prescription calls for "Guaifenesin c Codeine 5 cc q 4 h po prn"?
    a. 120 mL
    b. 150 mL
    c. 450 mL
    d. 480 mL

21. Which of the following topical corticosteroid dosage forms is more potent?
    a. Cream
    b. Gel
    c. Lotion
    d. Ointment

22. How often is a biennial inventory taken in a pharmacy?
    a. Monthly
    b. Twice per year
    c. Yearly
    d. Every 2 years

23. Which of the following is not used to treat depression?
    a. Antipsychotics
    b. MAO inhibitors
    c. SSRIs
    d. TCAs

24. What size container would you use in dispensing 240 mL of a liquid medication?
    a. 2 oz
    b. 4 oz
    c. 6 oz
    d. 8 oz

25. You have received a medication order for Lasix 40 mg bid for 10 days. You prepare a unit dose of Lasix suspension (10 mg/mL). How much would you dispense for a unit dose?
    a. 4 mL
    b. 8 mL
    c. 10 mL
    d. 18 mL

26. The pharmacy technician receives a prescription for Flexeril 10 mg and the instructions read "i po tid." What is the total daily dose?
    a. 10 mg
    b. 20 mg
    c. 30 mg
    d. 40 mg

27. What is the generic name for Patanol?
    a. Brimonidine
    b. Ciprofloxacin
    c. Latanoprost
    d. Olopatadine

28. Which schedule of medications has no medical use in the United States and possess an extremely high potential for abuse?
    a. Schedule I
    b. Schedule II
    c. Schedule III
    d. Schedule IV

29. Which of the following is not a disadvantage of an oral dosage form?
    a. Delayed onset of action
    b. Ease of administration
    c. First pass metabolism
    d. Taste of medication

30. What hospital committee is responsible for creating and maintaining the drug formulary?
    a. Infection Control Committee
    b. Nursing and Pharmacy Committee
    c. Pharmacy and Therapeutics Committee
    d. Product Evaluations Committee

31. A 10-year-old child weighs 90 lb. How much medication should the child receive using Young's formula if the adult dose is 30 mg?
    a. 13 mg
    b. 18 mg
    c. 50 mg
    d. 66 mg

32. What are the two methods of pharmacy claims submission to third-party payers?
    a. Electronic and e-mail
    b. Electronic and fax
    c. Electronic and FedEx
    d. Electronic and hard copy

33. How many tablets should be given to a patient with the following prescription?
    Hctz 50 mg one month supply
    1 tab po qod
    ref × 6

    a. 15 tablets
    b. 30 tablets
    c. 90 tablets
    d. 180 tablets

34. If the patient is to receive 2.4 g of medication/day and the drug is available in 600-mg tablets, how many tablets are needed for a day's dose?
    a. 0.5
    b. 1
    c. 4
    d. 8

35. Which of the following is true about generically equivalent drugs?
    a. Chemically different, but are expected to produce the same therapeutic outcome and toxicity
    b. Chemically identical in strength, concentration, dosage form, and route of administration
    c. Contain different active ingredients
    d. Priced exactly the same as brand name drugs

36. How many 30-mg KMNO4 (potassium permanganate) tablets are needed to prepare the following solution?
    KMNO4   1:5000   600 mL

    a. 2 tablets
    b. 3 tablets
    c. 4 tablets
    d. 6 tablets

37. A child weighs 30 kg and is prescribed a 10 mg/kg dose of amoxicillin tid. The pharmacy stocks 50 mg/mL. How much medication (in mL) would the patient receive in each day?
    a. 3
    b. 6
    c. 13
    d. 18

38. What does "NPO" mean on a prescription?
    a. Do not refill
    b. Do not place in mouth
    c. Do not repeat
    d. Nothing by mouth

39. What is the generic name for Zyprexa?
    a. Donepezil
    b. Metaxalone
    c. Olanzapine
    d. Risperidone

40. What is the correct interpretation of the following signa: 10 mg MS IM q 4 h prn pain?
    a. Inhale 10 mg of morphine sulfate every 4 hours as needed for pain
    b. Insert 10 mL of morphine sulfate intramuscularly every 4 hours as needed for pain
    c. Inject 10 mg of morphine sulfate intravenously every 4 hours as needed for pain
    d. Inject 10 mg of morphine sulfate intramuscularly every 4 hours as needed for pain

41. How would a patient take a medication if the directions read "prn"?
    a. As directed
    b. As needed
    c. By mouth
    d. By rectum

42. How many milliliters of water should be added to 1 L of 70% isopropyl alcohol to prepare a 30% solution?
    a. 2.33 mL
    b. 42.86 mL
    c. 1333 mL
    d. 2.33 L

43. How many days would a prescription of 30 tablets last if the directions were "i tab tid ac"?
    a. 3
    b. 6
    c. 8
    d. 10

44. How many grams of a 10% and 1% ointment should be used to make 45 g of a 2% ointment?
    a. 5 g of the 1%; 40 g of 2%
    b. 5 g of the 1%; 40 g of the 10%
    c. 5 g of the 10%; 40 g of the 2%
    d. 5 g of the 10%; 40 g of the 1%

45. Which of the following drugs would use "pulse dosing"?
    a. Clotrimazole
    b. Fluconazole
    c. Itraconazole
    d. Ketoconazole

46. Which of the following interpretations of the signa "i cap qid ac and hs" is correct?
    a. Take 1 caplet by mouth 1 hour before meals and at bedtime
    b. Take 1 capsule by mouth 1 hour before meals and bedtime
    c. Take 1 capsule by mouth after meals and before bedtime
    d. Take 1 capsule by mouth four times a day before meals and at bedtime

47. Which DAW code is used when the physician writes "Brand Name Only" on the prescription?
    a. 0
    b. 1
    c. 2
    d. 3

48. What term refers to a pharmacy receiving a predetermined amount of money for a patient regardless of the number of prescriptions filled or the value of the prescriptions each month?
    a. Capitation
    b. Copayment
    c. Deductible
    d. Fee for service

49. What is the meaning of the term "non rep"?
    a. Do not repeat
    b. No known allergies
    c. Nothing by mouth
    d. Refill

50. Cephalexin is to cephalosporin as ciprofloxacin is to _____?
    a. Macrolide
    b. Penicillin
    c. Quinolone
    d. Tetracycline

51. What is the meaning of AAC?
    a. Actual acquisition cost
    b. Average acquisition cost
    c. Average assessed cost
    d. Average acquisition cost containment

52. Which of the following drugs is not available in a transdermal dosage form?
    a. Clonidine
    b. Estradiol
    c. Fentanyl
    d. Fexofenadine

53. What is the generic name for Zestril?
    a. Enalapril
    b. Fosinopril
    c. Lisinopril
    d. Quinapril

54. How many milliliters of water should be added to 100 mL of 10% stock solution of sodium chloride to prepare a 0.9% solution of sodium chloride?
    a. 10.1
    b. 101
    c. 1011
    d. 1111

55. Which of the following drugs, if expired, can result in a fatality?
    a. Amoxicillin
    b. Cephalexin
    c. Clarithromycin
    d. Tetracycline

56. What term refers to the processes involved in the preparation of sterile products to prevent contamination of the product?
    a. Aseptic technique
    b. Extemporaneous compounding
    c. Geometric dilution
    d. Levigation

57. Why is it important to follow the procedures of an institution?
    a. Following procedures will result in a promotion
    b. Following procedures will result in a pay increase
    c. Procedures are established that will prevent errors from occurring in a pharmacy
    d. The PTCB and State Boards of Pharmacy follow-up with pharmacy technicians to ensure that they are following procedures. Failure to follow procedures may result in either a suspension or revocation of their certification

58. What is the meaning of the prefix "osteo-"?
    a. Bone
    b. Cell
    c. Lymph
    d. Muscle

59. How much medication should a 40-lb child receive if the adult dose is 25 mg?
    a. 5.66 mg
    b. 6.66 mg
    c. 7.66 mg
    d. 8.66 mg

60. Which body system is affected by "GERD"?
    a. Cardiovascular
    b. Endocrine
    c. Gastrointestinal
    d. Pulmonary

61. How many times a day would a patient take his or her medication if it is "tid"?
    a. 1
    b. 2
    c. 3
    d. 4

62. What should a pharmacy technician do while processing a prescription if he or she receives a contraindication message on the pharmacy terminal screen?
    a. Bypass the screen and continue to process the prescription
    b. Contact the physician and ask that a different drug be prescribed
    c. Inform the patient that you cannot fill the prescription because the physician made an error
    d. Inform the pharmacist of the message

63. Which of the following side effects may be attributed to an overdosage of salicylates?
    a. GI upset
    b. Platelet changes
    c. Tinnitus
    d. All of the above

64. Which of the following are indications for NSAIDs?
    a. Analgesic
    b. Anti-inflammatory
    c. Antipyretic
    d. All of the above

65. What is the generic name for the beta-blocker Tenormin?
    a. Atenolol
    b. Metoprolol
    c. Propranolol
    d. Nadolol

66. What type of drug recall occurs when a drug is not likely to cause a temporary adverse health consequence?
    a. Class I recall
    b. Class II recall
    c. Class III recall
    d. No recall is required

67. At which part of the liquid does one look when measuring liquids?
    a. A point between the bottom and top of the meniscus
    b. Bottom of the meniscus
    c. Top of the meniscus
    d. None of the above

68. Where should used needles be placed after use?
    a. In a biohazard container
    b. In a red plastic bag
    c. In a sharps container
    d. With normal trash

69. What temperature is considered room temperature?
    a. 8°C
    b. 8–15°C
    c. 15–30°C
    d. 30–40°C

70. What do the first five digits of an NDC number represent?
    a. Drug item
    b. Drug manufacturer
    c. Drug package
    d. None of the above

71. A patient receives 5 mL of a 15% solution of a drug. What is the drug dose?
    a. 75 mg
    b. 750 mg
    c. 7.5 g
    d. 75 g

72. Which of the following is a local anesthetic?
    a. Benzocaine
    b. Butorphanol
    c. Neostigmine
    d. Zolmitriptan

73. What form must be submitted to the DEA to destroy controlled substances?
    a. Form 41
    b. Form 49
    c. Form 224
    d. Form 225

74. How many grams of a 10% and 2% ointment should be used to make 25 g of a 5% ointment?
    a. 2%-9.4 g; 10%-15.6 g
    b. 2%-10 g; 10%-15 g
    c. 2%-12.5 g; 10%-12.5 g
    d. 2%-15.6 g; 10%-9.4 g

75. Amitriptyline is to TCA as venlafaxine is to _____.
    a. Calcium channel blocker
    b. H2 antagonist
    c. Protease inhibitor
    d. SSRI

76. In what schedule is methylphenidate classified?
    a. Schedule I
    b. Schedule II
    c. Schedule III
    d. Schedule IV

77. What type of pharmacy balance is required in all pharmacies?
    a. Class A
    b. Class B
    c. Electronic
    d. Triple beam

78. Which of the following drugs is a calcium channel blocker?
    a. Carvedilol
    b. Nadolol
    c. Nifedipine
    d. Valsartan

79. What is a common side effect of ACE inhibitors?
    a. Anaphylaxis
    b. CNS stimulation
    c. Cough
    d. Respiratory depression

80. What are the four elements of medical and pharmaceutical nomenclature?
    a. Prefixes, suffixes, root words, and combining vowels
    b. Prefixes, suffixes, key words, and combining vowels
    c. Prefixes, suffixes, key words, and combining consonants
    d. Prefixes, suffixes, root words, and combining consonants

81. How many milliliters of a 10% stock solution of an ingredient are needed to prepare 120 mL of a solution containing 10 mg of the ingredient per milliliter?
    a. 0.12
    b. 1.2
    c. 12
    d. 120

82. What advice should be given to a patient taking metronidazole?
    a. Avoid alcohol
    b. Take with food
    c. Take all of the medication
    d. All of the above

83. How many days will the following prescription of 60 tablets last if the directions read "i–ii tabs po q 4–6 h"?
    a. 5
    b. 7
    c. 10
    d. 15

84. Which of the following medications should not be given to individuals younger than age 18?
    a. Cephalexin
    b. Ciprofloxacin
    c. Clarithromycin
    d. Clindamycin

85. Which dosage form is an aqueous solution with sucrose?
    a. Emulsion
    b. Solution
    c. Suspension
    d. Syrup

86. How many 10-gr tablets are required to make 1000 mL of a 1:1000 solution?
    a. ½
    b. 1
    c. 1½
    d. 2

87. Which law ensures a safe environment for employees?
    a. ADA
    b. Any Willing Provider
    c. OBRA
    d. OSHA

88. What condition may result if a child takes aspirin after being exposed to chickenpox?
    a. Glaucoma
    b. Herpes zoster
    c. Reye syndrome
    d. Toxic shock syndrome

89. How many grams of dextrose are in 1 L of D5W?
    a. 50 mcg
    b. 50 mg
    c. 5.0 g
    d. 50 g

90. Which of the following is an example of drug duplication?
    a. Aldactone and Coreg
    b. Calan and Isoptin
    c. Coumadin and Zetia
    d. Dyazide and Vasotec

91. Which dosage form is defined as a clear, sweetened, flavored hydroalcoholic, containing water and alcohol, which may be either medicated or not?
    a. Elixir
    b. Emulsion
    c. Enema
    d. Syrup

92. When would you take a medication if the directions stated "ac"?
    a. After a meal
    b. At bedtime
    c. Before a meal
    d. In the morning

93. What is the maximum number of refills allowed for a prescription of oxycodone + APAP if authorized by the prescriber?
    a. 0
    b. 5
    c. 12
    d. Unlimited

94. What is the meaning of the prefix "intra-"?
    a. Below
    b. Between
    c. Equal
    d. Within

95. How much Demerol would be given to a patient if the dose on hand was 50 mg/mL and the patient is to receive 75 mg?
    a. 0.5 mL
    b. 1.0 mL
    c. 1.5 mL
    d. 2.0 mL

96. Which dosage form would use the process of inunction to be absorbed into the body?
    a. Capsules
    b. Inhalants
    c. Ointments
    d. Suppositories

97. Which auxiliary label should be affixed to a container of tetracycline?
    a. Avoid sunlight
    b. Take 1 hr before or 2 hr after taking dairy products or antacids
    c. Take all medication
    d. All of the above

98. Which of the following is the Federal Legend that must appear on all prescriptions?
    a. "Caution: Federal Law prohibits dispensing without a prescription"
    b. "Caution: Federal Law prohibits the transfer of this prescription to anyone other than the intended"
    c. "Package Not Child Resistant"
    d. "Warning—May be habit forming"

99. Which of the following is not an automated dispensing system?
   a. JCAHO
   b. Pyxis
   c. Robot Rx
   d. SureMed

100. What is the meaning of "D5W"?
   a. 5% distilled water
   b. 5% dextrose in water
   c. Discontinue 5% water
   d. Dispense for 5 weeks

101. What is another term for suggested retail price?
   a. Discounted price
   b. List price
   c. Net price
   d. Sale price

102. A pharmacy must ensure that its pharmacy records are "readily retrievable" for a pharmacy inspector. How much time is this?
   a. 24 hr
   b. 48 hr
   c. 72 hr
   d. 96 hr

103. Which of the following can be used to treat asthma?
   a. Beta 2 agonists
   b. Cromolyn
   c. Corticosteroids
   d. All of the above

104. To which organization would an individual report a medication error?
   a. DEA
   b. FDA
   c. Med Watch
   d. State Board of Pharmacy

105. Which of the following drug classifications does not interact with phenobarbital?
   a. Beta-blockers
   b. H2 antagonists
   c. TCAs
   d. Warfarin

106. What is the meaning of "prn"?
   a. As needed
   b. Per rectal needs
   c. Practical registered nurse
   d. Physician requires notice

107. Which dosage form consists of a solute and a solvent?
   a. Emulsion
   b. Solution
   c. Suspension
   d. Syrup

108. What factor(s) influence the effect of a drug on an individual?
     a. Age
     b. Disease
     c. Gender
     d. All of the above

109. Which schedule of medication may be purchased as an "exempt narcotic"?
     a. Schedule II
     b. Schedule III
     c. Schedule IV
     d. Schedule V

110. Which body system would be affected by an anaphylactic reaction?
     a. Digestive
     b. Endocrine
     c. Respiratory
     d. Skeletomuscular

111. Which of the following medication(s) should not be taken with phenytoin?
     a. Fluoxetine
     b. Oral contraceptives
     c. Theophylline
     d. All of the above

112. Where does one obtain a nosocomial infection?
     a. At home
     b. At a hospital
     c. At school
     d. At work

113. Which of the following tasks do computers perform?
     a. Communication
     b. Input and output
     c. Processing and storage
     d. All of the above

114. What does a red C indicate on a prescription?
     a. Prescription has been canceled by the physician
     b. Prescription has been copied and transferred to another pharmacy
     c. Prescription has been processed by the pharmacy and has been picked up by the patient
     d. Prescription is a controlled substance

115. Which of the following is the generic name for Capoten?
     a. Captopril
     b. Carvedilol
     c. Clonidine
     d. Clopidogrel

116. What is glaucoma?
     a. A bacterial infection of the eye
     b. A fungal infection of the eye
     c. A viral infection
     d. Increased pressure within the eye

117. Which of the following is not available as an OTC product?
    a. Chlorpheniramine
    b. Diphenhydramine
    c. Fexofenadine
    d. Loratadine

118. Which of the following classifications does not have a drug interaction with oral contraceptives?
    a. Antibiotics
    b. Anticonvulsants
    c. Antifungals
    d. Antihypertensives

119. Which type of diabetes can be controlled through exercise and diet?
    a. Gestational diabetes
    b. Secondary diabetes
    c. Type I diabetes
    d. Type II diabetes

120. What is another term for a "crash cart"?
    a. Code blue cart
    b. Code orange cart
    c. Code red cart
    d. Code yellow cart

121. Which form is used to document medication being administered to a patient?
    a. MAR
    b. MDR
    c. POS
    d. TAR

122. What document must be completed for every employee hired by a pharmacy?
    a. Application
    b. Background check
    c. I-9
    d. Reference check

123. What is a medication order called when it is presented to a community pharmacy?
    a. Inscription
    b. MAR
    c. Patient profile
    d. Prescription

124. What type of unit dose system is referred to as "punch cards, bingo cards, or blister packs"?
    a. Blended unit-dose system
    b. Modified unit-dose system
    c. Modular cassette
    d. Multiple medication packages

125. What part of the laminar flow hood is responsible for removing contaminants?
    a. The blower
    b. The HEPA filter
    c. The recovery vent
    d. The side walls

126. What medication could be prescribed for a patient experiencing a "UTI"?
    a. AZT
    b. HCTZ
    c. NTG
    d. SMZ-TMP DS

127. Depakote is to anticonvulsants as Celebrex is to _____
    a. Antibiotic
    b. Antifungal
    c. Estrogen
    d. NSAID

128. What is the generic name for Prevacid?
    a. Esomeprazole
    b. Lansoprazole
    c. Omeprazole
    d. Pantoprazole

129. What is another name for a troche?
    a. Effervescent tablet
    b. Gelatin capsule
    c. Granule
    d. Lozenge

130. Which law is being violated if a pharmacist prepares a medication under unsanitary conditions?
    a. DSHEA of 1994
    b. FDCA of 1938
    c. OBRA-90
    d. HIPAA

131. Which of the following is not a sulfa drug?
    a. Azulfidine
    b. Azactam
    c. Bactrim
    d. Gantrisin

132. Which reference book is included in the USP DI Volume III and contains the FDA's approved drug products?
    a. American Drug Index
    b. Blue Book
    c. Orange Book
    d. Red Book

133. If one gram of dextrose provides 3.4 kcal, how many kcal will 200 mL of a 25% dextrose solution provide?
    a. 17
    b. 170
    c. 340
    d. 680

134. Which of the following is not a reason for a third-party claim to be rejected by an insurance carrier?
    a. Drug not covered
    b. Invalid identification number
    c. Generic drug dispensed
    d. Refill too soon

135. What term refers to fragments of a vial closure that contaminate a parenteral solution?
    a. Bevel
    b. Coring
    c. Hub
    d. Lumen

136. What is the brand name for lorazepam?
    a. Ativan
    b. Dalmane
    c. Klonopin
    d. Valium

137. What term describes directions to a pharmacist on a prescription?
    a. DAW indicator
    b. Inscription
    c. Subscription
    d. Signa

138. The larger the needle gauge, the _____ the diameter of the needle.
    a. Larger
    b. Longer
    c. Smaller
    d. Shorter

139. Which of the following terms is a set amount of money that must be paid by the patient before the insurer will cover additional expenses?
    a. Coinsurance
    b. Copay
    c. Deductible
    d. Maximum allowable cost

140. What is the correct meaning for signa in the following prescription:
    Timoptic 0.25%   15 mL
    i gtt ou bid

    a. Instill 1 drop in each ear twice per day.
    b. Instill 1 drop in each eye twice per day.
    c. Instill 1 drop in left eye twice per day.
    d. Instill 1 drop in left ear twice per day.

PRACTICE EXAMINATION IV

Select the response that best answers the question.

1. You have received a medication order to prepare a 250 mL bag of NS with 1 g of Kefzol. The patient is to receive a 250-mg dose per hour. The infusion is calibrated at 10 gtt/mL. What flow rate is needed to deliver the dose?
    a. 1 gtt/min
    b. 10 gtt/min
    c. 15 gtt/min
    d. 20 gtt/min

2. Which classification of drug recall occurs if the patient experiences a reversible side effect?
    a. Class I
    b. Class II
    c. Class III
    d. Class IV

3. What is the generic name for Zestril?
   a. Benazepril
   b. Enalapril
   c. Lisinopril
   d. Prinivil

4. What is the basic reimbursement formula for pharmacies?
   a. Copayment
   b. Drug cost × standard markup rate
   c. Drug cost + dispensing fee
   d. Drug cost + dispensing fee – deductible

5. How many milliliters are in 1 L?
   a. 1
   b. 100
   c. 1,000
   d. 1,000,000

6. Which route of administration should be used in taking nitroglycerin?
   a. Buccal
   b. Oral
   c. Rectal
   d. Sublingual

7. What is meant by the half-life of a drug?
   a. The amount of time it takes to dissolve a substance
   b. The amount of time it takes to dispense a package or container of medication
   c. The amount of time necessary to process one half of the number of prescriptions in a given day
   d. The amount of time it takes to eliminate one half of the drug in circulation

8. Which of the following duties may the pharmacy technician not perform?
   a. Labeling medication doses, preparing intravenous admixtures, and maintaining the cleanliness of the laminar flow hood.
   b. Maintaining patient records, filling and dispensing routine orders for stock supplies, and preparing routine compounding.
   c. Prepackaging drugs in single dose or unit-of-use, maintaining inventories of drug supplies, and completing insurance forms.
   d. Providing clinical counseling, providing clinical information to medical staff, and providing patient medical history data to requestors.

9. Which of the following drug classifications can be used to treat chronic pain?
   a. H2 blockers
   b. MAOIs
   c. SSRIs
   d. TCAs

10. If 500 mL of D5W is to be infused over 6 hr and the drop factor is 15 gtt/mL, what will the rate in gtt/min be?
    a. 1
    b. 2
    c. 10
    d. 20

11. Which of the following is considered a solid dosage form?
    a. Cream
    b. Emulsion
    c. Suspension
    d. Tablet

12. You have received a prescription for amoxicillin 500 mg po. The patient is unable to chew or swallow capsules or tablets. How many milliliters should be given in each dose if the concentration is 125 mg/5 mL?
    a. 5
    b. 10
    c. 15
    d. 20

13. Which of the following is a calcium channel blocker?
    a. Atenolol
    b. Carvedilol
    c. Diltiazem
    d. Lisinopril

14. Which of the following interpretations of the signa "ii gtt bid os" is correct?
    a. Instill 2 drops in right ear twice per day
    b. Instill 2 drops in left ear twice per day
    c. Instill 2 drops in right eye twice per day
    d. Instill 2 drops in left eye twice per day

15. Which of the following respiratory medications is not a combination product?
    a. Advair
    b. Allegra D
    c. Combivent
    d. Singulair

16. Which of the following auxiliary labels should be placed on a prescription container of antianxiety, antidepressant, or anticonvulsant medication?
    a. Avoid dairy products
    b. May cause drowsiness
    c. Refrigerate
    d. Shake well

17. When a pharmacy technician is performing geometric dilution, when does the technician add the most potent ingredient, which may also have the smallest weight or smallest volume, to the mortar?
    a. Anytime
    b. As the first ingredient
    c. As the last ingredient
    d. Intermittently during the compounding process

18. What term describes the willingness of the patient to take a drug in the amounts and on schedule as prescribed?
    a. Compliance
    b. Ease of administration
    c. First-pass effect
    d. Second-pass effect

19. Which of the following is not required on a prescription label?
    a. Expiration date of prescription
    b. Patient's name
    c. Physician's DEA number
    d. Physician's name

20. Which process is the reducing of a substance to small, fine particles?
    a. Blending
    b. Comminution
    c. Sifting
    d. Tumbling

21. How much codeine is contained in one tablet of Tylenol #3?
    a. ¼ gr
    b. ½ gr
    c. ¾ gr
    d. 1 gr

22. Which of the following drugs is the generic name for Micronase?
    a. glimepiride
    b. glipizide
    c. glyburide
    d. lispro

23. What is the generic name for Fosamax?
    a. alendronate
    b. calcitonin-salmon
    c. etidronate
    d. raloxifene

24. Which term encompasses the absorption, distribution, metabolism, and elimination of a drug?
    a. Pharmacokinetics
    b. Pharmacognosy
    c. Pharmacology
    d. Pharmacopeia

25. Which of the following is not an example of a dispersion?
    a. Emulsion
    b. Lotion
    c. Ointment
    d. Suppository

26. What is the generic name for Dilantin?
    a. Divalproex
    b. Gabapentin
    c. Phenytoin
    d. Valproic acid

27. What is the meaning of "URI"?
    a. Upper respiratory infection
    b. Urethral and rectal infection
    c. Urine receptacle infection
    d. Upper respiratory influenza

28. What temperature is equivalent to 98.6°F?
    a. 35°C
    b. 36°C
    c. 37°C
    d. 38°C

29. How much medication should a 9-year-old child receive if the adult dose is 50 mg?
    a. 19.4 mg
    b. 21.4 mg
    c. 24.4 mg
    d. 26.4 mg

30. Which of the following drugs is the generic name for Glucotrol?
    a. Glimepiride
    b. Glipizide
    c. Glyburide
    d. Metformin

31. Which of the following drugs is not an SSRI?
    a. Fluoxetine
    b. Paroxetine
    c. Risperidone
    d. Sertraline

32. Which of the following natural supplements might be used to treat depression?
    a. Camomile
    b. Ginger
    c. Ginkgo
    d. St. John's wort

33. What is the generic name for Zyprexa?
    a. Nefazodone
    b. Olopatadine
    c. Olanzapine
    d. Trazodone

34. A patient presents a prescription to the pharmacy for Ceclor 125 mg/5 mL with the directions of 1 tsp po tid × 10 d. How much should be dispensed to the patient?
    a. 75 mL
    b. 100 mL
    c. 150 mL
    d. 200 mL

35. What is the meaning of DAW 2 in billing a prescription to an insurance carrier?
    a. Brand dispensed as a generic
    b. Physician approved the use of a generic drug
    c. Physician approved the use of a generic drug; the patient requested brand name
    d. Physician requested brand name

36. What is the sensitivity for a Class A Balance?
    a. 1 mg
    b. 6 mg
    c. 10 mg
    d. 20 mg

37. Which of the following should be used in lifting pharmacy weights to be placed on a balance?
    a. Filter paper
    b. Forceps
    c. Latex gloves
    d. Weighing papers

38. Which dosage form is produced by compression?
    a. Capsule
    b. Lozenge
    c. Suppository
    d. Tablet

39. Which of the following may be used to treat sleep disorders?
    a. Chromium picolinate
    b. Ginseng
    c. Glucosamine
    d. Melatonin

40. What is the maximum number of refills for a Schedule IV drug if authorized by the physician?
    a. 0
    b. 5
    c. 12
    d. Unlimited

41. What auxiliary label should be affixed to a prescription of ibuprofen?
    a. Avoid sunlight
    b. For external use
    c. Take on an empty stomach
    d. Take with food

42. Which of the following products is used for emesis?
    a. Emetrol
    b. Ipecac
    c. PEG
    d. Simethicone

43. What is the meaning of the abbreviation "qs ad"?
    a. A sufficient quantity for the left ear
    b. A sufficient quantity for the right ear
    c. A sufficient quantity for the right eye
    d. A sufficient quantity to make up to

44. What is the purpose of a loading dose of medication?
    a. To control costs
    b. To improve compliance
    c. To obtain a therapeutic level of the medication in the bloodstream as soon as possible
    d. To reduce side effects

45. What is the meaning of "w/v"?
    a. Number of g/1 mL
    b. Number of g/100 mL
    c. Number of mcg/100 mL
    d. Number of mg/100 mL

46. How is insulin administered?
    a. ID
    b. IM
    c. IV
    d. SQ

47. What drug is abbreviated "HCTZ"?
    a. Hycomine
    b. Hycodan
    c. Hydrochlorothiazide
    d. Hydrea

48. What is the percent equivalent of a 1:20 ratio?
    a. 0.05%
    b. 0.5%
    c. 5.0%
    d. 50%

49. What is the minimum amount of time that a patient must wait before purchasing another bottle of an exempt narcotic?
    a. 24 hr
    b. 48 hr
    c. 72 hr
    d. 96 hr

50. Which of the following products is not used to treat hyperlipidemia?
    a. Aspirin
    b. Fibric acid derivatives
    c. HMG-CoA reductase inhibitors
    d. Metamucil

51. A pharmacy technician is preparing heparin 25,000 units in 500 mL of D5W. What concentration should be on the label?
    a. 50 units/mL
    b. 75 units/mL
    c. 100 units/mL
    d. 125 units/mL

52. Which vitamin deficiency would result in rickets?
    a. Vitamin A
    b. Vitamin B1
    c. Vitamin C
    d. Vitamin D

53. What is the meaning of "CSAR"?
    a. Controlled Studies Are Reviewed
    b. Controlled Substance Administration Record
    c. Controlled Substance Audit and Review
    d. Cost, Sales, Allocation, and Resources

54. Which of the following drugs does not require blood work from a patient?
    a. Lithium
    b. Phenytoin
    c. Sulfasalazine
    d. Warfarin

55. Which of the following statements is not true concerning insulin?
    a. Glargine insulin should not be mixed with any other insulins
    b. Injection sites need to be rotated
    c. Regular and Lente insulins do not mix
    d. When mixing insulin, regular insulin should be drawn up after the first insulin in the syringe

56. Zidovudine is to AZT as lamivudine is to _____.
    a. a4c
    b. ddi
    c. d4t
    d. 3TC

57. How often must an inventory of controlled substances be taken?
    a. Weekly
    b. Monthly
    c. Yearly
    d. Every 2 years

58. If 5,000 mL of a substance weighs 6,565 g, what is the specific gravity of the substance?
    a. 0.76
    b. 0.95
    c. 1.31
    d. 1.5

59. What is the meaning of the Latin abbreviation "Rx" on a prescription?
    a. Insigna
    b. Sig
    c. Take
    d. Write on label

60. What does "U&C" mean when billing prescriptions?
    a. Unusual customer
    b. Unusual and customary
    c. Usual customer
    d. Usual and customary

61. Who may recommend an OTC product to a patient?
    a. All pharmacy technicians
    b. All PTCB-certified technicians
    c. All technicians who have completed continuing education in OTC products
    d. None of the above

62. What does the root word "derm" mean?
    a. Brain
    b. Skin
    c. Skull
    d. Tooth

63. Which of the following drugs is not a selective 5-HT receptor agonist used to treat migraine headaches?
    a. Imitrex
    b. Maxalt
    c. Midrin
    d. Zomig

64. Which of the following is a federal program for patients older than 65 or with certain diseases?
    a. ADC
    b. Medicaid
    c. Medicare
    d. Worker's Compensation

65. Which reference book contains the USP and NF drug standards and dispensing requirements?
    a. Drug Topics Orange Book
    b. Drug Topics Red Book
    c. USP DI Volume I
    d. USP DI Volume III

66. Which of the following symptoms may indicate digoxin toxicity?
    a. Arrhythmias
    b. Auditory disturbances
    c. Fever
    d. Hypotension

67. Who makes notations and signs Medication Administration Records (MARs) in an institution?
    a. Doctors
    b. Nurses
    c. Pharmacists
    d. Pharmacy technicians

68. You have received a prescription for Robitussin AC and the signa is "1 tsp qid for 10 days." How much would you dispense?
    a. 50 mL
    b. 100 mL
    c. 150 mL
    d. 200 mL

69. What assumption should a pharmacy technician make if he or she observes a white, fluffy precipitate in a 250-mL bag of D5W?
    a. The solution has been contaminated
    b. The solution has been exposed to the cold
    c. The solution has been exposed to bright light
    d. The solution should be shaken to disperse the precipitate before dispensing

70. How many units of heparin are in 50 mL of 100,000 units/L?
    a. 50 units
    b. 500 units
    c. 5,000 units
    d. 50,000 units

71. For which of the following drugs is it mandatory that a customer receive a PPI?
    a. Amoxicillin
    b. Lithonate
    c. Premarin
    d. Synthroid

72. Which of the following would require a potassium supplement?
    a. Aldactone
    b. Dyazide
    c. Dyrenium
    d. Lasix

73. Which of the following drugs is not used for asthma?
    a. Albuterol
    b. Ipratropium
    c. INH
    d. Salmeterol

74. What is the percentage strength of cocaine hydrochloride of 40 mg/mL?
    a. 0.04
    b. 0.4
    c. 4
    d. 40

75. How many milliliters are in 1 pint?
    a. 120
    b. 240
    c. 480
    d. 960

76. Levothyroxine is to hypothyroidism as glyburide is to _____.
    a. ACE inhibitor
    b. Beta-blocker
    c. Oral hyperglycemic agent
    d. Oral hypoglycemic agent

77. How many milligrams are gr iss?
    a. 32.5
    b. 65
    c. 97.5
    d. 130

78. How many days will the following prescription last?
    Ampicillin 250 mg #40
    1 cap po qid
    Ref x ii

    a. 4
    b. 10
    c. 20
    d. 30

79. How would one administer an "ung"?
    a. Orally
    b. Rectally
    c. Sublingually
    d. Topically

80. A potassium chloride solution has a concentration of 1.5 mEq/mL. How many milliliters contain 30 mEq?
    a. 0.05
    b. 15
    c. 20
    d. 45

81. How many milliliters of a D10W solution contain 100 g of dextrose?
    a. 0.01 L
    b. 0.1 L
    c. 1 L
    d. 2 L

82. Which of the following must appear on a unit dose product label?
    a. Dose strength of the medication
    b. Expiration date of the medication
    c. Medication name
    d. All of the above

83. Which of the following terms is an indication for a potassium chloride supplement?
    a. Hyperkalemia
    b. Hypoglycemia
    c. Hypokalemia
    d. Hyponatremia

84. Which classification of medications may yield side effects such as dry eyes, dry mouth, or difficult urination or defecation?
    a. Alpha-blockers
    b. Anticholinergics
    c. Beta-blockers
    d. Cephalosporins

85. Where would oxycodone with acetaminophen be stored in the pharmacy?
    a. In the refrigerator
    b. In the pharmacy safe
    c. With the "fast movers"
    d. With the pills and tablets

86. You have a solution of heparin 100,000 units/L, with an infusion apparatus labeled 60 gtt/mL. What is the flow rate to deliver a dose of 20 units/minute?
    a. 3 gtt/min
    b. 12 gtt/min
    c. 15 gtt/min
    d. 20 gtt/min

87. Which of the following is not an advantage of a plastic bag IV parenteral system?
    a. The plastic bag is light and cheap to transport
    b. The plastic bag takes less room for storage and disposal
    c. The quantity remaining in the bags are easy to read
    d. All of the above

88. What does an 80/20 report tell a pharmacist or pharmacy technician?
    a. Products that have a 80% gross profit
    b. Products that have a 20% gross profit
    c. Drug products that reflect 80% of your purchasing dollars
    d. Controlled substances that represent 20% of the total number of prescriptions filled

89. Which of the following is not a required text in a pharmacy?
    a. A copy of the Controlled Substance Act
    b. NF
    c. PDR
    d. USP

90. Which of the following drugs is not a beta-blocker?
    a. Coreg
    b. Inderal
    c. Procardia
    d. Tenormin

91. What is not found in a total nutrient admixture?
    a. Amino acid
    b. Dextrose
    c. Lipids
    d. Protein

92. What units are used to measure electrolytes?
    a. mEq
    b. mg
    c. mL
    d. units

93. Which of the following terms does not mean a "proprietary" drug?
    a. Brand
    b. Generic
    c. Patented
    d. Trade

94. Where would you prepare hazardous drugs in a pharmacy?
    a. In a biological safety hood
    b. In a horizontal laminar airflow hood
    c. In a vertical laminar airflow hood
    d. On an ointment slab

95. A 180-lb male is to receive 1.75 mg/kg/day of tobramycin. The pharmacy technician is to prepare the tobramycin in 100 mL of D5W and it is to be given three times per day. The drug is available in a 40-mg/mL vial and is to be administered over 30 min. How much medication will the patient receive each day?
    a. 48 mg
    b. 96 mg
    c. 143 mg
    d. 315 mg

96. What type of drug requires a DEA number?
    a. Controlled substance
    b. Investigational drug
    c. Legend drug
    d. OTC

97. What type of solution has greater osmolarity than blood?
    a. Hypertonic
    b. Hypotonic
    c. Isotonic
    d. Pyrogenic

98. Rx: Codeine phosphate   30 mg/tsp
           Tussin syrup   30 mL
           Elixophyllin qs   240 mL
           Sig: 5 mL qid pc hs

    If 5 mL of Tussin syrup contains 100 mg of guaifenesin, how many milligrams of the drug would be taken daily?
    a. 2.5
    b. 5
    c. 10
    d. 50

99. What is the route of administration for a prescription with the following directions: "i supp pr q 6 h prn"?
    a. Orally
    b. Rectally
    c. Urethrally
    d. Vaginally

100. What type of solution is a total parenteral solution?
    a. Dialysis solution
    b. Hypotonic solutions
    c. Hypertonic solutions
    d. Isotonic solutions

101. What organ would be affected if a patient was experiencing "rhinitis"?
    a. Bladder
    b. Ear
    c. Eye
    d. Nose

102. What volume does a small-volume parenteral contain?
    a. 100
    b. 250 mL
    c. 500 mL
    d. All of the above

103. What process occurs when a drug blocks the activity of metabolic enzymes in the liver?
    a. Additive effects
    b. Inhibition
    c. Potentiation
    d. Synergism

104. The pharmacist asks you to prepare 250 mL of a 25% acetic acid solution. How much acetic acid would you need to make this preparation?
    a. 62.5 mg
    b. 6250 mg
    c. 62.5 g
    d. 6,250 g

105. Which of the following dosage forms could a diabetic patient receive?
    a. Elixir
    b. Emulsion
    c. Spirits
    d. Syrups

106. Which organ can be affected by a condition of flutter?
    a. Esophagus
    b. Heart
    c. Intestine
    d. Kidneys

107. Which of the following auxiliary labels would not be appropriate for a prescription of sulfasalazine?
    a. Avoid sunlight
    b. Drink plenty of water
    c. Keep refrigerated
    d. May discolor urine

108. A pharmacy has 300 mL of a 50% solution; 200 mL is added to this solution to decrease the concentration. How many grams of active ingredient would be in the diluted solution?
    a. 7.5
    b. 30
    c. 150
    d. 300

109. How much of a 10% and 60% dextrose solution should be mixed to prepare 1 L of a 40% dextrose solution?
    a. 10%-600 mL; 60%-400 mL
    b. 10%-500 mL; 60%-500 mL
    c. 10%-400 mL; 60%-600 mL
    d. 10%-300 mL; 60%-700 mL

110. When opening a glass ampoule always use a gauze swab
    a. To protect your finger from cuts.
    b. To prevent contamination of the product inside the ampoule.
    c. To disinfect the ampoule.
    d. None of the above.

111. How many inventory turns would a pharmacy experience if their initial inventory of the accounting period was $225,000, the final inventory of the period was $250,000, and they had sales of $2.75 million?
    a. 12.22 turns
    b. 11.58 turns
    c. 11.00 turns
    d. 5.79 turns

112. A solution of haloperidol contains 2 mg/mL of active ingredient. How many grams are in 1 pint of this solution?
    a. 0.00946
    b. 0.0946
    c. 0.946
    d. 9.46

113. How often should a patient change his or her Catapres TTS patch?
    a. Once per day
    b. Every other day
    c. Weekly
    d. Monthly

114. Which of the following is the generic name for Percocet?
    a. Acetaminophen + codeine
    b. Acetaminophen + hydrocodone
    c. Acetaminophen + oxycodone
    d. Acetaminophen + propoxyphene

115. A 44-lb child is to receive 4 mg of phenytoin per kilogram of body weight daily as a anticonvulsant. How many milliliters of pediatric phenytoin suspension containing 30 mg/5 mL should the child receive?
    a. 13.3 mL
    b. 50 mL
    c. 80 mL
    d. 176 mL

116. Which organization is concerned about employee safety?
    a. HIPAA
    b. JCAHO
    c. OBRA
    d. OSHA

117. Which dosage form is a clear, sweetened, flavored hydroalcoholic solution containing water and ethanol?
    a. Collodion
    b. Elixir
    c. Suspension
    d. Syrup

118. The following abbreviation "ou" is found on a prescription. What does it mean?
    a. Both ears
    b. Both eyes
    c. Both feet
    d. Both hands

119. The product *Infants Mylicon Drops* contains 2 g of simethicone in a 30-mL container. How many milligrams of the drug are contained in each teaspoonful dose?
    a. 0.33
    b. 33
    c. 333
    d. 1000

120. What is another term for hyperalimentation?
    a. Aseptic technique
    b. Dietary supplementation
    c. Extemporaneous compounding
    d. TPN

121. Which of the following ophthalmic products should be refrigerated?
    a. Apraclonidine
    b. Brimonidine
    c. Brinzolamide
    d. Latanoprost

122. What is the generic name for Avapro?
    a. Candesartan
    b. Irbesartan
    c. Losartan
    d. Valsartan

123. In how many direction(s) does air flow in a laminar flow hood?
     a. 1
     b. 2
     c. 3
     d. 4

124. New OTC drugs are required to go through necessary phases. Which phase occurs when a final review is done on the ingredients of the agent in question and the public is able to give feedback?
     a. Phase I
     b. Phase II
     c. Phase III
     d. Phase IV

125. What is the generic name for Glucophage?
     a. Glimepiride
     b. Glipizide
     c. Glyburide
     d. Metformin

126. What factors should be considered when dealing with elderly patients?
     a. Auditory issues
     b. Chronic conditions
     c. Multiple medications
     d. All of the above

127. Which of the following drugs is available as both a tablet and an IV solution?
     a. Accupril
     b. Capoten
     c. Monopril
     d. Vasotec

128. What should one tell a patient with a prescription of griseofulvin suspension?
     a. Be careful of sunlight; it may cause photosensitivity
     b. Shake well
     c. Store at room temperature
     d. All of the above

129. Which of the following products is not available as a transdermal patch?
     a. Catapres
     b. Duragesic
     c. Nitroglycerin
     d. Tegretol

130. What is the nonproprietary name for Deltasone?
     a. Lithium
     b. Methylprednisolone
     c. Prednisolone
     d. Prednisone

131. Which answer best describes the information that should be included in a Schedule V sale log for C-V drugs sold without a prescription?
    a. Dispensing date, printed name, signature and address of buyer, name and quantity of the product sold, and the pharmacist's signature
    b. Dispensing date, signature and phone number of the buyer, product name, and product company with lot number
    c. Dispensing date, signature of the buyer, name and quantity of product sold, price of the product sold, and the lot number of the product sold
    d. Dispensing date, buyer signature, pharmacist signature, product name and amount, and the expiration date of the product

132. What should be done in preparing a prescription for etoposide?
    a. Flush the remaining contents down a sink or toilet
    b. Wear protective clothing if you are allergic to etoposide
    c. Place labels on the container so it has a professional appearance
    d. Prepare it in a biological safety cabinet

133. Which of the following drugs is not an MAO inhibitor?
    a. Bupropion
    b. Phenelzine
    c. Selegiline
    d. Tranylcypromine

134. What would be the infusion rate for a 50 mg/mL magnesium sulfate solution to provide 1.2 g/hr?
    a. 0.4 mL/hr
    b. 2.5 mL/hr
    c. 20 mL/hr
    d. 24 mL/hr

135. Which of the following is not a cardiovascular medication?
    a. Coreg
    b. Diovan
    c. Evista
    d. Plavix

136. What is another term for a Master Formula Sheet?
    a. MAR
    b. MSDS
    c. Pharmacy compounding log
    d. Record log sheet

137. What body organ would be affected by hepatoxicity?
    a. Intestines
    b. Kidneys
    c. Liver
    d. Thyroid

138. How would a prescriber write a prescription for "Zolpidem 5 mg at bedtime if needed"?
    a. Zolpidem 5 mg q hs prn
    b. Zolpidem 5 mg q hs ad
    c. Zolpidem 5 mg q 9 PM ad Lib
    d. Zolpidem 5 mg q hs qs

139. What does ASHP mean?
     a. American Schools of Health Practices
     b. American Society of Health-Systems Pharmacists
     c. American Society of Hospital Pharmacists
     d. Association of Specialty Health Practitioners

140. What type of hypersensitivity reaction occurs when circulating antibodies of the IgG, IgM, or IgA class react with an antigen associated with a cell membrane?
     a. Type I
     b. Type II
     c. Type III
     d. Type IV

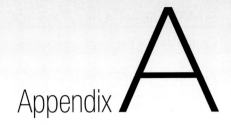

Appendix A

Pharmacy Technician Certification Examination Information

Certification is the process by which a nongovernmental association or agency grants recognition to an individual who has met certain predetermined qualifications specified by that association or agency. The goal of the PTCB's certification program is to enable pharmacy technicians to work more effectively with pharmacists to offer greater patient care and service. The PTCB is responsible for the development and implementation of policies related to national certification for pharmacy technicians.

PROFESSIONAL EXAMINATION SERVICE

The Professional Examination Service (PES), the PTCB's contracted testing company, is a nonprofit testing company founded in 1941. The PES specializes in the development and administration of national certification and licensure examinations. The PES's primary operating principle is to develop examinations of the highest quality and reliability. Examinations are developed using the standards established by the National Commission for Certifying Agencies, the American Psychological Association, and the U.S. Equal Employment Opportunity Commission as guidelines.

CERTIFICATION

There are two parts to being a certified pharmacy technician (CPhT). First, pharmacy technicians must sit for and pass the national PTCE. After a pharmacy technician has passed the exam, he or she may use the designation of CPhT. Second, to continue to hold certification, a CPhT is required to obtain 20 hr of continuing education for recertification within 2 years of original certification or previous recertification. For more information regarding certification please visit the PTCB web site (www.ptcb.org).

RECERTIFICATION

Renewal of certification is required every 2 years. During the 2-year certification period, a CPhT must earn 20 hr of pharmacy-related continuing education; 1 of the 20 hours must be in pharmacy law. Approximately 60 days before the recertification date, the PTCB will mail a recertification packet to the candidate's mailing address on file. For more information on recertification visit www.ptcb.org and download a copy of *PTCB's Recertification Requirements and Guidelines.*

ELIGIBILITY REQUIREMENTS

You must have received a high school diploma, a GED, or the foreign equivalent by the application receipt deadline and have never been convicted of a felony to sit for the PTCB Examination.

227

STATEMENT OF CONFIDENTIALITY

On the day of the exam, you will be asked to read and sign the following statements.

PTCE CANDIDATE ATTESTATION

1. This examination and the test questions contained herein are the exclusive property of the Pharmacy Technician Certification Board.
2. This examination and the items contained herein are protected by copyright law.
3. No part of this examination may be copied or reproduced in part or whole by any means whatsoever, including memorization.
4. The theft or attempted theft of an examination booklet is punishable as a felony.
5. My participation in any irregularity occurring during this examination, such as giving or obtaining unauthorized information or aid, as evidenced by observation or subsequent analysis, may result in termination of my participation, invalidation of the results of my examination, or other appropriate action.
6. Future discussion or disclosure of the contents of the examination orally, in writing, or by any other means is prohibited.
7. My signature below indicates that I have read and understood the statement of confidentiality. Failure to comply can result in termination of my participation, invalidation of the results of my examination, or other appropriate action.
8. I understand that during this examination, I may NOT communicate with other candidates, refer to any materials other than those provided to me, or assist or obtain assistance from any person. Failure to comply with these requirements may result in the invalidation of my examination results as well as other appropriate action.
9. Under penalty of perjury, I declare that the information provided in my examination application and any required accompanying documentation is true and complete. I also declare that I have received a high school diploma (or GED certificate) by the application deadline for this examination, and, further, that I have never been convicted of a felony.
10. I agree that in the event my answer materials are damaged or lost, any claim I may have will not exceed the amount of my application fee for this examination.

My signature below and/or on my answer sheet for this examination indicates that I have read and understood the attestation statement. I am aware that failure to comply with the outlined requirements will result in serious consequences, including the invalidation of my examination results.

REVOCATION POLICY

Basis for revocation: The certification of an individual may be revoked by the PTCB for any of the following reasons:
- documented, material deficiency in the current knowledge base necessary to achieve pharmacy technician certification;
- documented, gross negligence or intentional misconduct in the performance of services as a pharmacy technician;
- conviction of a felony or a crime involving moral turpitude (including but not limited to the illegal sale, distribution, or use of controlled substances and other prescription drugs);
- irregularity in taking, cheating on, or failing to abide by the rules regarding confidentiality of the Pharmacy Technician Certification Examination (including postexamination conduct);
- failure to cooperate with the PTCB during the investigation of another certified pharmacy technician;
- making false or misleading statements in connection with certification or recertification.

For additional information on the procedure for Revocation of Certification, contact the PTCB at (202) 429-7576, www.ptcb.org, or 2215 Constitution Avenue, NW, Washington, DC 20037.

AMERICANS WITH DISABILITIES ACT

Arrangements for persons with disabilities will be provided on request, in conformance with the Americans with Disabilities Act (ADA). Physicians or other professionals submitting documentation in support of your request for accommodation may be contacted by the PTCB for clarification of any information provided in regard to your testing needs. If you have a documented disability (including a visual, orthopedic, or hearing impairment; health impairment; learning disability; emotional disability; or multiple disabilities) and need modification to the usual testing conditions, you may request special testing accommodations (e.g., magnifying lens) to take the national PTCE. You will still be required to take the exam on regularly scheduled national test dates.

On the application, fill in the appropriate space in Box 18 that identifies the accommodation you are requesting, including extra time if needed. If you are requesting an accommodation other than those listed on the application, fill in the space for "Other" and provide a specific description of your needs. Appropriate documentation must be enclosed with your application and must sufficiently explain your disability and the need for the accommodation(s). You may include a letter from an appropriate professional (e.g., physician, psychologist, occupational therapist, educational specialist) or evidence of prior diagnosis or accommodation (e.g., special education services). Previous school records may also be submitted to document your disability. Any professional providing documentation should know of your disability, have diagnosed or evaluated you, or have provided the accommodation for you.

The documentation letter you obtain from that professional must be on official stationery and include the following information:

1. identification of the specific disability/diagnosis;
2. the approximate date when the disability was first diagnosed/identified;
3. a brief history of the disability;
4. identification of the tests/protocols used to confirm the diagnosis;
5. a brief description of the disability;
6. a description of past accommodations made for the disability;
7. an explanation of the need for the testing accommodation(s); and
8. signature and title of the professional.

If you have been diagnosed as having an emotional disability, your letter from the appropriate professional should include identification of the DSM-IV classification of the diagnosis.

Your request for special accommodations will be reviewed, and the PES will notify you of the status/disposition of your request at least 5 weeks before the examination date. If you have specific questions regarding the provisions of a testing accommodation, please contact the PES at 475 Riverside Drive, New York, NY 10115 or at (877) 782-2888 for details.

If you do not notify the PES of needed accommodations at the time of application, the accommodations will not be available at the time of the examination.

The PTCB acknowledges the provisions of the ADA and will offer the examination in a center and manner that is accessible to persons with disabilities or offer alternative arrangements for candidates with disabilities.

AFFIRMATIVE ACTION

The PTCB does not discriminate against any individual because of race, gender, age, religion, disability, veteran status, or national origin. The PTCB and PES endorse the principles of equal opportunity. Eligibility criteria for examination and certification under the national pharmacy technician certification program are applied equally to all applicants regardless of race, religion, sex, national origin, veteran status, age, or disability.

ADMISSION TO THE EXAMINATION

If your application was received and processed by the stated receipt deadline, you will be sent an admission ticket approximately **3 weeks** before the test date. The admission ticket will contain the name of the test, the date on which the test will be given, the address of the test center, the time you are to report to the test center, and your name and identification number. For directions to your test center, please contact the testing location. If you lose your admission ticket or have not received an admission ticket 1 week before the test date, you should contact PES at **(877) 782-2888**.

To be admitted to the examination, PTCE candidates are required to present one of the following: valid passport, driver's license with photograph (or non–driver's identification issued by the Department of Motor Vehicles), or US Armed Forces photo identification. Your government-issued photo identification must be clear and legible. Your name must appear as it is on your admission ticket. Your address can be different however please contact the PES at (877) 782-2888 with your correct address.

If you arrive at the test center without your photo identification (see acceptable forms of identification above) and your admission ticket, you will not be permitted to enter the test center. Also, if your name on your photo identification does not match the name on your admission ticket, you will not be permitted to test. In either instance, you will forfeit your exam fee exam.

DAY OF THE EXAMINATION CHECKLIST

• Arrive at the test center between 7:30 AM and 8:00 AM.
• Bring a clear and legible government-issued photo identification (your name on the identification and the admission ticket must match).
• Bring your admission ticket (this will be sent 3 weeks before the exam).
• Bring several sharpened #2 pencils.
• Bring a silent, hand-held, nonprogrammable, battery-operated or solar-powered calculator.

   Reference materials, books, or papers are not allowed in the examination room. Your examination booklet will serve as scratch paper. Candidates who arrive after the start of pretest instructions and candidates without the proper identification or admission ticket will not be admitted to the exam and their fees will be forfeited.

DAY OF THE EXAMINATION SCHEDULE

You must arrive at the test center at or before the 8:00 AM reporting time indicated on your admission ticket. If you are traveling to an unfamiliar area, allow adequate time to locate the test center. Seating of candidates, distribution of test materials, and testing instructions will begin shortly thereafter.

   The total testing time is 3 hr. Additional time has been allowed for instructions. You can expect to leave the test center around noon.

   Candidates who arrive after the chief examiner has started pretest instructions and candidates without proper government-issued photo identification (such as a driver's license or passport) or an admission ticket will not be admitted to the examination and their fees will be forfeited.

7:30 AM–8:00 AM	Report to the test center. Bring admission ticket, government-issued photo identification, several sharpened #2 pencils, and a calculator.
8:30 AM	Instruction and examination begin.
12:00 PM	Examination ends.

PROCEDURES FOR THE EXAMINATION

You should bring several sharpened #2 pencils with erasers. No reference materials, books, or papers are allowed in the examination room. No test materials, documents, or memoranda of any sort may be taken from the examination room. Your test booklet will serve as scratch paper for the examination.

   No questions concerning the content of the examination may be asked during the testing period. Listen carefully to instructions given by the chief examiner and read the directions in the test booklet.

   You will be given the opportunity to comment in writing on any question contained in the examination that you believe is misleading or deficient in accuracy or content. A form for this purpose will be provided. After the exam, each comment will be reviewed by the PTCB Certification Council. However, responses to individual comments will not be provided.

   You also may comment in writing about test center facilities, test supervision, or any other matter related to the testing program to the PES within 2 weeks after the day of the examination.

   Chief examiners are authorized to maintain a secure and proper test administration environment, including relocation of candidates. Candidates may not communicate with other candidates during the examination. Candidates will be inspected for recording devices such as hand-held scanners, cameras, tape recorders, or other recording devices. Areas around the testing room (e.g., hallways, restrooms, telephone stalls) are monitored throughout the examination for security purposes.

ABSENCE FOR THE EXAMINATION

WITHDRAWALS

If you must withdraw your application from the examination, fax or send by certified mail a written withdrawal request before the withdrawal receipt deadline (see Examination Schedule) to:

Professional Examination Service
475 Riverside Drive
New York, NY 10115

If you fax your request, be sure to obtain a fax confirmation receipt.

Checks for partial refunds ($105) will be issued 4 weeks after the withdrawal deadline; a $15 administrative fee applies. If you do not withdraw your application before the deadline, you will forfeit the entire $120 fee. Withdrawal requests will only be accepted from candidates. Employers or family members may not request withdrawal on behalf of candidates. **Your application fee cannot be applied to a future examination date.**

MEDICAL AND PERSONAL EMERGENCIES

Requests for medical and personal emergency withdrawals after the withdrawal deadline are handled by the PTCB on a case-by-case basis. Emergency withdrawals are granted for medical emergencies or deaths in the immediate family. Please mail or fax a letter to the PTCB describing your situation. Include:

- full name and signature;
- examination date;
- test center location;
- social security number;
- method of payment (e.g., corporate check, money order);
- copy of admission ticket; and
- documentation such as emergency room form, letter from physician, funeral notice, etc.

  Send no later than 7 days after the examination to:

  PTCB
  2215 Constitution Avenue, NW
  Washington, DC 20037
  Fax: (202) 429-7596

INCLEMENT WEATHER

The safety of all candidates is of utmost concern. In the event of inclement weather, the PES will coordinate with their onsite chief examiners and proctors to determine conditions at affected test centers. Cancellation will be recommended by the PES if any one of the following conditions exists:

- a state of emergency has been declared for the test center area;
- the test center facility has been closed; or
- the chief examiner cannot travel to the test center and indicates severe weather conditions at the test center.

  If any one of these conditions exists, the PES and PTCB will cancel the test administration at that center. The PES will work through the chief examiner to place notices with local news services indicating the examination cancellation. No alternate date will be scheduled.

  Affected candidates will be allowed to sit for the examination on the next test date and will be contacted at a later date with information on any procedures that need to be followed. Visit the PTCB's web site (www.ptcb.org) 2 days before the exam for test center address changes or cancellations.

OTHER ABSENCES

If you withdraw or are absent from the PTCE and wish to take the exam at a future date, you must obtain a new application or register online and apply as before. Fees for missed examinations are nonrefundable and non-transferable. **There are no exceptions.**

RECEIPT OF SCORES

The PES will mail score reports approximately **60 days** or sooner after the examination. Neither the PTCB nor the PES will report individual scores by telephone, fax, or e-mail. Candidates who do not receive score reports within **60 days after the test date should contact the PES immediately in writing,** and a duplicate score report will be issued at no cost. Written requests for duplicate score reports should be sent to:

Professional Examination Service
475 Riverside Drive
New York, NY 10115
Fax: (212) 367-4266

DUPLICATE SCORE REPORTS

Requests for duplicate score reports received more than 90 days after the examination date will require a $15 processing fee. Please contact the PES for more information.

HAND SCORING

If you receive a failing score on the test, you may request a hand score of your answer sheet. Requests for hand scoring must be made in writing to PES within 90 days of the test date and must include the following information: social security number; test date, and signature. An administrative fee of $50 (certified check or money order in US dollars, payable to "Professional Examination Service") will be charged for each hand score request. Do not request hand scoring services until you have received your score report from the PES.

REEXAMINATION

The PTCE may be taken by eligible candidates as many times as needed to earn a passing score. A new application including appropriate documentation and $120 in fees must be submitted each time to the PES.

Applications are available from the PTCB using the Ask PTCB page or from your state pharmacy organization. Candidates may also complete an application via the Internet.

PASSING SCORE

A panel of content experts establishes a passing score for the national the PTCE using appropriate standard setting procedures, under the guidance of PES. The passing score for the PTCE is criterion referenced rather than normative; that is, it is based on a standard of performance that experts in the profession have determined to be acceptable for certification. It is not based on a "curve" as are some academic tests.

Candidates must obtain a scaled score of at least 650 to pass the PTCE. The passing score was established by a panel of content experts who used the modified-Angoff method. Using this method, each question is individually evaluated and rated by the panelists. Panelists estimate the percentage of qualified candidates who will answer each item correctly. The overall passing score is computed by averaging the panelists' ratings. The PTCB Certification Council recommends the passing score to the Board of Governors.

To ensure the security and integrity of the PTCE, multiple forms of the examination with different questions are used in different years. The passing score is not set as a specific raw score or number of questions answered correctly because some of these exam forms may be slightly easier or more difficult than other forms. Because of the variations in difficulty, the PTCE is equated. After the test forms have been equated, the raw scores are converted to scaled scores, which are equivalent for all administrations of the PTCE. Thus a given scaled score reflects the same level of ability regardless of the form of the PTCE that was taken. The range of total scaled scores for the PTCE is 300–900.

Equating is a statistical process by which scores on different forms of the PTCE are calibrated onto a common scale. Equating ensures that candidates of comparable proficiency will be likely to obtain approximately the same-scaled scores regardless of fluctuations in the overall difficulty level from one examination administration to another.

After each examination administration, individual test items are evaluated for their performance. Items identified as being ambiguous may be scored with multiple correct answers with no penalty to the candidates.

Many quality control procedures are used during the scoring process to ensure the accuracy of score reports. Answer sheets are electronically scored and the data stored on computer files from which score reports are generated. A preliminary item analysis is conducted and reviewed by the PTCB Certification Council to make sure that the examination items perform as expected and are psychometrically sound. In addition, comments from candidates on exam questions are considered at this time. This review allows for adjustments to scoring if there are flawed test items. All the answer sheets are scored following the production of a final scoring key. Score reports are then printed and mailed.

Each candidate will receive a score report that will provide feedback from the three main function areas of the examination content outline. This is done to give the candidate an idea of how well he or she performed in each area and to identify areas of weakness. The passing score, however, is based on the candidate's performance on all questions. There is no passing score for each of the functions.

RECOGNITION OF CERTIFICATION

After you have met all eligibility requirements and have passed the national PTCE, you may use the designation "CPhT" after your name. CPhTs have demonstrated their knowledge and skills related to the work of pharmacy technicians. A certificate and wallet card will be sent to newly certified pharmacy technicians approximately 60 days after sitting for the certification examination. Certification is valid for 2 years. CPhT designation lapel pins and uniform patches may also be purchased.

A listing of CPhTs will be maintained by the PTCB and may be reported in its publications.

CONFIDENTIALITY OF SCORES

The application to take the national PTCE constitutes written authorization for the test developer to release that candidate's scores to the PTCB and to the candidate only. Access to candidate scores is limited to those staff members at the PTCB and PES who are involved in the production and mailing of these reports. Group performance data will be used by the PES, the PTCB, or others designated by the PTCB for purposes of research and development and reporting to the profession. Individual test scores are provided to the candidate only.

RECERTIFICATION

If you successfully sit for and pass the PTCE, you may use the designation CPhT. PTCB certification is valid for 2 years. CPhTs are required to complete 20 hr of pharmacy-related continuing education (1 hr must be in pharmacy law) during their 2-year certification period. For more information regarding the recertification process, download a copy *PTCB's Recertification Requirements and Guidelines*.

PERSONAL INFORMATION UPDATE

Each exam candidate must notify the PES in writing of any changes in name or address. Changes in name must be accompanied by appropriate documentation (e.g., notarized copy of marriage certificate, divorce decree). The PES cannot notify you of exam admission or test results if your information is not current.

EXAMINATION FORMAT

The PTCE contains 125 multiple-choice questions plus an additional 15 nonscored questions, for a total of 140 questions. The 15 additional nonscored questions are pretest questions and are not used in calculating your score. The pretest questions provide statistical information for possible use on future examinations; this information is vital in building a quality test. The pretest questions are randomly placed throughout the exam. Candidates are encouraged to answer all questions. Each exam question provides four choices, with only ONE designated as the correct or best answer. The questions from the three functions tested are distributed randomly throughout the total exam. It is to your advantage to answer every question on the exam because the final score is based on the total number of questions answered correctly.

The PTCE samples your knowledge and skill base for activities performed in the work of pharmacy technicians. Each question is carefully written, referenced, and validated to determine its accuracy and correctness. The Certification Council and Pharmacy Technician Resource Panel (composed of pharmacists, CPhTs, and pharmacy technician educators drawn from various practice settings and geographic areas) have developed the actual test items under the direction of PES testing experts. In addition, the content framework of the entire examination is supported by a nationwide study of the work pharmacy technicians perform in a variety of practice settings including community and institutional pharmacies. The content outline of the exam, the knowledge statements required to perform activities associated with each function area of the exam, and a full-length practice test are available on the PTCB web site (www.ptcb.org).

The content of the exam is characterized under three function areas:

Assisting the pharmacist in serving patients: 64% of exam

Maintaining medication and inventory control systems: 25% of exam

Participating in the administration and management of pharmacy practice: 11% of exam

PREPARING FOR THE EXAMINATION

The national PTCE applies to all practice settings. In preparing for the national PTCE, familiarity with the material contained in any basic pharmacy technician training manuals or books may be helpful. Your supervising pharmacist may also be helpful in designing a study plan. The PTCB does not endorse, recommend, or sponsor any review course, manuals, or books for the PTCB examination.

The PTCB encourages pharmacy technicians to visit the "Exam Information" portion of the PTCB web site (www.ptcb.org). Candidates are able to access a full-length practice test, a list of texts used to assist in writing questions for the exam, and a "Useful Numbers" section that provides the contact numbers for publishers of exam study materials.

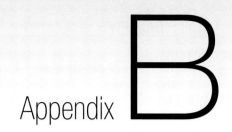

Pharmaceutical Conversions

METRIC PREFIXES

Nano: 1/1,000,000,000 of the unit of measure
Micro: 1/1,000,000 of the unit of measure
Milli: 1/1,000 of the unit of measure
Kilo: 1,000 × the unit of measure
Another way to understand this relationship is the following:

Nano- (smallest)	Micro-	Milli-	Unit	Kilo- (largest)

To move from a smaller unit to a larger unit, divide in multiples of 1,000. To move from a larger unit to a smaller unit, multiply in multiples of 1,000.

METRIC UNITS OF MEASURE

Weight: gram (g or gm), basic unit
Volume: liter (L)

HOUSEHOLD UNITS OF MEASURE

Volume:
  5 mL = 1 teaspoon (tsp)
  3 tsp = 1 tablespoon (tbsp)
  2 tbsp = 1 fluid ounce (fl oz)
  8 fl oz = 1 cup
  2 cups = 1 pint (pt)
  2 pt = 1 quart (qt)
  4 qt = 1 gallon (gal)

mL (smallest)	tsp	tbsp	oz	cup	pint	quart	gallon (largest)

Weight:
  1 pound (lb) = 16 oz

APOTHECARY

Volume:
   1 fluid dram (fl dr) = 1 tsp
   3 fl dr = 1 tbsp
Weight:
   28.35 grams (g) = 1 ounce (oz)
   16 oz = 1 lb
   2.2 lb = 1 kilogram (kg)

MILITARY TIME

Standard Time	Military Time
1:00 AM	0100
2:00 AM	0200
3:00 AM	0300
4:00 AM	0400
5:00 AM	0500
6:00 AM	0600
7:00 AM	0700
8:00 AM	0800
9:00 AM	0900
10:00 AM	1000
11:00 AM	1100
NOON	1200
1:00 PM	1300
2:00 PM	1400
3:00 PM	1500
4:00 PM	1600
5:00 PM	1700
6:00 PM	1800
7:00 PM	1900
8:00 PM	2000
9:00 PM	2100
10:00 PM	2200
11:00 PM	2300
MIDNIGHT	2400

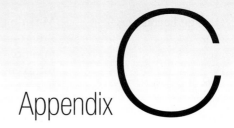

Pharmaceutical Abbreviations

Amounts	Meaning
aa	of each
ad	up to, so as to make
cc	cubic centimeter (mL)
dtd	dispense such doses or give of such doses
Eq	equivalent
g	gram
gal	gallon
gr	grain
gtt	drop(s)
h	hour
hr	hour
kg	kilogram
L	liter
lb	pound
mcg	microgram
mEq	milliequivalent
mg	milligram
mg/kg	milligram of drug per kilogram of body weight
mL	milliliter (cc)
mOsmol	milliosmole
#	number
qs	a sufficient quantity
qs ad	a sufficient quantity to make up to
pt	pint
qt	quart
ss	one-half
tbsp	tablespoonful
tsp	teaspoonful
U	unit

Dosage Forms	Meaning
amp	ampule
cap	capsule
ECT	enteric-coated tablet
elix	elixir
fl	fluid

237

Dosage Forms	Meaning
fl oz	fluid ounce
inj	injection
IV	intravenous
IVP	intravenous push
IVPB	intravenous piggyback
MDI	metered-dose inhaler
oint	ointment
sol	solution
supp	suppository
susp	suspension
syr	syrup
tab	tablet
TDS	transdermal delivery system
TPN	total parenteral nutrition
ung	ointment

Solutions	Meaning
D5LR	5% dextrose in lactated Ringer's solution
D5NS	5% dextrose in normal saline solution
DW	distilled water
D5W	5% dextrose in water
D10W	10% dextrose in water
D20W	20% dextrose in water
NS	normal saline (0.9% sodium chloride)
1/2NS	half-strength normal saline (0.45%)
O/W	oil-in-water
RL	Ringer's lactate solution
R/L	Ringer's lactate solution
SWFI	sterile water for injection
W/O	water-in-oil

Sites of Administration	Meaning
abd	abdomen
ad	right ear
as	left ear
au	each ear
buc	in the cheek
IA	intra-arterial
ID	intradermal
IM	intramuscular
IT	intrathecal
IV	intravenous
npo	nothing by mouth
od	right eye
os	left eye
ou	each eye
per	by or through
po	by mouth
pr	by rectum
R	rectum
pv	by vagina
SC, SQ, subq	subcutaneous (under the skin)
SL	sublingual (under the skin)

Sites of Administration	Meaning
top	topical
vag	vaginal

Time of Administration	Meaning
a	before
ac	before meals
ad lib	at pleasure, freely
am	morning, before noon
ATC	around the clock
bid	twice per day
h, hr	hour
hs	at bedtime
noct	at night
p	after
pc	after meals
pm	evening, afternoon
post-op	postoperative
pp	after meals
prn	as needed
q	each, every
qd	every day
qh	every hour
q4h	every 4 hr
q6h	every 6 hr
q8h	every 8 hr
qid	four times per day
qod	every other day
tid	three times per day
wk	week

Medications	Meaning
ABC	abacavir
APAP	acetaminophen (Tylenol)
ASA	aspirin
ATV	atazanavir
AZT	zidovudine (Retrovir)
BCP	birth control pill
CBV	zidovudine/lamivudine
ddC	zalcitabine
ddi	didanosine (Videx)
d4t	stavudine (Zerit)
DES	diethylstilbestrol
DLV	delavirdine
EES	erythromycin ethylsuccinate
EFV	efavirenz
FPV	fosamprenavir
FTC	emtricitabine
HC	hydrocortisone
HCTZ	hydrochlorothiazide (Diuril)
HRT	hormone replacement therapy
IDV	indinavir
INH	isoniazid

Medications	Meaning
LPV/r	lopinavir with ritonavir
MOM	Milk of Magnesia
MS	morphine sulfate
MTX	methotrexate
MVI	multiple vitamins
NFV	nelfinavir
NTG	nitroglycerin
NVP	nevirapine
PCN	penicillin
PTU	propylthiouracil
RTV	ritonavir
SMZ/TMP	sulfamethoxazole/trimethoprim (Bactrim or Septra)
SQV-HGC	saquinavir
SQV-SGC	saquinavir
T-20	enfuvirtide
TDF	tenofovir DF
TRZ	zidovudine/lamivudine/abacavir
TVD	emtricitabine
ZnO	zinc oxide
3TC	lamivudine (Epivir)
5FU	fluorouracil (Efudex)

Body Conditions	Meaning
AIDS	acquired immunodeficiency syndrome
BM	bowel movement
BP	blood pressure
BPH	benign prostatic hypertrophy
BS	blood sugar
CA	cancer
CAD	coronary artery disease
CHF	congestive heart failure
COPD	chronic obstructive pulmonary disease
CP	chest pain
CVA	cardiovascular accident
DT	delirium tremens
DJD	degenerative joint disease
DM	diabetes mellitus
GERD	gastroesophageal reflux disease
GI	gastrointestinal
GT	gastrostomy tube
GU	genitourinary
HA	headache
HBP	high blood pressure
HIV	human immunodeficiency virus
HR	heart rate
HT, HTN	hypertension
JRT	juvenile rheumatoid arthritis
NKA	no known allergies
NKDA	no known drug allergies
N&V, N/V	nausea and vomiting
OA	osteoarthritis
OCD	obsessive compulsive disease
P	pulse

Body Conditions	Meaning
PTT	prothrombin time
PVC	premature ventricular contractions
RA	rheumatoid arthritis
RBC	red blood cells
SCT	sickle-cell trait
SOB	shortness of breath
SX	symptoms
TED	thromboembolic disease
Tx	treatment
UA	uric acid, urinalysis
URI	upper respiratory infection
UTI	urinary tract infection
VS	vital signs
WBC	white blood cells

Miscellaneous Pharmacy Abbreviations	Meaning
C	Celsius
c	with
DAW	dispense as written
D/C	discontinue or discharge
dil	dilute, dissolve
disp	dispense
div	divide
F	Fahrenheit
KVO	keep vein open
m ft	mix and make
non rep	do not repeat
NR	no refill
RN	registered nurse
Rx	take
s	without
sig	write on label
T	temperature
ut dict	as directed
ud	as directed

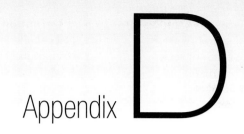

Appendix D

Drug Nomenclature— Stems Used by the USAN Council

Stem Examples	Definition
-ac	anti-inflammatory
-actide	synthetic corticotrophin
-adol or -adol-	analgesic
-adox	quinolone antibacterial
-aj-	antiarrhythmic
-aldrate	antacid aluminum salt
-alol	combined alpha- and beta-blocker
-amivir	neuraminidase inhibitor
-andr-	androgen
-anserin	serotonin 5-HT receptor antagonist
-antel	anthelmintic
-arabine	antineoplastic
-aril, -aril-	antiviral
-arit	antirheumatic
-arol	anticoagulant
-arot-	arotinoid
arte-	antimalarial
-ase	enzyme
-ast	antiasthmatic
-astine	antihistamine
-atadine	tricyclic antiasthmatic
-azenil	benzodiazepine receptor agonist/antagonist
-azepam	antianxiety agent
-azepide	cholecystokinin
-azocine	narcotic antagonist
-azoline	antihistamine or local vasoconstrictor
-azosin	antihypertensive
-bactam	beta-lactamase inhibitor
-bamate	tranquilizer
-barb or -barb-	barbituric acid derivative
-bendazole	anthelmintic
bol- or -bol-	anabolic steroid
-butazone	anti-inflammatory

243

Stem Examples	Definition
-caine	local anesthetic
calci- or -calci-	vitamin D analog
-camsule	camphor sulfonic acid derivative
-carbef	carbacephem antibiotic
cef-	cephalosporin
-cept	receptor
-cic	hepatoprotective
-cidin	natural antibiotic
-cillin	penicillin
-citabrine	nucleoside antiviral/antineoplastic
-clidine	muscarinic agonist
-clone	hypnotic tranquilizer
-cog	blood coagulation factor
-conazole	systemic antifungal
-cort-	cortisone derivative
-crinat	diuretic
-crine	acridine derivative
-cromil	antiallergic
-curium	neuromuscular blocking agent
-cycline	tetracycline antibiotic
-dan	positive isotropic agent
-dapsone	antimicrobacterial
-dar	multidrug inhibitor
-dil, dil-, or -dil-	vasodilator
-dipine	phenyl pyridine
-dismase	superoxide dismutase activity
-ditan	antimigraine 5-HT receptor agonist
-dopa	dopamine receptor agonist
-dralazine	antihypertensive
-dronate	calcium metabolism receptor
-ectin	antiparasitic
-entan	endothelin receptor antagonist
-erg-	ergot alkaloid derivative
-eridine	analgesic
-ermin	growth factor
estr- or -estr-	estrogen
-etanide	diuretic
-ezolid	oxazolidinone antibacterial
-fenamate	fenamic acid ester or salt
-fenin	diagnostic aid
-fenine	analgesic
-fentanil	narcotic analgesic
-fiban	fibrinogen receptor antagonist
-fibrate	clofibrate type compound
-filcon	hydrophilic contact lens material
-fingol	sphingosine
-flapon	5-lipoxygenase activating protein inhibitor
-flurane	general inhalation anesthetic
-focon	hydrophobic contact lens material
-formin	oral hypoglycemic agent
-fradil	calcium channel blocker
-fungin	antifungal antibiotic
-fylline or -phylline	theophylline derivative
-gab-	GABA mimetic

Stem Examples	Definition
-gado-	gadolinium derivative
-ganan	antibacterial
-gest	progestin
-giline	MAO inhibitor
-gillin	antibiotic
gli-	oral hypoglycemic agent
-glitazone	antidiabetic
-gramostim	granulocyte macrophage colony-stimulating factor
-grastim	granulocyte colony-stimulating factor
-grel- or -grel	platelet antiaggregant
guan-	antihypertensive
-icam	anti-inflammatory agent
-ifen	antiestrogens
-ilide	Class III antiarrhythmic
-imex	immunostimulant
-imib	Acyl-CoA:cholesterol acetyltransferase (ACAT) inhibitor
-imode	immunomodulator
-imus	immunosuppressive
io-	iodide-containing contrast media
-irudinm	anticoagulant
-isomide	antiarrhythmic
-iurn	quaternary ammonium derivative
-kacin	antibiotic
-kalant	potassium channel agonist
-kef- or -keph-	encephalin agonist
-kin	interleukin type substance
-kinra	interleukin receptor antagonist
-kiren	renin inhibitor
-lazad	lipid peroxidation inhibitor
-leukin	interleukin-2 type compound
-lubant	leukotriene antagonist
-lukast	leukotriene receptor antagonist
-lutamide	antiandrogen
-mab	monoclonal antibody
-mantadine or -mantine-	adamantine derivative
-mastat	antineoplastic
-meline	cholinergic agonist
-mer	polymer
-mesine	sigma receptor ligand
-mestane	antineoplastic
-metacin	anti-inflammatory substance
-micin	aminoglycoside antibiotic
-monam	monobactam antibiotic
-mostim	monocyte macrophage colony-stimulating factor
-motine	antiviral
-moxinm	monoamine oxidase inhibitor
-mustine	antineoplastic agent
-mycin	macrolide antibiotic
-nab or -nab-	cannabinol derivative
nal-	narcotic agonist/antagonist
-navir	HIV protease inhibitor
-nidap	nonsteroidal anti-inflammatory agent
-nidazole	antiprotozoal agent
nifur-	5-nitrofuran derivative

Stem Examples	Definition
-nixin	anti-inflammatory agent
-olol	beta-blocker
-olone	steroid
-onoide	topical steroid
-orex	anorexiant
-orphan	morphinan derivative
-oxacin	quinolone antibiotic
-oxan	alpha-adrenoreceptor antagonist
-oxanide	antiparasitic agent
-oxef	antibiotic
-oxetine	antidepressant
-pafant	platelet activating factor antagonist
-pamide	diuretic
-pamil	coronary vasodilator
-pamine	dopaminergic
-parcil	antithrombotic
-parcin	glycopeptide antibiotic
-parin	heparin derivative
-paroid	heparinoid type substance
-penem	antibiotic
perfl(u)-	per-fluoro chemical
-peridol	antipsychotic
-pirox	antimycotic pyridine derivative
-plact	platelet factor 4 analog
-planin	antibacterial
-platin	antineoplastic
-plon	non-benzodiazepine anxiolytic
-poetin	erythropoietin
-porfin	benzoporphyrin
-pramine	imipramine type antidepressant
-prazole	antiulcer
pred-, -pred-, or -pred	prednisone derivative
-pressin	vasoconstrictor
-priode	antipsychotic
-pril	antihypertensive agent
-prilat	antihypertensive agent
-prim	antibacterial
-profen	anti-inflammatory agent
-prost or -prost-	prostaglandin derivative
-queside	cholesterol sequestrant
-ractam	nootrope substance
-relin	prehormone
-relix	hormone release inhibiting agent
-renone	aldosterone antagonist
-restat- or -restat	aldose-reductase inhibitor
-retin	retinol derivative
-ribine	ribofuranil
rifa-	antibiotic
-rinone	cardiotonic agent
-rozole	aromatase inhibitor
-rubicin	antineoplastic antibiotic
-sal, -sal-, or sal-	salicylic acid derivative
-sartan	angiotensin II receptor antagonist
-semide	diuretic

Stem Examples	Definition
-serpinme	derivatives of Rauwolfia alkaloid
-setron	serotonin (5-HT3) antagonist
-sidomine	antianginal
som-	growth hormone derivative
som-, -bove	bovine somatotropin derivative
som-, por-	porcine somatotropin derivative
-spirone	anxiolytic
-sporin	immunosuppressant
-stat or -stat-	enzyme inhibitor
-ster-	steroid (androgens, anabolic)
-steride	testosterone reductase inhibitor
-stigmine	anticholinesterase
-stinmel	NMDA receptor antagonist
sulfa-	sulfonamide antibacterial
-sulfan	antineoplastic alkylating agent
-tant	tachykinin receptor antagonist
-tecan	antineoplastic
-tepa	antineoplastic
-teplase	tissue-type plasminogen activator
-terol	bronchodilator
-tesinol	thymidylate synthetase inhibitor
-thiazide	diuretic
-tiapine	antipsychotic
-tiazem	calcium channel blocker
-tibant	antiasthmatic
-tide	peptide
-tidine	H2 receptor antagonist
-tocin	oxytocin derivative
-toin	antiepileptic
-trexate	folic acid analog
-trexed	antineoplastic agent
-tricin	antibiotic
-triptan	antidepressant
-triptyline	antidepressant
-troban	antithrombotic
-trodast	thromboxane A receptor antagonist
-troline	antipsychotic
trop- or -trop-	atropine derivative
-udine	antineoplastic
-uplase	urokinase-type plasminogen activator
-uracil	uracil derivatives used as thyroid antagonists and as antineoplastic
-uridine	uridine derivatives used as antiviral agents and as antineoplastic
-vastatin	antihyperlipidemic
-verine	spasmolytic agent
vin- or -vin-	vinca alkaloid
-vir-, -vir, or vir-	antiviral substance
-virsen	antisense
-vudine	antineoplastic/antiviral agent
-xanox	antiallergic respiratory tract drug
-zolamide	carbonic anhydrase inhibitor
-zolast	benzoxazole antiasthmatic

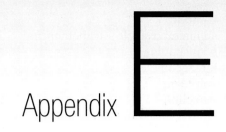

Appendix E

Top 200 Prescription Drugs and Classification

Generic	Brand	Drug Classification
amoxicillin trihydrate	Amoxil	Antibiotic (penicillin)
amoxicillin trihydrate	Trimox	Antibiotic (penicillin)
hydrocodone + APAP	Lortab	Analgesic
levothyroxine sodium	Levoxyl	Hormone (thyroid replacement)
levothyroxine sodium	Synthroid	Hormone (thyroid replacement)
azithromycin	Zithromax	Antibiotic (macrolide)
albuterol	Proventil	Anti-asthmatic
atorvastatin	Lipitor	Hyperlipidemia (HMG CoA reductase)
conjugated estrogens	Premarin	Hormone replacement
cephalexin	Keflex	Cephalosporin
atenolol	Tenormin	Cardiac (beta-blocker)
alprazolam	Xanax	Antianxiety
propoxyphene	Darvocet-N	Narcotic analgesic
amoxicillin + clavulanate	Augmentin	Combination antibiotic
loratadine	Claritin	H1 antihistamine
furosemide	Lasix	Loop diuretic
ibuprofen	Motrin	NSAID
omeprazole	Prilosec	Proton pump inhibitor
amlodipine	Norvasc	Calcium channel blocker
APAP + codeine	Tylenol c Codeine	Narcotic analgesic
celecoxib	Celebrex	Cox-2 inhibitor
metformin	Glucophage	Biguanide oral hypoglycemic
sertraline	Zoloft	SSRI antidepressant
paroxetine	Paxil	SSRI antidepressant
†rofecoxib	Vioxx	Cox-2 inhibitor
hydrochlorothiazide	HydroDIURIL	Thiazide diuretic
lansoprazole	Prevacid	Proton pump inhibitor
fluoxetine	Prozac	SSRI antidepressant
prednisone	Deltasone	Corticosteroid
oxycodone + acetaminophen	Percocet	Narcotic analgesic
warfarin sodium	Coumadin	Anticoagulant
simvastatin	Zocor	HMG-CoA reductase inhibitor
lisinopril	Zestril	ACE inhibitor
cetirizine	Zyrtec	H1 blocker
ciprofloxacin	Cipro	Quinolone antibiotic

†This drug is no longer available.

Generic	Brand	Drug Classification
sulfamethoxazole + trimethoprim	Bactrim	Sulfa antibiotic
fexofenadine	Allegra	H1 blocker
lorazepam	Ativan	Benzodiazepine antianxiety
zolpidem	Ambien	Hypnotic
penicillin	Penicillin VK	Penicillin antibiotic
ethinyl estradiol + norgestimate	Ortho Tri-Cyclen	Oral contraceptive
medroxyprogesterone + conjugated estrogens	Prempro	Hormone replacement
insulin	Humulin	Hormone
digoxin	Lanoxin	Antiarrhythmic
levofloxacin	Levaquin	Quinolone antibiotic
ranitidine	Zantac	H2 blocker
trazodone	Desyrel	Antidepressant
citalopram	Celexa	SSRI antidepressant
cyclobenzaprine	Flexeril	Skeletal muscle relaxant
amitriptyline	Elavil	Tricyclic antidepressant
tramadol	Ultram	Analgesic
naproxen	Naprosyn	NSAID
glipizide	Glucotrol	Hypoglycemic
fluconazole	Diflucan	Antifungal
metoprolol	Toprol XL	Beta-blocker
gabapentin	Neurontin	Anticonvulsant
sildenafil	Viagra	Erectile dysfunction
fluticasone	Flonase	Allergy
metoprolol	Lopressor	Beta-blocker
clarithromycin	Biaxin	Macrolide antibiotic
bupropion	Wellbutrin	Antidepressant
clonazepam	Klonopin	Anticonvulsant
quinapril	Accupril	ACE inhibitor
pravastatin	Pravachol	HMG-CoA reductase inhibitor
alendronate	Fosamax	HMG-CoA reductase inhibitor
enalapril	Vasotec	ACE inhibitor
promethazine	Phenergan	Antiemetic
venlafaxine	Effexor	SSRI antidepressant
montelukast	Singulair	Antiasthmatic-leukotriene inhibitor
diazepam	Valium	Skeletal muscle relaxant
methylprednisone	Medrol	Corticosteroid
fluticasone	Flovent	Anti-asthmatic
triamterene + hydrochlorothiazide	Dyazide	Thiazide diuretic
allopurinol	Zyloprim	Gouty arthritis
estradiol	Estrace	Estrogen
triamterene + hydrochlorothiazide	Maxzide	Thiazide diuretic
amphetamine + dextroamphetamine	Adderall	Attention deficit disorder
propranolol	Inderal	Beta-blocker
mometasone furoate monohydrate	Nasonex	Allergy
doxazosin	Cardura	Cardiovascular alpha-blocker
oxycodone	OxyContin	Narcotic analgesic
medroxyprogesterone	Provera	Progestin hormone
risperidone	Risperdal	Antipsychotic
divalproex	Depakote	Bipolar disease
methylphenidate	Ritalin	Attention deficit disorder
diltiazem	Cardizem	Calcium channel blocker
verapamil	Isoptin	Calcium channel blocker
glyburide	Micronase	Sulfonylurea oral hypoglycemic

Generic	Brand	Drug Classification
carisoprodol	Soma	Skeletal muscle relaxant
cefprozil	Cefzil	Cephalosporin antibiotic
benazepril	Lotensin	ACE inhibitor
folic acid	Folic Acid	Supplement
ramipril	Altace	ACE inhibitor
clopidogrel	Plavix	Fibrinolytic agent
norethindrone + ethinyl estradiol + ferrous fumarate	Loestrin FE	Oral contraceptive
hydroxyzine HCl	Atarax	Antihistamine
cefuroxime	Ceftin	Cephalosporin antibiotic
doxycycline	Vibramycin	Tetracycline antibiotic
fexofenadine + pseudoephedrine	Allegra-D	Antihistamine/decongestant
meclizine	Antivert	Antiemetic
olanzapine	Zyprexa	Antipsychotic
isosorbide mononitrate	Imdur	Cardiovascular vasodilator
gemfibrozil	Lopid	Antihyperlipidemia
pantoprazole	Protonix	Proton pump inhibitor for gastrointestinal disease
losartan	Cozaar	Angiotensin II receptor antagonists
terazosin	Hytrin	Cardiovascular alpha-blocker
norgestrel + ethinyl estradiol	Ovral; Lo/Ovral	Oral contraceptive
triamcinolone	Kenalog	Corticosteroid
spironolactone	Aldactone	Potassium-sparing diuretic
rosiglitazone	Avandia	Glitazone oral hypoglycemic
norethindrone + ethinyl estradiol	Ortho-Novum	Oral contraceptive
metoclopramide	Reglan	Antiemetic
minocycline	Minocin	Tetracycline antibiotic
amlodipine + benazepril	Lotrel	Cardiovascular
latanoprost	Xalatan	Prostaglandin for glaucoma
famotidine	Pepcid	H2 blocker
clonidine	Catapres	Alpha-blocker
lisinopril + hydrochlorothiazide	Zestoretic	Cardiovascular
valsartan	Diovan	Angiotensin II receptor antagonist
nitrofurantoin	Macrobid	Antibiotic
levonorgestrel + ethinyl estradiol	Alesse	Oral contraceptive
nifedipine	Procardia	Calcium channel blocker
mupirocin	Bactroban	Topical antibiotic
temazepam	Restoril	Benzodiazepine
acyclovir	Zovirax	Antiviral
valsartan + hydrochlorothiazide	Diovan – HCT	Cardiovascular
fosinopril	Monopril	ACE inhibitor
captopril	Capoten	Beta-blocker
norgestimate + ethinyl estradiol	Ortho-Cyclen	Oral contraceptive
pioglitazone	Actos	Glitazone oral hypoglycemic
acetaminophen + butalbital + caffeine	Fioricet	Narcotic analgesic
esterified estrogens + methyltestosterone	Estratest	Hormone
clotrimazole + betamethasone	Lotrisone	Topical antifungal/steroid
methylphenidate	Concerta	Attention deficit disorder
raloxifene	Evista	Hormone for osteoporosis
promethazine + codeine	Phenergan c Codeine	Expectorant/antitussive
albuterol + ipratropium	Combivent	Anti-asthmatic–bronchodilator
budesonide	Rhinocort	Anti-asthmatic–corticosteroid

Generic	Brand	Drug Classification
glyburide + metformin	Glucovance	Combination oral hypoglycemic
phenytoin	Dilantin	Anticonvulsant
irbesartan	Avapro	Angiotensin II receptor antagonist
clindamycin	Cleocin	Antibiotic
glimepiride	Amaryl	Sulfonylurea oral hypoglycemic
levonorgestrel + ethinyl estradiol	Triphasil	Oral contraceptive
desogestrel + ethinyl estradiol	Mircette	Oral contraceptive
tolterodine	Detrol	Competitive muscarinic receptor
metronidazole	Flagyl	Antibiotic
sumatriptan	Imitrex	Migraine analgesic
rabeprazole	Aciphex	Proton pump inhibitor for gastrointestinal disease
buspirone	BuSpar	Antianxiety
losartan + hydrochlorothiazide	Hyzaar	Cardiovascular
bisoprolol + hydrochlorothiazide	Ziac	Cardiovascular
nefazodone	Serzone	Antidepressant
fluvastatin	Lescol	HMG-CoA reductase inhibitor for hyperlipidemia
tamsulosin	Flomax	Alpha-blocker for benign prostatic hypertrophy
nortriptyline	Pamelor	Tricyclic antidepressant
esomeprazole	Nexium	Proton pump inhibitor for gastrointestinal disease
fenofibrate	TriCor	Fibric acid derivative for hyperlipemia
tamoxifen	Nolvadex	Hormone for chemotherapy
diltiazem	Tiazac	Cardiovascular-calcium channel blocker
felodipine	Plendil	Cardiovascular-calcium channel blocker
valacyclovir	Valtrex	Antiviral
mirtazapine	Remeron	Antidepressant
tetracycline	Sumycin	Tetracycline antibiotic
metaxalone	Skelaxin	Skeletal muscle relaxant
tobramycin + dexamethasone	TobraDex	Ophthalmic antibiotic/steroid
cimetidine	Tagamet	H2 blocker for gastrointestinal disease
nabumetone	Relafen	NSAID
hydrocodone + ibuprofen	Vicoprofen	Analgesic
mometasone	Elocon	Topical steroid
fluticasone + salmeterol	Advair	Antiasthma
benzonatate	Tessalon	Cough suppressant
phenobarbital	Phenobarbital	Anticonvulsant
erythromycin	Erythromycin	Macrolide antibiotic
triamcinolone	Nasacort	Antiasthmatic corticosteroid
phenazopyridine	Pyridium	Urinary tract analgesic
neomycin, polymyxin, and hydrocortisone	Cortisporin Otic	Antibiotic
hydrocodone + chlorpheniramine	Tussionex	Antitussive
hyoscyamine	Levsin	Gastrointestinal disease
nitroglycerin	Nitrostat	Cardiovascular vasodilator
quetiapine	Seroquel	Antischizophrenic agent
insulin lispro, rDNA	Humalog	Hormone
ipratropium	Atrovent	Bronchodilator for asthma
methocarbamol	Robaxin	Skeletal muscle relaxant
donepezil	Aricept	Alzheimer's disease
diclofenac	Voltaren	NSAID
dicyclomine	Bentyl	Gastrointestinal disease

Generic	Brand	Drug Classification
calcitonin-salmon	Miacalcin	Hormone to treat osteoporosis
doxepin	Sinequan	Tricyclic antidepressant
brimonidine	Alphagan	Alpha 2 agonist for glaucoma
naproxen sodium	Anaprox	NSAID
carbamazepine	Tegretol	Anticonvulsant
nifedipine	Adalat	Calcium channel blocker
carvedilol	Coreg	Beta-blocker
indomethacin	Indocin	NSAID
fentanyl	Duragesic	Narcotic analgesic
gatifloxacin	Tequin	Quinolone antibiotic
olopatadine	Patanol	Mast cell stabilizer
oxybutynin	Ditropan	Urinary antispasmodic agent

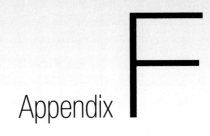

Vitamins

Vitamin	Name	Use
A	Retinol	Retinal function and bone growth
B1	Thiamine	Carbohydrate metabolism
B2	Riboflavin	Tissue respiration
B3	Niacin	Lipid metabolism
B6	Pyridoxine	Amino acid metabolism
B9	Folic acid	Red blood cell formation
B12	Cyanocobalamin	Red blood cell formation
C	Ascorbic acid	Collagen formation, tissue repair
D2	Ergocalciferol	Absorption and utilization of calcium and phosphate
D3	Cholecalciferol	Absorption and utilization of calcium and phosphate
E		Antioxidant
K1	Phytonadione	Blood clotting
K3	Menadione	Blood clotting

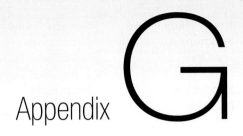

Appendix

Common OTC Products

Brand Name	Generic Name	Classification
Actifed	pseudoephedrine, triprolidine	Decongestant
Advil	ibuprofen	Analgesic, antipyretic
Afrin	oxymetazoline	Decongestant
Aleve	naproxen sodium	Analgesic
Anbesol	benzocaine, phenol	Topical anesthetic
Aspercreme	trolamine salicylate	Topical analgesic
Bayer Aspirin	aspirin	Analgesic, antipyretic, anti-inflammatory,
Benadryl	diphenhydramine	Antihistamine
Benylin	diphenhydramine	Antitussive
Betadine	povidone iodine	Topical antiseptic
Bonine	meclizine	Antiemetic
Bufferin	aspirin	Analgesic, antipyretic, anti-inflammatory
Caladryl	pramoxine, camphor, calamine	Protectant
Carmex	menthol, camphor, alum, salicylic acid	Protectant
Cépastat	phenol	Anesthetic
Chlor-Trimeton	chlorpheniramine	Antihistamine
Chloraseptic	benzocaine, menthol	Topical anesthetic
Citrucel	methylcellulose	Laxative
Colace	docusate sodium	Stool softener
Compound W	salicylic acid	Keratolytic
Cortaid	hydrocortisone	Allergic reactions
Delsym	dextromethorphan	Antitussive
Dimetapp	brompheniramine	Antihistamine
Donnagel	attapulgite	Antidiarrheal
Doxidan	docusate calcium	Stool softener
Dramamine	dimenhydrinate	Antiemetic
Dulcolax	bisacodyl	Laxative
DuoFilm	salicylic acid	Keratolytic
Ecotrin	aspirin	Analgesic, antipyretic, anti-inflammatory
Emetrol	phosphorated carbohydrates	Antiemetic
Excedrin	acetaminophen, aspirin, caffeine	Analgesic
Fibercon	polycarbophil	Laxative
Femstat 3	butoconazole	Antifungal
Gas-X	simethicone	Antiflatulent
Gaviscon	aluminum hydroxide, magnesium trisilicate	Antacid
Gly-Oxide	carbamide peroxide	Topical anesthetic
Gyne-Lotrimin	clotrimazole	Antifungal

Brand Name	Generic Name	Classification
Imodium AD	loperamide	Antidiarrheal
Ivy Dry	tannic acid, benzocaine, menthol, camphor	Astringent
Kaopectate	attapulgite	Antidiarrheal
Lactinex	lactobacillus	Lactose intolerance
Listerine	thymol, eucalyptol, methyl salicylate, menthol	Oral antiseptic
Lotrimin AF	clotrimazole	Antifungal
Maalox	aluminum and magnesium hydroxide	Antacid
Metamucil	psyllium hydrophilic mucilloid	Laxative
Micatin	miconazole	Antifungal
Mineral Ice	menthol	Topical muscle relaxant
Monistat	miconazole	Antifungal
Motrin	ibuprofen	Analgesic, antipyretic
Motrin IB	ibuprofen	Analgesic
Mylanta	aluminum and magnesium hydroxide	Antacid
Mylanta Gas	simethicone	Antiflatulent
Mylicon Drops	simethicone	Antiflatulent
Myoflex	trolamine salicylate	Topical analgesic
Naphcon A	pheniramine, naphazoline	Decongestant
NasalCrom	cromolyn sodium	
Neo-Synephrine	phenylephrine	Decongestant
Neosporin	polymyxin B sulfate, neomycin, bacitracin	Topical antibiotic
Nicoderm	nicotine transdermal	Smoking cessation
Nicorette	nicotine polacrilex	Smoking cessation
Nicotrol	nicotine transdermal	Smoking cessation
Nix	permethrin	Pediculule
Nodoz	caffeine	CNS stimulant
Ocean	normal saline	Nasal moisturizer
Orabase-B	benzocaine	Oral anesthetic
Orajel	benzocaine	Oral anesthetic
Orudis KT	ketoprofen	Analgesic
Oxy 5/Oxy 10	benzoyl peroxide	Acne agent
Pepcid AC	famotidine	Antiulcer
Pepto-Bismol	bismuth subsalicylate	Gastrointestinal distress
Percogesic	phenyltoloxamine citrate, acetaminophen	Analgesic
Peri-Colace	docusate sodium, casanthranol	Stool softener and laxative
Peroxyl	hydrogen peroxide	Topical antiseptic
Phazyme	simethicone	Antiflatulent
Phillips Milk of Magnesia	magnesium hydroxide	Laxative
Primatene Mist	epinephrine	Bronchodilator
RID	pyrethrin	Pediculule
Riopan	hydroxymagnesium, simethicone	Antacid
Robitussin	guaifenesin	Expectorant
Rogaine	minoxidil	Hair replacement
Senokot	senna concentrate	Laxative
Sominex	diphenhydramine	Sleep
Sucrets	hexylresorcinol, dyclonine	Oral anesthetic
Sudafed	pseudoephedrine	Decongestant

Brand Name	Generic Name	Classification
Tagamet	cimetidine	Antiulcer
Tums	calcium carbonate	Antacid
Tavist-D	clemastine fumarate, pseudoephedrine	Antihistamine and decongestant
Tears Naturale	hydroxypropyl methylcellulose	Lubricant
Tinactin	tolnaftate	Antifungal
Tylenol	acetaminophen	Analgesic, antiinflammatory
Zantac 75	ranitidine	Antiulcer
Zilactin	tannic acid	Cold sores
Zostrix	capsaicin	Topical muscle relaxant

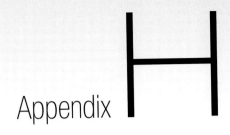

Appendix H

Laboratory Values

The normal ranges are for reference only.

Serum Plasma

Albumin	3.2–5 g/dL
Bicarbonate	19–25 mEq/L
BUN/creatinine ratio	10:1–20:1
Calcium	8.6–10.3 mg/dL
Chloride	98–108 mg/L
Creatinine	0.5–1.4 mg/dL
Creatinine clearance	75–125 mL/min
Glucose	80–120 mg/dL
Hemoglobin	4–8%
Magnesium	1.6–2.5 mg/dL
Potassium	3.5–5.2 mEq/L
Sodium	134–149 mEq/L
Urea nitrogen (BUN)	7–20 mg/dL

Cholesterol

Total	<200 mg/dL
LDL	65–170 mg/dL
HDL	40–60 mg/dL
Triglycerides	45–150 mg/dL

Liver Enzymes

GGT

Male	11–63 IU/L
Female	8–35 IU/L
SGOT (AST)	<35 IU/L (20–48)
SGPT (ALT)	(10–35) <35 IUL

CBC

Hgb (hemoglobin)

Male	13.5–16.5
Female	12.0–15.0

Hct (hematocrit)

Male	41–50
Female	36–44

State Boards of Pharmacy

Alabama State Board of Pharmacy
Jerry Moore, Executive Director
1 Perimeter Park South, Suite 425 South, Birmingham, AL 35243
(205) 967-0130
www.albop.com

Alaska Board of Pharmacy
Deborah Stovern, Licensing Examiner
P.O. Box 110806, Juneau, AK 99811-0806
(907) 465-2589
www.dced.state.ak.us/occ/ppha.htm
(through the Division of Occupational Licensing)

Arizona State Board of Pharmacy
Llyn A. Lloyd, Executive Director
4425 W. Olive Avenue, Suite 140, Glendale, AZ 85302
(623) 463-2727
www.pharmacy.state.az.us
E-mail: *info@azsbp.com*

Arkansas State Board of Pharmacy
Charles S. Campbell, Executive Director
101 E. Capitol, Suite 218, Little Rock, AR 72201
(501) 682-0190
www.state.ar.us/asbp
E-mail: *sheila.castin@mail.state.ar.us*

California State Board of Pharmacy
Patricia F. Harris, Executive Officer
400 R Street, Suite 4070, Sacramento, CA 95814
(916) 445-5014
www.pharmacy.ca.gov

Colorado State Board of Pharmacy
Susan L. Warren, Program Administrator
1560 Broadway, Suite 1310, Denver, CO 80202
(303) 894-7750
www.dora.state.co.us/pharmacy
E-mail: *kent.mount@dora.state.co.us*

Connecticut Commission of Pharmacy
Michelle Sylvestre, Board Administrator
State Office Building, 165 Capitol Avenue, Room 147
Hartford, CT 06106
(860) 713-6070
Fax: (860) 713-7242
E-mail: michelle.sylvestre@po.state.ct.us
www.ctdrugcontrol.com/rxcommision.htm

Delaware State Board of Pharmacy
David W. Dryden, Executive Secretary
P.O. Box 637, Dover, DE 19901
(302) 739-4798

District of Columbia Board of Pharmacy
Graphelia Ramseur, Health Licensing Specialist
825 N. Capitol Street, N.E., Room 2224, Washington, DC 20002
(202) 442-9200
Fax: (202) 442-9431

Florida Board of Pharmacy
John D. Taylor, Executive Director
4052 Bald Cyress Way, Bin #C04, Tallahassee, FL 32399-3254
(850) 245-4292
http://www.doh.state.fl.us/mqa/pharmacy/ph_home.html

Georgia State Board of Pharmacy
Anita O. Martin, Executive Director
237 Coliseum Drive, Macon, GA 31217-3858
(478) 207-1686
www.sos.state.ga.us/ebd-pharmacy

Guam Board of Examiners for Pharmacy
Teresita Villagomez, Acting Administrator
P.O. Box 2816, Hagatna, GU 96932
(671) 475-0251

Hawaii State Board of Pharmacy
Lee Ann Teshima, Executive Officer
P.O. Box 3469, Honolulu, HI 96801
(808) 586-2694
www.state.hi.us/doca.pvl

Idaho Board of Pharmacy
Richard "Mick" Markuson, Executive Director
PO Box 83720, Boise, ID 83720-0067
(208) 334-2356
www.state.id.us/bop

Illinois Department of Professional Regulation
Kim Scott, Pharmacy Coordinator
320 W. Washington Street, Third Floor, Springfield, IL 62786
(217) 785-8159
www.dpr.state.il.us
(through Department of Professional Regulation)

Indiana Board of Pharmacy
Mark Bina, Director
402 W. Washington Street, Room 041, Indianapolis, IN 46204-2739
(317) 234-2067
www.in.gov/hpb/boards/isbp/

Iowa Board of Pharmacy Examiners
Lloyd K. Jessen, Executive Secretary/Director
400 S.W. Eighth Street, Ste. E, Des Moines, IA 50309-4688
(515) 281-5944
www.state.ia.us/ibpe

Kansas State Board of Pharmacy
Susan Linn, Executive Director
Landon State Office Building, 900 Jackson, Room 513, Topeka, KS 66612
(785) 296-4056
www.ink.org/public/pharmacy

Kentucky Board of Pharmacy
Michael A. Moné, Executive Director
23 Millcreek Park, Frankfort, KY 40601-9230
www.state.ky.us.boards/pharmacy

Louisiana Board of Pharmacy
Malcolm J. Broussard, Executive Director
5615 Corporate Boulevard, Suite 8E, Baton Rouge, LA 70808-2537
(225) 925-6496
www.labp.com

Maine Board of Pharmacy
Geraldine "Jeri" Betts, Board Administrator
35 State House Station, Augusta, ME 04333
(207) 624-8603
Direct line: (207) 624-8625
Fax: (207) 624-8637
www.maineprofessionalreg.org

Maryland Board of Pharmacy
LaVerne George Nasea, Executive Director
4201 Patterson Avenue, Baltimore, MD 21215-2299
(410) 764-4755
www.dhmh.state.md.us/pharmacyboard/
E-mail: *md_pharmacy_board@yahoo.com*

Massachusetts Board of Registration in Pharmacy
Charles R. Young, Executive Director
239 Causeway Street, Boston, MA 02113
(617) 727-9953
www.state.ma.us/reg/boards/ph
E-mail: *charles.r.young@state.ma.us*

Michigan Board of Pharmacy
Cathy Seyka, Licensing Manager
611 W. Ottawa, First Floor, P.O. Box 30670, Lansing, MI 48909-8170
(517) 373-9102
www.cis.state.mi.us

Minnesota Board of Pharmacy
David E. Holmstrom, Executive Director
2829 University Avenue S.E., Suite 530,
Minneapolis, MN 55414-3251
(612) 617-2201
www.phcybrd.state.mn.us
E-mail: *pharmacy.board@state.mn.us*

Mississippi State Board of Pharmacy
William L. "Buck" Stevens, Executive Director
P.O. Box 24507, Jackson, MS 39225-4507
(601) 354-6750
www.mbp.state.ms.us

Missouri Board of Pharmacy
Kevin E. Kinkade, Executive Director
P.O. Box 625, Jefferson City, MO 65102
(573) 751-0091
www.ecodev.state.mo.us/pr/pharmacy
E-mail: *kkinkade@mail.state.mo.us*

Montana Board of Pharmacy
Rebecca Deschamps, RPh, Executive Director
P.O. Box 200513, 111 N. Jackson, Helena, MT 59620-0513
(406) 841-2356
Fax: (406) 841-2343
discoveringmontana.com/dli/bsd/license/bsd_boards/pha_board/board_page.html

Nebraska Board of Examiners in Pharmacy
Becky Wisell, Executive Secretary
P.O. Box 94986, Lincoln, NE 68509
(402) 71-2115
www.hhs.state.ne.us

Nevada State Board of Pharmacy
Keith W. Macdonald, Executive Secretary
555 Double Eagle Court, Ste. 1100, Reno, NV 89511-8991
(775) 850-1440
www.state.nv.us/pharmacy

New Hampshire Board of Pharmacy
Paul G. Boisseau, Executive Secretary
57 Regional Drive, Concord, NH 03301-8518
(603)271-2350
www.state.nh.us/pharmacy
E-mail: *nhpharmacy@nhsa.state.nh.us*

New Jersey State Board of Pharmacy
Deborah (Debbie) Whipple, Executive Director
P.O. Box 45013, Newark, NJ 07101
(973) 504-6450
www.state.nj.us/lps/ca/brief/pharm.htm

New Mexico Board of Pharmacy
Jerry Montoya, Chief Inspector/Director
1650 University Boulevard N.E., Suite 400B, Albuquerque, NM 87102
(505) 841-9102
www.state.nm.us/pharmacy
E-mail: *nmbop@nm-us.campuscwix.net*

New York Board of Pharmacy
Lawrence H. Mokhiber, Executive Secretary
89 Washington Avenue, 2nd Floor West, Albany, NY 12234-1000
(518) 474-3817 ext. 130
Fax: (518) 473-6995
www.nysed.gov/prof/pharm.htm
E-mail: *pharmbd@mail.nysed.gov*

North Carolina Board of Pharmacy
David R. Work, Executive Director
P.O. Box 459, Carrboro, NC 27510-0459
(919) 942-4454
www.ncbop.org

North Dakota State Board of Pharmacy
Howard C. Anderson, Jr., Executive Director
P.O. Box 1354, Bismarck, ND 58502-1354
(701) 328-9535

Ohio State Board of Pharmacy
William T. Winsley, Executive Director
77 S. High Street, Room 1702, Columbus, OH 43215-6126
(614) 466-4143
www.state.oh.us/pharmacy
E-mail: *exec@bop.state.oh.us*

Oklahoma State Board of Pharmacy
Bryan H. Potter, Executive Director
4545 Lincoln Boulevard, Suite 112, Oklahoma City, OK 73105-3488
(405) 521-3815
www.pharmacy.state,ok.us
E-mail: *pharmacy@oklaosf.state.ok.us*

Oregon State Board of Pharmacy
Gary A. Schnabel, Executive Director
800 N.E. Oregon Street, #9, State Office Building, Room 425, Portland, OR 97232
(503) 731-4032
www.pharmacy.state.or.us
E-mail: *pharmacy.board@state.or.us*

Pennsylvania State Board of Pharmacy
Melanie Zimmerman, Executive Secretary
124 Pine Street, P.O. Box 2649, Harrisburg, PA 17105-2649
(717) 783-7156
www.dos.state.pa.us/bpoa/phabd/mainpage.htm

Puerto Rico Board of Pharmacy
Beverly Davila Morales, Executive Director
800 Avenida Robert T. Todd, Office #201, Stop 18, Santurce, PR 00908
(787) 725-8161

Rhode Island Board of Pharmacy
Richard A. Yacino, Chief
3 Capitol Hill, Room 205, Providence, RI 02908
(401) 222-2837

South Carolina Board of Pharmacy
Cheryl A. Ruff, Administrator
P.O. Box 11927, Columbia, SC 29211-1927
(803) 896-4700
www.llr.state.sc.us

South Dakota State Board of Pharmacy
Dennis M. Jones, Executive Secretary
4305 S. Louise Avenue, Suite 104, Sioux Falls, SD 57106
(605) 362-2737
Fax: (605) 362-2738
www.state.sd.us/dcr/pharmacy

Tennessee Board of Pharmacy
Kendall M. Lynch, Director
Second Flr., Davy Crockett Tower, 500 James Robertson Pkwy, Nashville, TN 37243
(615) 741-2718
www.state.tn.us/commerce/boards/pharmacy/

Texas State Board of Pharmacy
Gay Dodson, Executive Director/Secretary
333 Guadalupe, Tower 3, Suite 600, Box 21, Austin, TX 78701-3942
(512) 305-8000
www.tsbp.state.tx.us
E-mail: *kay.wilson@tsbp.state.tx.us*

Utah Board of Pharmacy
Diana L. Baker, Bureau Director
160 E. 300 South, P.O. Box 146741, Salt Lake City, UT 84114-6741
(801) 530-6767
www.commerce.state.ut.us/dopl/dopl1.htm
(through Division of Occupational and Professional Licensing)

Vermont Board of Pharmacy
Carla Preston, Staff Secretary
26 Terrace Street, Drawer 09, Montpelier, VT 05609-1106
(802) 828-2875
www.vtprofessionals.org/pharmacists
E-mail: *cpreston@sec.state.vt.us*

Virgin Islands Board of Pharmacy
Lydia T. Scott, Commissioner of Health
Roy L. Schneider Hospital, 48 Sugar Estate, St. Thomas, VI 00802
(340) 774-0117

Virginia Board of Pharmacy
Elizabeth Scott Russell, Executive Director
6606 W. Broad Street, Suite 400, Richmond, VA 23230-1717
(804) 662-9911
www.dhp.state.va.us/levelone/pharm.htm
(or through Department of Health Professions at: *www.dhp.state.va.us*)
 E-mail: *pharmbd@dhp.state.va.us*

Washington State Board of Pharmacy
Donald H. Williams, Executive Director
P.O. Box 47863, Olympia, WA 98504-7863
(360) 236-4825
www.doh.wa.gov/pharmacy
(through Department of Health) *www.doh.wa.gov*
E-mail: *Don.Williams@doh.wa.gov*

West Virginia Board of Pharmacy
William T. Douglass, Jr., Executive Director
232 Capitol Street, Charleston, WV 25301
(304) 558-0558

Wisconsin Pharmacy Examining Board
Patrick D. Braatz, Director
1400 E. Washington, P.O. Box 8935, Madison, WI 53708
(608) 266-2812
www.state.wi.us/agencies/drl.
E-mail: *dorl@mail.state.wi.us*

Wyoming State Board of Pharmacy
James T. Carder, Executive Director
1720 S. Poplar Street, Suite 4, Casper, WY 82601
(307) 234-0294
pharmacyboard.state.wy.us
E-mail: *pharmbd@trib.com*

Technician Organizations

PROFESSIONAL MEMBERSHIP ORGANIZATIONS

American Association of Colleges of Pharmacy
American Association of Pharmacy Technicians
American Pharmacists Association
American Society of Health-System Pharmacists
APhA-Pharmacist.com
Canadian Association of Pharmacy Technicians
Joint Commission on Accreditation of Healthcare Organizations
National Pharmacy Technician Association

ANSWERS

CHAPTER 1 PRETEST ANSWERS

1. c—Nitrostat is available as a sublingual dosage form.
2. a—Solve using a proportion: 0.5 mcg/2 mL = 0.125 mcg/X mL, where X = 0.5 mL.
3. c—An individual experiencing nausea and vomiting may have difficulty taking an oral and keeping it down. Nausea and vomiting would not affect a person using a suppository. Unfortunately, not many products are available as a suppository.
4. d—HIPAA does not discuss consequences for violations of the law.
5. c—Normal saline is a 0.9% (w/v) solution. %w/v is the number of grams/100 mL × 100.
6. b—Because of the acidic nature of both fruit juices and colas, penicillin is inactivated by both of them.
7. c—The problem can be solved by using the following formula: final volume × % (expressed as a decimal) = amount of active ingredient (g). The final volume is 30 mL and 1:200 can be expressed as 1/200 or 0.005. The answer is 0.15 g. Multiplying 0.15 g × 1000 mg/g will yield 150 mg.
8. c—Rhinitis medicamentosa is a rebound effect caused by nasal decongestants.
9. d—Remeron (mirtazapine) is not a combination product. Estratest (esterified estrogens + methyl testosterone), Hyzaar (losartan + hydrochlorothiazide), and Lotrel (amlodipine + benazepril).
10. b—IVs go directly into the bloodstream, bypassing the absorption of the product into the bloodstream. IVs do not undergo the first-pass effect.
11. b—Specific gravity is a ratio between the weight of a substance and the weight of an equal volume of water. 1 mL water weighs 1 g; 4 fl oz = 120 mL. Therefore, 0.84 = wt of substance/120 g.
12. b—Concerta (methylphenidate) is used in the treat ADHD and ADD. Proton pump inhibitors are used to treat ulcers and gastroesophageal reflux disease.
13. b—A diagnostic agent is used in making a diagnosis of a condition.
14. c—1 kg = 2.2 lb; therefore, 154 lb = 70 kg. Set up a proportion: 12 mg/1 kg = X mg/70 kg. Multiply the number of milligrams × 5 days and the answer will be 4.2 g.
15. b—Add the totals of all of the different ingredients and you will have 2,270 mg. One must divide 2,270 mg/tablet by 1,000 mg/g to determine the number of grams.
16. d—The patient is receiving 4 doses (4 doses/day × 5 mL/dose = 20 mL/day). Next, multiply the amount per day (20 mL) × duration (10 days) = 200 mL.
17. b—Discrimination occurs when a decision is made based on an individual's age, gender, race, or sexual preference.
18. a—According to the Controlled Substances Act of 1970, meperidine (Demerol) is a Schedule II drug.
19. c—The Controlled Substances Act requires that all prescribers and dispensers of controlled substances have a DEA number. The requirement of having the physician's DEA number on a prescription shows the pharmacist that the physician has the authority to prescribe controlled substances.
20. c—The prescribed dose is 500 mg three times per day. Because the pharmacy stocks 250-mg capsules, a proportion is set up: 250 mg/1 cap = 500 mg/X caps. Every 500 mg dose would require two 250-mg capsules. 2 250-mg caps/dose × 3 doses/day × 10 days = 60 caps.
21. a—Diovan (valsartan) is an angiotensin II receptor antagonist. Isoptin (verapamil), Plendil (feldopine), and Tiazac (diltiazem) are calcium channel blockers.

22. c—The symptoms of glycosuria, polydipsia, and polyuria are characteristic signs of diabetes.
23. b—Pharmacy technicians perform technical duties. This is an example of a judgmental activity performed by pharmacists.
24. b—With any insurance plan, a formulary will be set up stating which drugs will be covered or excluded under the plan. "NDC not covered" means that the product is not recognized by the insurance plan.
25. c—Convert the weight in pounds to kg (187 lb/2.2 lb per kg = 85 kg). Multiply the daily dose by the weight of the individual (50 mg/kg/day × 85 kg = 4,250 mg/day). Multiply the daily amount by the length of therapy (4250 mg × 10 days = 42,500 mg). Calculate the number of capsules by dividing the total weight by the weight per capsule (42,500 mg/250 mg per capsule = 170 capsules).
26. c—Set up a proportion (1 g/1,000,000 mcg = 0.12 g/X g, where X = 120,000 mcg). Divide the total weight by the weight per capsule (120,000 mcg/150 mcg per capsule = 800 capsules).
27. c—Convert the ratio to a fraction; divide the fraction and multiply the answer by 100. (1:1500 > 1/1500; 1/1500 × (100 = 0.067%).
28. d—Nitrostat is taken sublingually to obtain a therapeutic effect quickly. Nitrostat is rapidly absorbed into the bloodstream by placing it under the tongue to avoid a first-pass effect.
29. d—All the information should be collected to ensure the patient profile is accurate and to reduce the possibility of drug interactions and contraindications associated with medications.
30. b—A rapid onset is beneficial because a therapeutic level and response occur more quickly in the body.
31. a—Celexa (citalopram), Nardil (phenelzine), Eldepryl (selegiline), and Parnate (tranylcypromine).
32. b—Doxepin is found in the topical product Zonalon.
33. a—Multiply the total weight of the compound by the percentage of each ingredient expressed as a decimal (HC:60 g × 0.01 = 0.6 g; precipitated sulfur: 560 g × 0.2 = 12 g).
34. b—Calculate the number of mg by multiplying the number of grains × 65 mg/g and divide by 1,000. (30 g × 65 mg/g = 1,950 mg; 1,950 mg/1,000 mg/g = ~1.95–2.0 g).
35. b—Lorazepam is a Schedule IV drug and can have up to five refills within 6 months of the date it was written by the prescriber.
36. b—Rotating medications is an inventory management tool and is done to minimize obsolescence of a medication.
37. c—According to the Controlled Substances Act, a physician has up to 7 days to provide a pharmacy a handwritten prescription for a Schedule II medication if it was called into the pharmacy. The quantity prescribed should only be enough until the patient can see the physician.
38. c—Drug Topics Orange Book discusses therapeutic equivalences of drug products; Drug Topics Red is concerned with pharmaceutical pricing and reimbursements.
39. c—MERF stands for Medication Error Reporting Form, which informs manufacturers of errors caused by commercial packaging and labeling. USP-ISMP stands for the Institute for Safe Medication Practices. MedWatch is the FDA Medical Products Reporting Program.
40. c—The basic formula is the ingredient cost + a dispensing fee. The ingredient cost can be calculated using actual acquisition cost (AAC), average wholesale price (AWP), or maximum allowable cost (MAC). A third-party contract can state what cost is to be used.
41. c—NACDS stands for the National Association of Chain Drug Stores.
42. c—Serevent (salmeterol), Proventil or Ventolin (albuterol), Vanceril or Vancenase (beclomethasone), and Azmacort (triamcinolone).
43. b—Paxil (paroxetine), Effexor (venlafaxine), Prozac (fluoxetine), and Zoloft (sertraline) are the brand name/generic names of these products.
44. b—Injectable diazepam is the drug of choice for status epilepticus. If results are not obtained, phenytoin may be used.
45. d—Solve using a proportion: (2 mEq/mL = 40 mEq/mL, where X = 20 mL).
46. b—Calculate the number of grams, which should be in the final solution (X g/500 mL = 1 g/500 mL, where X = 1 g). Determine the amount of concentrate needed to contain the desired amount of grams (1 g/X mL = 80 g/100 mL, where 1.25 mL is equal to the amount of concentrate required).
47. a—A total nutrient admixture consists of amino acids, dextrose, and lipids.
48. d—Anturane (sulfinpyrazone), Colchicine (colchicine), Col-Probenecid (probenecid-colchicine), and Zyloprim (allopurinol).
49. a—Folic acid is also known as vitamin B9 and is necessary for the creation of new cells.
50. d—Nasonex is a topical corticosteroid to treat respiratory allergies.

51. a—Adderall (amphetamine-dextroamphetamine), Norpramin (desipramine), and Ritalin (methylphenidate) are used to treat ADHD. Even though amitriptyline is a tricyclic antidepressant as is desipramine, amitriptyline is not used for ADHD.

52. b—Lodine (etodolac), Dolobid (diflunisal), Motrin (ibuprofen), and Daypro (oxaprozin) are the correct brand/generic names of these products.

53. a—Amantadine (Symmetrel) is used in the prevention of influenza and the treatment of Parkinson's disease.

54. c—Nifedipine (Procardia or Adalat) is a calcium channel blocker.

55. b—Ultralente has a duration of 18–20 hr; NPH, 10–16 hr; Regular, 5–6 hr; and Humalog, 1 hr.

56. c—Lindane (Kwell) and Permethrin (Elimite) require a prescription.

57. c—Using the formula (IS)(IV) = (FS)(FV), where the initial strength is 17%, the final strength is 1:750 or 0.13%, and the final volume is 1 gallon or 128 fl oz. Solving for the initial volume will result in 1 fl oz being required to make this dilution.

58. a—1 lb = 454 g, and the amount of active ingredient required can be found using the following equation: final weight (454 g) × %[(expressed as a decimal) 0.0025] = 1.14 g.

59. c—Losartan is an angiotensin II receptor antagonist, acebutolol is a beta-blocker, clonidine is a central acting medication, and terazosin is an alpha-blocker.

60. b—Net profit = selling price – acquisition price – expenses: ($55.00 – $3.75 – $45.00 = $6.25).

61. a—Chocolate or regular milk and orange juice may be mixed with Sandimmune at room temperature. Carbonated beverages should not be mixed with Sandimmune.

62. c—Misoprostol (Cytotec is a prostaglandin E analog), alginic acid (Gaviscon—coating agent), mesalamine (Rowasa or Asacol are anti-inflammatory agents), and sucralfate (Carafate—coating agent).

63. c—1 tsp = 5 mL; therefore, total quantity (120 mL)/dose quantity (5 mL/tsp) = 24 tsp. Solve using the following proportion: 15 mg/1 tsp = X mg/24 tsp, where X = 360 mg. To calculate the number of tablets, divide the total weight of codeine (360 mg)/weight per tablet (30 mg per tablet) = 12 tablets.

64. d—The suffix "-dipsia" means thirst and is found in terms such as polydipsia.

65. a—"ut dict" is from the Latin term "ut dictum," meaning as directed.

66. d—The Prescription Drug Marketing Act of 1987 prevents reimportation of pharmaceutical products into the United States from other markets.

67. d—Beta-blockers should not be used because they will reduce the action of the heart and cause a pooling of blood in the lower chambers.

68. b—Intron (interferon alfa 2b), interferon alfa 2a (Roferon), interferon beta-1a (Avonex), and interferon beta-1b (Betaseron).

69. d—Solve using the alligation method, where 95% is the highest concentration, 30% is the lowest concentration, and you are making a 50% solution. Calculate the number of parts of each solution needed for this compound. Next, calculate the volume by using proportions.

70. b—ACPE stands for the American College of Pharmacy Education.

71. c—Estrace is an estrogen hormone.

72. c—Solve using the following equation: final volume × percentage (expressed as a decimal) = amount of active ingredient. (10 mL × 0.004 = 0.04 g). Convert grams to milligrams by multiplying by 1,000: (0.04 g × 1,000 mg/g = 40 mg).

73. c—The Physicians' Desk Reference (PDR) is not a required text to be maintained in a pharmacy, but it may be used as a reference.

74. d—Number of tablets/day × 14 days per person × 2 persons: (4 tablets/day × 14 days/person × 2 persons = 112 tablets).

75. c—Lisinopril is an ACE inhibitor and is not indicated in the treatment of angina. Isosorbide dinitrate, isosorbide mononitrate, and nitroglycerin are nitrates used to treat angina.

76. a—The generic name for Augmentin is amoxicillin+ clavulanate.

77. b—D5W and 0.9% NS are the two most common intravenous vehicles.

78. d—Gross profit = selling price – cost: ($226.50 – $172.44 = $54.06).

79. d—Theophylline is a xanthine derivative.

80. c—An individual should be tapered off of prednisone, a corticosteroid, because of the adverse effects that may occur.

81. c—Medicare is a federally funded program for senior citizens and patients with permanent disabilities. Infants are not covered under Medicare. They may be covered under Medicaid.

82. b—Convert 143 lb to kg (143 lb × 1 kg/2.2 lb). Multiply patient weight in kilograms by dosage by the number of minutes in 1 hr: (65 kg × 5 mcg/kg/min × 60 min/hr = 19,500 mcg). Convert mcg to mg (19,500 mcg × 1 mg/1,000 mcg = 19.5 mg).
83. d—Insulin syringes are available as 30 units/mL, 50 units/mL, and 100 units/mL.
84. b—Robitussin AC in the original manufacturer's bottle of 4 oz may be purchased by an individual who is at least 18 years of age and has not purchased another bottle within the past 48 hr.
85. d—15 g (approximately 4 oz) is the maximum weighable amount on a Class A (III) balance.
86. d—The therapeutic window shows the optimum range of therapeutic effects, whereas underdosing produces very few effects and overdosing can lead to severe side effects or even toxicity.
87. b—Tylenol with codeine (acetaminophen + codeine) is a Schedule III medication.
88. b—Class A balances have a sensitivity of 6 mg.
89. d—Use the following formula: (IS)(IV) = (FS)(FV) or [(100%)(X mL) = (2%)(1,000 mL)]. One will need 20 mL of the 100% solution. The amount of diluent needed can be calculated by subtracting the initial volume from the final volume (1,000 mL – 20 mL = 980 mL of diluent).
90. d—Acyclovir (Zovirax) is an antiviral used to treat various viral infections such as genital herpes, herpes simplex, and herpes zoster.
91. b—Clark's rule calculates a child's dose based on weight using the following formula: child's dose = weight (lb)/150 × adult dose (54/150 × 650 = 234 mg). Because the problem is asking for the dose in milliliters, a proportion should be used: 160 mg/5 mL = 234 mg/X mL, where X = 7.31 mL.
92. c—Use the following formula: final volume (600 mL) × % expressed as a decimal (1:200 or 1/200) = amount of active ingredient (X grams).
93. c—5%w/v means 5 g are dissolved in 100 mL. The problem can be solved using a proportion: 5 g/100 mL = X g/1,000 mL, where X = 50 g.
94. d—Oral syringes are used to administer small volumes of oral solutions.
95. b—A filter needle prevents glass from entering the final solution when drawing from an ampoule. Depth filters trap particles as a solution moves through channels; filter straws are used for pulling medication from ampoules; and a final filter is used before the solution enters the patient's body.
96. a—Quinapril (Accupril) is an ACE inhibitor.
97. c—Singulair (Montelukast) is a leukotriene inhibitor.
98. c—Estrace is not a combination drug. Bactrim DS is sulfamethoxazole/trimethoprim; Dyazide is triamterene/hydrochlorothiazide; and Prempro is conjugated estrogens/medroxyprogesterone.
99. c—VIPPS stands for Verified Internet Pharmacy Practice, which is an accreditation awarded to Internet pharmacies that meet and maintain specific standards.
100. d—10 g (solute)/400 g (solvent) × 100% = 3%.
101. b—The problem can be solved using the following formula: (IS)(IV) = (FS)(FV), where 2 g/5 mL is the initial strength, 20 mL is the final volume, and 50 mg/mL is the final strength, which will yield an initial volume of 2.5 mL. Final volume (20 mL) – initial volume (2.5 mL) = amount of diluent (17.5 mL).
102. a—Solve using alligation, where D10W (10% dextrose in water) is the highest concentration; D6W (6% dextrose in water) is the desired concentration to be made; SWFI (sterile water for injection) has a 0% concentration and is the lowest strength.
103. c—Heparin is administered intravenously to dissolve blood clots.
104. b—Prevacid (lansoprazole) is an oral proton pump inhibitor. Ciloxan (ciprofloxacin), Xalatan (latanoprost), and Timoptic (timolol) are ophthalmic preparations.
105. a—A common side effect of aspirin, corticosteroids. and NSAIDs is stomach irritation; acetaminophen does not produce this side effect
106. b—Dyazide is a capsule.
107. c—OTC drugs do not require a prescription.
108. c—"DX" means diagnosis.
109. c—Amount per dose (1 tsp or 5 mL) × daily frequency (tid or 3 times a day) × duration (10 days) = 5 mL/dose × 3 doses/day × 10 days = 150 mL.
110. d—Normal saline is isotonic and has a concentration of 0.9%; a hypertonic solution has a concentration greater than 0.9%
111. b—Solve by using the following formula: (retail) – (% discount)(retail) = price after discount; $30.00 – (0.10)(30.00) = $27.00.

112. b—A flocculating agent is used to enhance particle "dispersability."
113. b—An order for non-schedule drugs, devices, and supplies that may be ordered electronically by fax, e-mail, or computer. A number assigned to the purchase order is to be used to track the order.
114. d—A PBM is a pharmacy benefit manager.
115. a—The smaller the gauge of the needle, the greater the possibility that coring will occur.
116. d—They sign the signature log, which verifies that they have received the medication and an offer to counsel was made. The signature log may be either paper or electronic.
117. c—HCFA stands for Health Care Financing Administration
118. d—INH is taken after a patient has been exposed to tuberculosis; amoxicillin may used prophylactically for dental work, chloroquine for malaria, and propranolol for migraines.
119. b—Using a proportion: 500 mL/4 hr = X mL/1 hr, X = 125 mL.
120. a—15% w/v means 15 g/100 mL and 1 L = 1,000 mL. Solve using a proportion: 15 g/100 mL = X g/1,000 mL, where X = 150 g.
121. c—Horizontal laminar flow hoods are used to prepare IVs and blow toward the operator; vertical laminar flow hoods are used to prepare chemotherapy agents and blow downward.
122. a—Mycelex troches are placed between the cheek and are a buccal dosage form.
123. a—Chiropractors are not medical doctors and are unable to prescribe medications; an ophthalmologist's specialty is eye diseases; psychiatrists are concerned with affective disorders; and veterinarians are medical doctors for animals.
124. c—PTU and methimazole are used to treat Graves' disease or hyperthyroidism, which may be caused by an excess of endogenous iodine from the intake of thyroid hormones or from an overproduction of thyroid-stimulating factor.
125. b—1 gr = 65 mg; using a proportion 1 gr/65 mg = 1/150 gr/X mg, which is equal to approximately 0.4 mg.
126. b—i (1) gtt (drop) ou (each eye) bid (twice per day).
127. a—Zithromax (azithromycin), Biaxin (clarithromycin), Dynabac (dirithromycin), and Ilosone (erythromycin estolate).
128. a—The monoamine oxidase inhibitors may interact with cured cheeses and red wines containing tyramine.
129. a—Darvon (propoxyphene), Demerol (meperidine), Dilaudid (hydromorphone), and Dolophine (methadone).
130. a—PCAs are used to infuse analgesics; a CADD Plus pump may be used for antibiotics; and CADD-TPN may be used to infuse TPNs.
131. a—Digibind is the antidote for an overdose of Lanoxin (digoxin); digitalis is derived from the foxglove plant, which is used to make digoxin. Digitoxin is a derivative of digoxin.
132. c—1 kg = 2.2 lb; 1 kg/2.2 lb = 80 kg/X lb.
133. c—Class A balances are also known as Class III balances; after tarring the balance with powder papers, the weights are placed on the right side of the balance using forceps and the item to be weighed is placed on the right hand pan.
134. b—Inpatient pharmacies provide pharmaceutical products to the patients of the hospital where a medication order has been written for the patient. An outpatient pharmacy provides medications for patients who present prescriptions to be filled.
135. c—A 1:25 ratio is converted to a percentage by dividing the first number of the ratio by the second number and multiplying the answer by 100.
136. c—The Prescription Drug Equity Act requires PBMs to have a "brick and mortar pharmacy" in addition to providing a mail-order pharmacy service. The Any Willing Provider Law allows any pharmacy to participate in an insurance plan as long as it is willing to meet the conditions of the contract; the Freedom of Choice Law allows participants to ask a pharmacy to participate in an insurance plan, but the pharmacy must agree to the conditions of the plan; and the Sherman Anti-trust Laws promote free trade.
137. d—Nitroglycerin does not need to be placed in a child-resistant container per the Poison Control Act of 1970.
138. b—Anabolic steroids are classified as a Schedule III medication.
139. b—Carbamazepine (Tegretol) is used to prevent convulsions.
140. a—Prozac (fluoxetine), AeroBid (flunisolide), Azmacort (fluocinonide), and Flovent or Flonase (fluticasone).

CHAPTER 2 REVIEW ANSWERS

ANSWERS TO REVIEW QUESTIONS

1. d—The Joint Commission on Accreditation of Healthcare Organizations (JCAHO) is a nonprofit organization whose standards are set to ensure quality services in hospitals and long-term care facilities. The Drug Enforcement Agency (DEA) was formed as a result of the Controlled Substance Act of 1970 and is part of the Department of Justice. The DEA is responsible for enforcing the Controlled Substance Act. The Environmental Protection Agency (EPA) is responsible for maintaining the environment and is concerned with pharmacy handling, storage, and destruction of substances such as hazardous waste and controlled substances. The Food and Drug Administration (FDA) is responsible that all medications, whether legend or OTC, are pure, safe, and effective for use in the United States.

2. b—Medicare is a federal health care coverage program for those 65 years of age and older, certain disabled persons, and persons with end-stage renal disease as mandated by Title XVIII of the Social Security of 1965. Parts A and B of Medicare cover both hospital care and outpatient services. In the future, Medicare will cover prescriptions also.

3. c—A deductible is a set amount that must be paid by the patient for each benefit period before the insurer will cover additional expenses. Per diem refers to a predetermined amount of money that is paid to an individual or institution for a daily service. Patient assistance programs are special programs offered by pharmaceutical manufacturers for patients with specific needs, who may be unable to afford their medication. A fixed copay is one in which the patient pays a fixed or set dollar amount on each prescription.

4. b—Documentation that provides detailed information on the hazards of a particular substance. Information found on a Material Safety Data Sheet includes composition of the substance, hazards identified, first aid measures, and toxicology. This document must be provided by the drug manufacturer.

5. d—Used syringes and needles should be placed in the red plastic sharps container to prevent an individual from being injured by a used needle.

6. c—Jewelry should not be worn while preparing IV admixtures because it may puncture the latex gloves.

7. c—Reconstitution involves mixing a liquid and solid to form a suspension or solution. Geometric dilution is a technique for mixing two powders of unequal quantity. Levigation is the mixing of particles with a base vehicle, in which they are insoluble, to produce a smooth dispersion of the drug by rubbing with a spatula on a tile. Trituration is the process of reducing the particle size and mixing one powder with another.

8. c—Absorption bases are characterized as being greasy, occlusive, difficult to spread, nonwashable, and anhydrous.

9. a—An automatic stop order can be found in both hospitals and long-term nursing facilities. The order will stop for a particular classification after a predetermined period unless otherwise specified by the physician. A STAT order needs to be filled as soon as possible—in a hospital, usually with 5–15 min; an ASAP order is not as urgent as a STAT order but takes priority over a incoming order; a prn order refers to an order that can be filled whenever needed by the patient.

10. b—Drug Topics Red Book provides information regarding drug costs, Orange Book provides information about therapeutic equivalence, National Formulary sets standards for pharmaceutical ingredients, and the United States Pharmacopoeia is an official compendium of monographs setting official national standards for drug substances and dosage forms.

11. c—A hermetic container is impervious to air under normal handling, shipment, storage, and distribution. A child-resistant container is a container that cannot be opened by 80% of the children younger than age 5, but can be opened by 90% of the adults. An EZ open container is one that has been requested by an individual or a physician. A light-resistant container protects the contents from light through the use of an opaque covering.

12. d—Room temperature is between 15 and 30°C (59–86°F); cold is not greater than 8°C (46°F); cool is between 8 and 15°C (46–59°F); and excessive heat is above 40°C (greater than 104°F).

13. c—A lot number identifies a particular batch or run of a specific medication. A drug schedule is assigned by the DEA based on a potential for abuse of the product. An UPC is a universal product code assigned to OTC drugs, which is similar to a NDC number. An NDC number identifies the drug manufacturer, the drug product, and the packaging of the product.

14. c—The lot number of the medication dispensed is not required on a prescription label. The following information is required: name of pharmacy, address of pharmacy, telephone number of pharmacy, prescriber's name, date prescription was filled, patient's name, name and strength of medication, quantity of medication, directions for use, refill information, and auxiliary labeling.

15. b—A Patient Package Insert is not required to be given to patients receiving prescriptions of antidepressants, but the FDA has recently announced that a "black box warning" must appear in the drug literature of various antidepressants.

16. b—Emulsions can be prepared by one of three methods, the Continental (dry gum method), the wet gum method, or the beaker method.

17. b—70% isopropyl alcohol should be used in cleaning the bench of either a vertical or horizontal laminar airflow hood.

18. c—Total parenteral solutions are composed of 50% dextrose, 20% fat, and 10% amino acids. Peripheral parenteral nutrition is composed of 25% dextrose, 10% amino acids, and 10% fat.

19. b—Geometric dilution is the mixing of two ingredients of unequal quantities. During geometric dilution, one begins with the smallest quantity of the ingredient and adds an equal quantity of the next substance in a mortar. Blending is the act of combining two ingredients; levigation is the process of reducing the particle size during the preparation of an ointment; and spatulation is the process of combining substances by way of a spatula.

20. d—A thickening agent is used in the preparation of a suspension to increase its viscosity; emulsifiers are stabilizers in emulsions; a flocculating agent is an electrolyte used in the preparation of an emulsion; and a mucilage is a wet, slimy liquid formed in the wet gum method of preparing an emulsion.

21. a—Aquaphor is an example of an absorbent base; hydrophilic ointment is an example of an oil/water base; Eucerin is an example of a water/oil base; and PEG is an example of a water-miscible base.

22. a—A fixed copay is a predetermined amount of money to be paid on each prescription; a percentage copay is a predetermined percentage of the negotiated price of a prescription; a variable copay is used when a prescription is not covered under the formulary or may be considered a "lifestyle drug," such as Retin-A, Renova, or Viagra.

23. b—The cost of a hazardous substance is not found on an MSDS form; accidental release measures, exposure controls/personal protection, and handling and storage are found on the MSDS form.

24. a—Absorption bases are anhydrous; water/oil emulsion bases, oil/water bases, and water-miscible bases are hydrous.

25. a—The drug manufacturer is responsible for providing the MSDS form to the purchaser.

26. b—Federal Law allows a pharmacy to transfer prescription for Schedules III–V medications to another pharmacy only once. The patient must have the remaining refills processed at the pharmacy to which it was transferred.

27. b—A therapeutic code of A means that the medication is therapeutically equivalent to other pharmaceutically equivalent product. B ratings mean the FDA does not consider the drug at this time to be therapeutically equivalent to other pharmaceutically equivalent products. AB ratings indicate that the product meets bioequivalence requirements. AA ratings state that the product does not present bioequivalence problems in conventional forms.

28. a—Angina occurs when an imbalance in oxygen supply and demand occurs; hypertension occurs when the systolic pressure is greater than 140 and diastolic pressure is greater than 90; myocardial infarction occurs when the heart is deprived of oxygen; and a stroke occurs when the brain is deprived of oxygen.

29. c—Potentiation occurs when one drug prolongs the effect of another drug; addition is the combined effect of two drugs; antagonism occurs when a medication works against another medication; and synergism occurs when the combined effect of two drugs is greater than the sum of both drugs.

30. d—Secondary diabetes is caused by another medication; gestational diabetes occurs during pregnancy; type I diabetes occurs when the body is unable to produce insulin; and type II diabetes occurs later in life and can be controlled by diet, exercise, and oral hypoglycemics.

31. a—A patient experiencing bipolar disease has periods of both depression and mania; an individual suffering from epilepsy will have abnormal electrical discharges occurring in the cerebral cortex; individuals afflicted with mania will have extreme excitement, hyperactivity, and possible increased psychomotor activity; people with schizophrenia exhibit extreme psychotic behavior.

32. b—Drug Facts and Comparisons have monthly updates issued, Drug Topics Red Book and the Physicians' Desk Reference (PDR) are updated yearly.

33. c—A physician DEA begins with two letters and is followed by seven numbers The first letter is either an A, B, F, or M. The second letter is the first letter of a physician's last name. If the sum of the first, third, and fifth numbers is added to twice the sum of the second, fourth, and sixth numbers, the total should be a number whose last digit is the same as the last digit of the DEA number.

34. b—Amoxicillin Pediatric drops is an oral suspension and can be administered to the patient using an oral syringe; a low dose and U-100 syringe are used to inject insulin; and tuberculin syringes are used to inject various parenteral substances into the body.

35. d—A sphygmomanometer is used to measure the vital capacity of an individual; nebulizers are used to generate very fine particles of liquid in a gas and are used in providing inhalation therapy; peak flow meters are used to measure and manage asthma in an individual; pneumograms are a two-channel recording of heart rate and respiration in the monitoring of apnea.

36. a—The CADD Prizm PCS Pump is an example of a patient-controlled analgesia (PCA) device, CADD Plus Pump is used to infuse antibiotics; CADD TPN is used to infuse total parenteral nutrition; and an elastometric balloon system is an infusion device where the medication is inside a pressurized balloon reservoir and is infused by deflating the balloon.

37. a—Glucometers are used by diabetics to measure glucose in the blood; echocardiogram and electrocardiogram are used in cardiac patients; and a syringe infusion system will contain medication in a special syringe and is infused by a special infusion pump.

38. c—A single-dose container is a single-unit container for parenteral administration only; a tight container protects the contents from contamination by liquids, other solids, or vapors during normal shipping, handling, storage, and distribution; a single-unit container holds a specific quantity of drug for one dose; and a unit-dose container contains articles for administration other than the parenteral dose, coming directly from the container.

39. b—Emulsions can be prepared using these methods.

40. c—Syrups can be made by the heat method; suppositories can be made by either the compression or fusion mold.

41. b—Suppositories can made either by the compression or fusion mold method.

42. b—White petrolatum is an oleaginous base.

43. d—Used needles and syringes should be placed in a sharps container; used gloves, gowns, and masks may be placed in a biohazard bag.

44. a—AAC is an abbreviation for actual acquisition cost, which is the price the pharmacy actually paid for a medication after receiving discounts and rebates; AWP stands for the average wholesale price; capitation is a type of reimbursement program; and MAC stands for maximum allowable cost, which is used in billing out generic medications.

45. d—A standing order is one in which the patient receives a medication at a specific time each day while they are in the hospital; an ASAP order is an urgent order, but not as urgent as a STAT order, which must be filled within 15 min of receiving it.

46. c—A warm temperature is between 30 and 40°C; a cool temperature is between 8 and 15°C; room temperature is between 15 and 30°C; and excessive heat occurs above 40°C.

47. c—Pyxis Medstation is an automated dispensing device kept on the nursing unit; Baker cells are used in an outpatient pharmacy; Omnilink RXC is a physician's order entry system; and Safety Pak is an automated bar code medication packaging system.

48. c—A medication number (prescription or serial number) is not required on a medication label.

49. b—Expiration dates and lot numbers of a medication are not found on a patient package insert.

50. a—A centralized pharmacy is one where all functions occur in the main area. Medications are transferred to the floors at predetermined times. Decentralized and satellite pharmacies are synonymous and are located near the nursing unit. A floor stock system places all responsibility on the nursing staff.

ANSWERS TO ABBREVIATIONS QUESTIONS

1. a. ac = before meals
    b. amp = ampoule
    c. bid = twice a day
    d. cap = capsule
    e. emuls = emulsion

f. hs = at bedtime or at hour of sleep
g. npo = nothing by mouth
h. oint = ointment
i. pc = after meals
j. po = by mouth
k. pr = per rectum
l. q4h = every 4 hr
m. q6h = every 6 hr
n. q8h = every 8 hr
o. qd = every or each day
p. qid = four times per day
q. qod = every other day
r. stat = immediately
s. supp = suppository
t. syr = syrup
u. tab = tablet
v. tid = three times per day

2. a. tsp = teaspoon
b. tbsp = tablespoon
c. qt = quart
d. pt = pint
e. oz = ounce
f. NS = normal saline (0.9%)
g. mL = milliliter
h. mg = milligram
i. mEq = milliequivalent
j. mcg = microgram
k. lb = pound
l. kg = kilogram
m. gr = grain
n. g = gram
o. gal = gallon
p. fl oz = fluid ounce
q. DW = distilled water
r. D5W = 5% dextrose in water
s. D5LR = 5% dextrose in lactated Ringer's solution
t. D20W = 20% dextrose in water
u. D10W = 10% dextrose in water
v. cc = cubic centimeter
w. ½ NS = ½ normal saline (0.45%)

3. a. APhA = American Pharmaceutical Association
b. ASAP = as soon as possible
c. AWP = average wholesale price
d. CMS = Centers for Medicare and Medicaid Services
e. DAW = dispense as written
f. DEA = Drug Enforcement Agency
g. EPA = Environmental Protection Agency
h. FDA = Food and Drug Administration
i. GERD = gastroesophageal reflux disease
j. GPO = Group Purchasing Organization
k. HIPAA = Health Insurance Portability and Accountability Act
l. JCAHO = Joint Commission of Accredited Healthcare Organizations
m. MI = myocardial infarction

     n. NABP = National Association of Boards of Pharmacy
     o. NF = National Formulary
     p. OSHA = Occupational Safety and Health Administration
     q. OTC = over the counter
     r. P & T Committee = Pharmacy and Therapeutics Committee
     s. PI = protease inhibitor
     t. U & C = usual and customary
     u. USP = United States Pharmacopeia

4. 3TC = lamivudine
   APAP = acetaminophen
   ASA = aspirin
   AZT = azidothymidine
   ddi = didanosine
   d4T = stavudine
   FeSo4 = ferrous sulfate
   HCTZ = hydrochlorothiazide
   INH = isoniazid
   KCl = potassium chloride
   MOM = Milk of Magnesia
   NTG = nitroglycerin
   Pb = phenobarbital
   PCN = penicillin
   SMZ-TMP = sulfamethoxazole/trimethoprim
   TCN = tetracycline

ANSWERS TO PRACTICE LAW QUESTIONS

1. b—The first five numbers identify the drug manufacturer, the middle four numbers identify the drug product, and the last two numbers identify the packaging.
2. b—The Food, Drug, and Cosmetic Act of 1938 defines adulteration and misbranding. Misbranding involves labeling.
3. b—The Occupational and Safety Act of 1970 requires that work sites are safe for the employees.
4. d—The Poison Prevention Act of 1970 requires that all prescriptions be prepared in child-resistant containers except in five different situations. The patient requesting an EZ open container is one of the situations.
5. b—This is an example of adulteration.
6. c—The Durham-Humphrey Act of 1950 allows for a noncontrolled substance to be telephoned in from a physician's office.
7. d—Nitroglycerin is one of the medications that does not need to be in a child-resistant container according to the Poison Control Act.
8. c—The Durham-Humphrey Act clearly defined legend and OTC medications.
9. c—The Durham-Humphrey Act stated that all legend medications must bear the following: Federal Law prohibits the dispensing of this medication without a prescription.
10. c—The Controlled Substance Act allows a DEA Form 222 to be valid for 60 days after it is signed by the pharmacist in charge or an individual with the power-of-attorney.
11. c—The Occupational and Safety Act of 1970 was written to protect the worker from hazards in the workplace. Material Safety Data Sheets are required to inform an individual of the hazards of handling a particular product and the appropriate treatment if one comes in contact with the substance.
12. b—The Controlled Substance Act allows for the partial filling of a Schedule II medication with the remaining medication to be provided to the patient within 72 hr or else the quantity becomes void.
13. d—The Controlled Substance Act allows for the partial filling of a Schedule III–V medication on the request of the patient. The remaining balance of medication can only be dispensed if the physician has indicated a refill on the prescription. The total number of units of medication or refills can not exceed what is indicated on the prescription.

14. a—The first letter of a physician's DEA number will be either an A, B, F, or M. The second letter is the first letter of the physician's last name at the time he or she applied for their DEA number. DEA numbers are required as a result of the Controlled Substance Act.
15. c—The Controlled Substance Act requires that a pharmacy use DEA Form 222 to purchase Schedule II medications. The DEA Form 222 issued to a pharmacy is specific to that pharmacy for the use of ordering or transferring Schedule II medications.
16. c—DEA Form 222 can be used to transfer Schedule II medications, such as Percocet, to another pharmacy.
17. b—On discovery of a theft of controlled substances, the local law enforcement agency needs to be notified and DEA Form 106 needs to be submitted.
18. c—HIPAA is concerned with insurance reform, patient confidentiality, and security of computer systems.
19. b—Centers for Medicare and Medicaid Services (CSM) oversees the operation and reimbursement of these two federal programs.
20. d—The Food, Drug, and Cosmetic Act (FDCA 1938) created the FDA and one of its duties was to review Investigational New Drug Applications.
21. d—Harrison Narcotic Act requires a prescription for opium-containing products.
22. b—Comprehensive Drug Abuse Prevention and Control Act.
23. c—Omnibus Reconciliation Act of 1990 (OBRA 90) requires drug utilization on all prescriptions/medication orders and an offer to counsel patients on their prescriptions. Failure to do may result in monetary penalties and the loss of Medicaid funds.
24. a—Durham-Humphrey Act allowed prescription to be called into the pharmacy from a physician's office.
25. c—Tax-free saving accounts were created under the Medicare Drug Improvement and Modernization Act of 2003.
26. c—The Omnibus Reconciliation Act of 1987 was concerned with care in long-term care facilities and one of the items it addresses is the use of unnecessary medications.
27. d—The Poison Control Act of 1970 allows certain medications to be dispensed without a child-resistant container.
28. d—Medicare Drug Improvement and Modernization Act of 2003 lowered the reimbursement rate for durable medical equipment.
29. d—The Prescription Drug Marketing Act prohibits the reimportation of medication back into the United States. This law is being examined.
30. d—The State Boards of Pharmacy oversee the practice of pharmacy in their respective states.

ANSWERS TO PHARMACOLOGY REVIEW QUESTIONS

1. a. Premarin = conjugated estrogens
   b. Lipitor = atorvastatin
   c. Norvasc = amlodipine
   d. Lanoxin = digoxin
   e. Zithromax = azithromycin
   f. Zocor = simvastatin
   g. Zestril = lisinopril
   h. Tenormin = atenolol
   i. Xanax = alprazolam
   j. Cardizem = diltiazem
   k. Glucotrol = glipizide
   l. Allegra = fexofenadine
   m. Procardia = nifedipine
   n. Dilantin = phenytoin
   o. Wellbutrin = bupropion
   p. Relafen = nabumetone
   q. Risperdal = risperidone
   r. Serevent = salmeterol
   s. Zantac = ranitidine
   t. Plavix = clopidogrel

u. Azmacort = triamcinolone
v. Amaryl = glimepiride
w. Phenergan = promethazine
x. Nolvadex = tamoxifen
y. Lasix = furosemide
z. Vasotec = enalapril

2. a. cephalexin = Keflex
    b. fluoxetine = Prozac
    c. paroxetine = Paxil
    d. mupirocin = Bactroban
    e. acetaminophen + codeine = Tylenol C Codeine
    f. propoxyphene N/APAP = Darvocet N
    g. triamterene/HCTZ = Dyazide or Maxzide
    h. alendronate = Fosamax
    i. losartan = Cozaar
    j. fluconazole = Diflucan
    k. amitriptyline = Elavil
    l. rosiglitazone = Avandia
    m. esomeprazole = Nexium
    n. olanzapine = Zyprexa
    o. montelukast = Singulair
    p. nefazodone = Serzone
    q. tolterodine = Detrol
    r. oxycodone = OxyContin
    s. acyclovir = Zovirax
    t. propranolol = Inderal
    u. doxycycline = Vibramycin
    v. nortriptyline = Pamelor
    w. etodolac = Daypro
    x. clindamycin = Cleocin
    y. metronidazole = Flagyl
    z. naproxen = Naprosyn

3. a. Vicodin: Do Not Drink Alcoholic Beverages
                          May Cause Drowsiness
                          Caution: Federal Law prohibits the transfer of this drug to any person
                              other than the patient for whom it was prescribed
    b. Glucophage: Do Not Drink Alcoholic Beverages
                          Take with Food or Milk
    c. Coumadin: Do Not Take with Aspirin
                          Take Exactly as Directed by Physician
                          Do Not Drink Alcoholic Beverages
    d. Cipro: Do not Take with Antacids
                          Avoid Sunlight
    e. Tetracycline: Avoid Sunlight
                          Do not take Dairy Products and Antacids 1 Hour Before Meals or
                              2 Hours after Meals
    f. Deltasone: Take with Food or Milk
                          Take Exactly as Directed by Physician
    g. Biaxin: Shake Well
                          Store at Room Temperature and Discard after 14 Days
    h. Ambien: Do Not Drink Alcoholic Beverages
                          May Cause Drowsiness

		Caution: Federal Law prohibits the transfer of this drug to any person other than the patient for whom it was prescribed.
i.	Motrin:	Take with Food or Milk
		Do Not Drink Alcoholic Beverages
		May Cause Drowsiness
j.	Depakote:	Take with Food or Milk
		May Cause Drowsiness
k.	Xalatan:	Refrigerate
		For Ophthalmic Use Only
l.	Antivert:	Do Not Drink Alcoholic Beverages
		May Cause Drowsiness
m.	Tobradex:	For Ophthalmic Use Only
n.	Proventil:	Shake Well
o.	Bactrim suspension:	Shake Well
		Avoid Sunlight
		Store at Room Temperature
p.	Augmentin:	Take with Food or Milk
q.	Benzamycin:	Keep refrigerated
		Discard after 3 months
r.	Minocin:	Avoid Sunlight
		Do Not Take Dairy Products and Antacids 1 Hour Before Meals or 2 Hours after Meals
s.	Amoxicillin Susp	Shake Well
		Refrigerate and Discard after 14 Days
t.	Lotrisone Cream:	For External Use Only
u.	Feldene:	Take with Food or Milk
		Do Not Drink Alcoholic Beverages
v.	Ritalin:	Caution: Federal Law prohibits the transfer of this drug to any person other than the patient for whom it was prescribed
w.	Vicoprofen:	Take with Food or Milk
		May Cause Drowsiness
		Caution: Federal Law prohibits the transfer of this drug to any person other than the patient for whom it was prescribed
x.	Hydrochlorothiazide:	Take with Orange Juice or Banana
y.	Ultram:	Take all Medication until completed.
z.	Humulin N:	Keep Refrigerated
		Shake Well

4. a. Premarin: hormone replacement
   b. Synthroid: hypothyroidism
   c. Lipitor: hyperlipidemia
   d. Prilosec: stomach ulcers
   e. Vicodin: analgesic
   f. Proventil: asthma
   g. Norvasc: hypertension
   h. Amoxil: antibiotic
   i. Prozac: depression
   j. Zoloft: depression
   k. Glucophage: diabetes
   l. Lanoxin: arrhythmias
   m. Prempro: hormone replacement
   n. Paxil: depression
   o. Zithromax: macrolide antibiotic
   p. Zestril: hypertension

q. Zocor: hyperlipidemia
r. Prevacid: stomach ulcers
s. Augmentin: antibiotic
t. Celebrex: analgesic
u. Coumadin: anticoagulant
v. Vasotec: hypertension
w. Lasix: diuretic
x. Cipro: antibiotic
y. Keflex: antibiotic
z. Deltasone: inflammation

5. a. pravastatin: hyperlipidemia
   b. clarithromycin: antibiotic
   c. norgestimate/ethinyl estradiol: birth control
   d. acetaminophen/codeine: analgesic
   e. atenolol: hypertension
   f. cetirizine: respiratory allergies
   g. zolpidem: hypnotic
   h. alprazolam: anxiety
   i. tramadol: analgesic
   j. quinapril: hypertension
   k. diltiazem: hypertension
   l. glipizide: diabetes
   m. fexofenadine: respiratory allergies
   n. triamterene/HCTZ: diuretic
   o. doxazosin: hypertension
   p. alendronate: osteoporosis
   q. benazepril: hypertension
   r. nifedipine: hypertension
   s. sildenafil citrate: erectile dysfunction
   t. ibuprofen: analgesic
   u. valproate: epilepsy
   v. phenytoin: epilepsy
   w. bupropion: depression; smoking cessation
   x. gabapentin: epilepsy
   y. losartan: hypertension
   z. fluconazole: fungus

6. a. sulfasalazine: sulfa drug
   b. erythromycin stearate: macrolide
   c. doxycycline: tetracycline
   d. ranitidine: H2 blocker
   e. ampicillin: penicillin
   f. acyclovir: antiviral
   g. lamivudine: NRTI
   h. promethazine: antiemetic
   i. azelastine: antihistamine
   j. codeine: narcotic analgesic
   k. carbamazepine: antiepileptic
   l. albuterol: bronchodilator
   m. beclomethasone: corticosteroid
   n. diphenoxylate + atropine: antidiarrheal
   o. simethicone: antiflatulent

    p. doxazosin: alpha-blocker

    q. quinidine: membrane stabilizing agent

    r. amlodipine: calcium channel blocker

    s. verapamil: calcium channel blocker

    t. captopril: ACE inhibitor

    u. HCTZ: thiazide diuretic

    v. lovastatin: HMG CoA reductase inhibitor

    w. sumatriptan: selective 5-HT receptor agonist

    x. estradiol: estrogen replacement

    y. fluconazole: antifungal

    z. terbinafine: antifungal

7. a. fluoxetine: SSRI

    b. omeprazole: proton pump inhibitor

    c. cephalexin: cephalosporin antibiotic

    d. pravastatin: HMG CoA reductase inhibitor

    e. celecoxib: COX 2 inhibitor

    f. sertraline: SSRI

    g. atenolol: beta-blocker

    h. furosemide: loop diuretic

    i. metformin: biguanide

    j. digoxin: cardiac glycoside

    k. sulfamethizole/trimethoprim: sulfa antibiotic

    l. ibuprofen: NSAID

    m. rosiglitazone: glitazone

    n. salmeterol: bronchodilator

    o. cefprozil: cephalosporin

    p. quinapril: ACE inhibitor

    q. amitriptyline: TCA

    r. lisinopril: ACE inhibitor

    s. imipramine: TCA

    t. fluvastatin: HMG CoA reductase inhibitor

    u. ciprofloxacin: quinolone antibiotic

    v. indomethacin: NSAID

    w. hydroxyzine HCl: antihistamine

    x. carbamazepine: antiepileptic

    y. diltiazem: calcium channel blocker

    z. triamcinolone: corticosteroid

8. To what drug classification does each drug belong?

    a. esomeprazole: proton pump inhibitor

    b. prednisone: corticosteroid

    c. acetaminophen + codeine: analgesic

    d. zolpidem: hypnotic

    e. alprazolam: antianxiety agent

    f. fexofenadine: antihistamine

    g. doxazosin: alpha-blocker

    h. citalopram: SSRI

    i. naproxen: NSAID

    j. oxycodone: narcotic

    k. carvedilol: beta-blocker

    l. etodolac: NSAID

    m. piroxicam: NSAID

    n. APAP + hydrocodone: analgesic
    o. levofloxacin: quinolone antibiotic
    p. enalapril: ACE inhibitor
    q. lansoprazole: proton pump inhibitor
    r. APAP + oxycodone: analgesic
    s. tramadol: analgesic
    t. clotrimazole: antifungal
    u. nelfinavir: protease inhibitor
    v. butalbital/codeine/APAP: analgesic
    w. ketoconazole: antifungal
    x. clonidine: CNS agent
    y. nadolol: beta-blocker
    z. doxycycline: tetracycline antibiotic

9. Identify one indication for the following herbal agents.
    a. aloe vera: wound and burn healing
    b. cascara Sagrada: laxative
    c. st. John's wort: depression
    d. melatonin: insomnia
    e. gingko biloba: memory
    f. glucosamine: osteoarthritis
    g. cranberry: urinary tract infection
    h. chondroitin: osteoarthritis
    i. goldenseal: antimicrobial
    j. echinacea: antiviral

ANSWERS TO PRACTICE MATH QUESTIONS
Conversions:
1. 1 kg = 2.2 lb
2. 5.5 kg = 5,500 g
3. 2,500 mg = 2.5 g
4. 350 mcg = 0.350 mg
5. 75 mL = 75 cc
6. 120 mL = 24 tsp
7. 6 tsp = 2 tbsp
8. 7.5 fl oz = 45 tsp
9. 1.5 cups = 12 fl oz
10. 2 gal = 8 qt
11. 6.5 qt = 13 pt
12. 7.5 gr = 487.5 mg
13. 2 g = 30.7 gr
14. 1 L = 200 tsp
15. 650 mg = 10 gr
16. 125 mg = 0.125 g
17. 2.4 g = 2,400,000 mcg
18. 12 tsp = 4 tbsp
19. 2.5 qt = 80 fl oz
20. 75 mg = 0.075 g
21. 2 gal = 7,680 mL
22. 8 cups = 0.5 gal
23. 1 lb = 454 g
24. 6 fl oz = 12 tbsp
25. 2 fl oz = 12 tsp

CALCULATIONS
Note: There may be more than one way to do many of these problems.

1. **Answer = 50,000 tablets**: Convert 30 g to mcg by multiplying by 1,000,000. Divide 30,000,000 mcg by 600 mcg/tablet.

2. **Answer = 200 mcg**: Convert mg to mcg by multiplying 0.2 mg by 1,000 mcg/mg.

3. **Answer = 25 mg**: Multiply 5 mg by 3 days. Multiply 2½ mg by 4 days. Add the sum of these two products.

4. **Answer = 50 mcg**: Convert 0.05 mg to micrograms. Multiply 0.05 mg by 1,000 mcg.

5. **Answer = 1.33 mL**: This is a proportion problem that uses both Arabic and Roman numerals (v = 5 and viiss = 7.5). Set the proportion up as 7.5 gr/2 mL = 5 gr/X mL.

6. **Answer = 6.25 g**: Multiply 250 mcg/tablet by 25,000 tablets. Divide the product 1,000,000 mcg/g.

7. **Answer = 0.4 mg**: 1 grain is equal 65 mg. Solve by using the following proportion: 65 mg/1 gr = X mg/1/150 gr.

8. **Answer = 3.0 g of antipyrine**: Using the following formula: final weight × % (expressed as a decimal) = amount of active ingredient, where 60 g is the final weight and 5% is equal to 0.05.

9. **Answer = 7 mL**: This problem can be solved by using the following proportion: 50 mg/5 mL = 70 mg/X mL.

10. **Answer = 5,000 mcg**: Solve using a proportion 20 mg/2 mL = X mg/0.5 mL, where X = 5 mg. Convert 5 mg to mcg by multiplying by 1,000 mcg/mg.

11. **Answer = 187.5–375 mg.** Convert pounds to kilograms (165 lb × 1 kg/2.2 lb). Multiply the weight in kilograms by 2.5 mg to obtain the lower dosage and multiply the weight in kilograms to obtain the upper dosage.

12. **Answer = 49 capsules.** Convert pounds to kilograms (154 lb × 1 kg/2.2 lb). Multiply the weight in kilograms by 25 mg/kg to obtain the dose per day. Multiply the daily dose by 7 days. Divide the total dose by 250 mg per capsule to obtain the number of capsules needed.

13. **Answer = 9.54 mL.** Convert pounds to kilograms (140 lb × 1 kg/2.2 lb). Multiple the weight in kilograms by 15 mg/kg to obtain the daily dosage required. To calculate volume desired, solve using a proportion: 100 mg/mL = daily dosage/X mL.

14. **Answer = 0.6 mL.** This can be solved using a proportion 250 mg/10 mL = 15 mg/X mL. Cross multiplying and dividing will provide you with the answer.

15. **Answer = 12.5 mg.** Convert weight in pounds to kilograms (55 lb × 1 kg/2.2 lb). Multiply weight in kilograms by 500 mcg/kg to obtain the correct dose in mcg. Convert mcg to mg by multiplying mcg by 1 mg/1,000 mcg.

16. **Answer = 0.5 mL.** The problem can be solved by using two proportions. First, convert 330 mcg to mg (1,000 mcg/1 mg = 330 mcg/ X mg, where X = 0.330 mg). Next, calculate the number of milliliters by using the following: 6.6 mg/mL = 0.330 mg/X mL).

17. **Answer = 0.58 mL.** This can be solved using proportions. 2.5 mg/2 mL = 0.725 mg/X mL.

18. **Answer = 1.2 mL.** This can be solved using a proportion. 80 mg/mL = 100 mg/X mL.

19. **Answer = 10 g.** Convert 20 mg to grams by using the following proportion: 1,000 mg/1 g = 20 mg/X g, where X = 0.02 g. Next, determine the number of mL in 0.5 L by using a proportion 1 L/1,000 mL = 0.5 L/X mL, where X = 500 mL. Next, use a proportion to solve for the number of grams: 0.02 g/1 mL = X g/500 mL, where X = 10 g.

20. **Answer = 32 doses.** One tablespoon is equal to 15 mL and 1 pint is equal to 480 mL. Solve using a proportion: 15 mL/1 dose = 480 mL/X doses, where X = 32 doses.

21. **Answer = 56 tablets.** Solve using the following proportion: 75 mg dose/1 tablet = 300 mg dose/X tablets, which is 4 tablets. "BID" means twice per day. Solve for the number of tablets: 4 tablets/dose × 2 doses/day × 7 days = 56 tablets.

22. **Answer = 4%.** Convert the ratio to a proportion (1:25 is equal to 1/25). Next, multiply 1/25 by 100 to obtain the answer of 4%.

23. **Answer = 0.5%.** Convert the ratio to a proportion (1:200 is equal to 1/200). Next, multiply 1/200 by 100 to obtain the answer of 0.5%.

24. **Answer = 77°F.** Solve by using the formula 9C = 5F – 160, where you substitute the C for 25: (9)(25) = (5)(F) – 160 and perform the necessary operations.

25. **Answer = 18.33°C.** Solve by using the formula 9C = 5F − 160, where you substitute the F for 65: (9)(C) = (5)(65) − 160 and perform the necessary operations.
26. **Answer = 104°F.** Solve by using the formula 9C = 5F − 160, where you substitute the C for 40: (9)(40) = (5)(F) − 160 and perform the necessary operations.
27. **Answer = 7°C.** Solve by using the formula 9C = 5F − 160, where you substitute the F for 45: (9)(C) = (5)(F) − 160 and perform the necessary operations.
28. **Answer = 0.48 mL.** This can be solved as a proportion using international units; 500,000 units/1.2 mL = 200,000 units/X mL.
29. **Answer = 1.0 mL.** This is a proportion problem. 50 units/2 mL = 25 units/X mL, where X = 1.0 mL.
30. **Answer = 3.5 mL.** This is a proportion problem. 50,000 units/ 1 mL = 175,000 units/X mL, where X = 3.5 mL.
31. **Answer = 3 packets.** This is a proportion problem using mEq. 20 mEq/1 packet = 60 mEq/X packets, where X = 3 packets.
32. **Answer = 7.5 mL.** Solve this problem using the following proportion: 40 mEq/tbsp = 20 mEq/X mL, where X = 7.5 mL.
33. **Answer = 800 doses.** Convert 0.120 g to mcg (1,000,000 mcg/1 g = X mcg/0.120 g, where X = 120,000 mcg). Calculate the number of doses using a proportion: 150 mcg/1 dose = 120,000 mcg/X doses, where X = 800 doses.
34. **Answer = 200 mL.** The patient is to take 250 mg four times per day for 10 days. 250 mg is contained in a 1 tsp (5 mL) dose: (5 mL/dose)(4 doses/day)(10 days) = 200 mL.
35. **Answer = 7.5 mL.** Convert 25 lb to kilograms using the following proportion: 2.2 lb/1 kg = 25 lb/X kg, where X = 11.36 kg. Multiply patient's weight (kg) by the dose (4 mg/kg) or (4 mg/kg)(11.36 kg) = 45.45 mg. Calculate the number of milliliters needed: 30 mg/5 mL = 45.45 mg/X mL, where X = 7.5 mL.
36. **Answer = 108 mg/kg.** Convert the weight of the child in pounds to kg by dividing 33 lb by 2.2 lb/kg, which equals 15 kg. Calculate the amount of aspirin the child consumed by multiplying 20 tablets by 81 mg/tablet, which equals 1,620 mg. Solve using a proportion: 1,620 mg/15 kg = X mg/1 kg, which equals 108 mg/kg.
37. **Answer = 166.67 mg/kg.** Calculate the weight in kilograms by dividing 44 lb by 2.2 lb/kg, which equals 20 kg. Calculate the number of milligrams per day by multiplying 25 mg/kg/day by 20 kg, which equals 500 mg. The patient is to receive three equal doses. Divide the total amount of medication by three doses (500 mg/3 doses = 166.67 mg/dose).
38. **Answer = 25 mg.** Solve using Young's rule. Young's rule = {age (in years)/[age (in years) + 12]} × adult dose. In this problem, the child is 4 years old and the adult dose is 100 mg. Substituting into the equation will result in the following: [4/(4+12)] × 100 mg = 25 mg.
39. **Answer = 50 mg.** Solve by using Young's rule. 36 months/12 months/year = 3 years. [(3)/(3+12)] × 250 mg = 50 mg.
40. **Answer = 17 mg.** Solve using Young's rule: [2.5/(2.5 +12)] × 100 mg = 17 mg.
41. **Answer = 15 mg.** Solve using Clark's rule. Clark's rule = [weight (lb)/150] × adult dose = amount of dose (45/150) × 50 mg = 15 mg.
42. **Answer = 5 mL.** Solve using Clark's rule: (50/150) × 15 mL = 5 mL.
43. **Answer = 200 mg.** Solve using Clark's rule: (60/150) × 500 mg = 200 mg.
44. **Answer = 16.5 mg.** Solve using Clark's rule. First convert kilograms to pounds: 1 kg/2.2 lb = 15 kg/X lb, in which X equals 33 lb. Substitute into the equation: (33/150) × 75 mg = 16.5 mg.
45. **Answer = 0.76.** Specific gravity (SG) = weight of a substance/weight of an equal volume of water, where 1 mL of water weighs 1 g. You have been given the weight (95 g) and volume of the substance (125 mL = 125 g). SG = 95/125 or 0.76.
46. **Answer = 76 mL.** Specific gravity = 1.05 and weight is 80 g. Substituting into the equation for specific gravity: 1.05 = 80/X, where X = 76 mL.
47. **Answer = 125 g.** Specific gravity is 1.25 and equal volume of liquid is 100 mL. Substituting into the equation for specific gravity: 1.25 = X/100, where X = 125 g.
48. **Answer = 0.8.** Weight of substance is 60 g and it occupies a volume of 75 mL. Substituting into the equation for specific gravity: SG = 60/75, where the SG = 0.8.
49. **Answer = 2.5 g.** 1 L = 1000 mL. Convert % to a decimal (%/100 or 0.25%/100 = 0.0025). Solve using the following equation: final volume (FV) × % (expressed as a decimal) = amount of active ingredient

(AI). 1,000 mL × 0.0025 = 2.5 g of silver nitrate. In this situation, because it is a solution (w/v), the AI will be expressed in g.

50. **Answer = 22.7 g.** 1 lb = 454 g. Convert the % (5%) to a decimal (0.05). Solve using the following equation: FW × % (decimal) = amount of AI (g) or 454 g × 0.05 = 22.7 g. The AI is expressed in g because it is a w/w problem.

51. **Answer = 1.125 g.** Convert % (0.45%) to a decimal (0.0045). Solve using the following equation: FV × % (decimal) = amount of AI (g) or 250 mL × 0.0045 = 1.125 g. The answer must be expressed in g because it is a w/v problem.

52. **Answer = 5 g.** 1:200 is a ratio. 1 L = 1,000 mL. Convert ratio (1:200) to a fraction (1/200) and express the answer as a decimal (0.05). This is a w/v problem and can be solved using the following: FV (1,000 mL) × percent as a decimal (0.005) = amount of AI (5 g).

53. **Answer = 10,000 mcg.** Convert ratio (1:100) to a fraction (1/100) to a decimal (0.01). In this problem, the FV (1.0 mL) × % as a decimal (0.01) = 0.01 g. One is asked to answer the problem in micrograms, which can be converted by (0.01 g) (1,000 mg/1 g) (1,000 mcg/1 mg) = 10,000 mcg.

54. **Answer = 4.88%.** This is a dilution problem and can be solved using the following equation: initial strength (IS) × initial weight (IW) = final strength (FS) × final weight (FW). IS = 5%, IW = 120 g, FS (unknown), FW = 123 g. (5%)(120 g) = (X%)(123 g), where X = 4.88%.

55. **Answer = 60 tablets.** 8 oz of ointment is approximately 240 g. The problem can be solved using the following equation: FW × % (decimal) = amount of AI (g) or 240 g × 0.15 = 36 g or 3,600 mg (36 g × 1,000 mg/g) of active ingredient. To calculate the number of tablets needed, divide the total amount of AI by the weight of one tablet, which is 36,000 mg/600 mg/tablet = 60 tablets.

56. **Answer = 30 mL.** This is a dilution problem and can be solved using (IS)(IV) = (FS)(FV), where IS (3%), IV (unknown), FS (1:200), and FV (6 oz). One needs to make sure that both the strengths and volumes are in common terms. Convert the ratio (1:200) to a fraction (1/200) to a decimal (0.005) to a percent (0.005 × 100 = 0.5%). Next, convert ounces (6 oz) to milliliters: (6 oz)(30 mL/oz) = 180 mL. Substitute into the following equation: (IS)(IV) = (FS)(FV) or (IV)(3%) = (0.5%)(180 mL), where IV is 30 mL.

57. **Answer = 64%.** This is a dilution problem and can be solved using the following: (IS) (IV) = (FS)(FV), where IS = unknown, IV = 2 oz, FS = 4%, and FV = 32 oz (4 bottles × 8 oz/bottle). (IS)(2 oz) = (4%)(32 oz), where IS = 64%.

58. **Answer = 6.67 mL.** This is a dilution problem and can be solved using (IS)(IV) = (FS)(FV), where IS = 75%, IV = unknown, FS = 4%, and FV = 125 mL: (75%)(IV) = (4%)(125 mL), where IV = 6.67 mL.

59. **Answer = 2.5%.** 1 L = 1,000 mL. This is a dilution problem, where IS = 25%, IV = 100 mL, FS = unknown, and FV = 1,000 mL: (25%)(100 mL) = (FS)(1,000 mL), where FV = 2.5%.

60. **Answer = 76.8 mL.** This is a dilution problem, where IS = 75%, IV = unknown, FS = 72%, and FV = 80 mL: (75%)(IV) = (72%)(80 mL), where IV = 76.8 mL.

61. **Answer = 476 mL.** 1 gallon = 3,840 mL. This is a dilution problem, where IS = 10%, IV = unknown, FS = 1.24%, and FV = 3,840 mL: (10%)(IV) = (1.24%)(3,840 mL), where IV = 476 mL.

62. **Answer = 51 g.** One ounce (wt) is approximately 30 g. This is a dilution problem, where IS = 10%, IW = 120 g (4 oz × 30 g/oz), FS = 7%, and FW = unknown: (10%)(120 g) = (75%)(FW) where FW = 171 g. The problem is asking for the amount of diluent to be added. FW – IW = amount of diluent or 171 g– 120 g = 51 g of diluent.

63. **Answer = 10 mL.** This is a dilution problem, where the concentrations are expressed as ratios, but can be solved in the same way. IS = 1:20, IV = unknown, FS = 1:100, and FV = 50 mL: (1:20)(IV) = (1:100)(50 mL), where IV = 10 mL.

64. **Answer = 91.94 mL.** This is a dilution problem using ratios as concentrations. IS = 1:6, IV = unknown, FS = 1:8, and FV = 125 mL: (1:6)(IV) = (1:8)(125 mL), where IV = 91.94 mL.

65. **Answer = 33 mL.** This is a dilution problem using ratios as concentrations. IS = 1:2, IV = unknown, FS = 1:3, and FV = 50 mL: (1:2)(IV) = (1:3)(50 mL), where IV = 33 mL.

66. **Answer = 25 mL.** 2 L = 2,000 mL (2 liters × 1000 mL/L). This is a dilution problem using ratios as concentrations. IS = 1:50, IV = unknown, FS = 1:4,000, and FV = 2,000 mL, where IV = 25 mL.

67. **Answer = 750 mL.** This is a dilution problem using ratios as concentrations. IS = 1:2,000, IV = 500 mL, FS = 1:5,000, and FV = unknown: (1:2,000)(500 mL) = (1:5,000)(FS), where FS = 1,250 mL. The problem is asking for the amount of diluent to be added and can be calculated by subtracting the initial volume from the final volume. 1,250 mL – 500 mL = 750 mL of diluent.

68. **Answer = 2,400 mL.** 1 quart = 960 mL. This is a dilution problem asking for the amount of diluent (water) to be added in preparing this compound. IS = 70%, IV = 960 mL, FS = 20%, and FV = unknown: (70%)(960 mL) = (20%)(FV), where FV = 3,360 mL. FV – IV = amount of diluent to be added or 3,360 mL – 960 mL = 2,400 mL.

69. **Answer = 1 mL.** This is a dilution problem using concentration expressed as mg/mL but can be solved the same way. IS = 5 mg/mL, IV = unknown, FS = 0.5 mg/mL, and FV = 10 mL: (5 mg/mL)(IV) = (0.5 mg/mL)(10 mL), where IV = 1 mL.

70. **Answer = 3.75 mL of cefazolin; 11.25 mL of diluent.** This is a dilution problem that can be solved using the following formula : (IS)(IV) = (FS)(FV), where the IS = 1 g/5 mL or (1,000 mg/5 mL), IV is unknown, the FS is 50 mg/mL, and the FV is 15 mL. (1,000 mg/5 mL)(IV) = (50 mg/mL)(15 mL), where the IV = 3.75 of cefazolin. The problem asks for the amount of diluent that is needed and can be solved using (FV) – (IV) = amount of diluent: (15 mL) – (3.75 mL) = 11.25 mL of diluent.

71. **Answer = 3 mL of vitamin B12 and 27 mL of diluent.** This is a dilution problem that can be solved using the following formula: (IS)(IV) = (FS)(FV), where the IS = 1 mg/mL or 1,000 mcg/mL, IV is unknown, FS = 100 mcg/mL, and FV = 30 mL: (1,000 mcg/mL)(IV) = (100 mcg/mL)(30 mL), where IV = 3 mL. The amount of diluent = FV – IV or 30 mL – 3 mL = 27 mL.

72. **Answer = 30 mL.** This is a dilution problem where concentrations are expressed as a concentration and a percentage. The concentrations need to be expressed in the same terms. Convert the ratio (1:4) to a percent (25%). This is a dilution problem that can be solved using the following formula: (IS)(IV) = (FS)(FV), where IS = 30%, IV is unknown, FS = 25%, and FV = 36 mL: (30%)(IV) = (25%)(36 mL), where IV = 30 mL.

73. **Answer = 0.35 mL.** This is a dilution where concentrations are expressed as both % and g/mL and therefore the concentrations must be expressed in the same terms; 28% means that that 28 g are in 100 mL of solution or 0.28 g/mL. IS = 42 g/mL, IV is unknown, FS = 0.28 g/mL, and FV = 52 mL: (42 g/mL)(IV) = (0.28 g/mL)(52 mL), where X = 0.35 mL.

74. **Answer = 1 mL.** This is a dilution problem with concentrations expressed as both % and a ratio. Convert 1:100,000 to a percent (0.001%); IS = 0.5%, IV is unknown, FS = 1/100,000, and FV = 500 mL: (0.5%)(IV) = (0.001%)(500 mL), where IV = 1 mL.

75. **Answer = 0.96 mL.** This is a dilution problem with strengths being expressed as both percents and mg/L. w/v% is the number of grams per 100 mL of solution. Convert 100 mg/1,000 mL to a percent, which is 0.01%.

76. **Answer = 379 mL.** This is a dilution problem with concentrations expressed in percents. IS = 95%, IV is unknown, FS = 75%, and the FV is 1 pint (480 mL): (95%) × (IV) = (75%) × (480 mL), where X = 379 mL.

77. **Answer = 95%-5:9; 50%-4:9.** This is an alligation problem. Draw a tic-tac-toe table, placing the highest concentration (95%) in the upper left hand corner, the desired is the concentration (75%) in the middle, and the lowest concentration (50%) in the bottom left hand corner. Subtract the concentrations in a diagonal manner and place the number opposite the remaining concentration. 95% – 75% = 20 parts of 50%. 75% – 50% = 25 parts of 95%. Total all of the parts (45); 95% will require 25/45 (5:9) and 50% will require 20/45 (4:9).

78. **Answer = 7.5%-55.6 mL; 1:2,000-64.4 mL.** This is an alligation problem. Convert 1:2,000 to a percent (0.5%). Draw a tic-tac-toe table, placing the highest concentration (7.5%) in the upper left hand corner, the desired concentration (3.5%) in the middle, and the lowest concentration in the bottom left hand corner (0.5%). Subtract the concentrations in a diagonal manner and place the number opposite the remaining concentration. Calculate the proportions of each needed and multiply by the quantity to be prepared. 7.5%: (3 parts/7 parts) × 120 mL = 55.6 mL; 0.5%: (4 parts/7 parts) × 120 mL = 64.4 mL.

79. **Answer = 2.5%-109 mL; 0.9%-391 mL.** This is an alligation problem. Draw a tic-tac-toe table, placing the highest concentration (2.5) in the upper left hand corner, the desired concentration (1.25) in the middle, and the lowest concentration (0.9%) in the bottom left hand corner. Subtract the concentrations in a diagonal manner and place the number opposite the remaining concentration. Calculate the proportions of each needed and multiply by the quantity to be prepared. 2.5%: (0.4 parts/1.65 parts) × 500 mL = 109 mL; 0.9%: (1.25 parts/1.65 parts) × 500 mL = 391 mL.

80. **Answer = 20%-250 mL; 10%-750 mL.** This is an alligation problem. Draw a tic-tac-toe table, placing the highest concentration (20%) in the upper left hand corner, the desired concentration (12.5%) in the middle, and the lowest concentration (10%) in the bottom left hand corner. Subtract the

concentrations in a diagonal manner and place the number opposite the remaining concentration. Calculate the proportions of each needed and multiply by the quantity to be prepared (1 L = 1,000 mL). 20%: (2.5 parts/10 parts) × 1,000 mL = 250 mL; 10%: (7.5 parts/10 parts) × 1,000 mL = 750 mL.

81. **Answer = 5%-1.5 parts; 1%-2.5 parts.** This is an alligation problem. Draw a tic-tac-toe table, placing the highest concentration (5%) in the upper left hand corner, the desired concentration (2.5%) in the middle, and the lowest concentration (1%) in the bottom left hand corner. Subtract the concentrations in a diagonal manner and place the number opposite the remaining concentration. Calculate the proportions of each needed. 5%: 1.5:4 and 1%: 2.5:4.

82. **Answer = 20%-112.5 mL; SWFI-187.5 mL.** This is an alligation problem using IV solutions. Draw a tic-tac-toe table, placing the highest concentration (20%) in the upper left hand corner, the desired concentration (7.5%) in the middle, and the lowest concentration (0%) in the bottom left hand corner. Subtract the concentrations in a diagonal manner and place the number opposite the remaining concentration. SWFI is sterile water for injection and has a concentration of 0%, and D20W means 20% dextrose in water. Calculate the proportions of each needed and multiply by the quantity to be prepared. 20%: (7.5 parts/20 parts) × 300 mL = 112.5 mL; SWFI: (12.5 parts/20 parts) × 300 mL = 187.5 mL.

83. **Answer = 20% and 5%-250 mL; 20%-125 mL, 10%-375 mL.** This problem can be prepared using two different combinations (20% and 5%; 20% and 10%) to prepare 500 mL of D12.5. In both situations, one must have a concentration above the desired concentration and one concentration below the desired concentration. Draw a tic-tac-toe table, placing the highest concentration (20%) in the upper left hand corner, the desired concentration (12.5%) in the middle, and the lowest concentration (5%) in the bottom left hand corner. Subtract the concentrations in a diagonal manner and place the number opposite the remaining concentration. Subtract the concentrations in a diagonal manner and place the number opposite the remaining concentration. Calculate the proportions of each needed and multiply by the quantity to be prepared. 20%: (7.5 parts/15 parts) × 500 mL = 250 mL; 5%: (7.5 parts/15 parts) × 500 mL. Draw a tic-tac-toe table, placing the highest concentration (20%) in the upper left hand corner, the desired concentration (12.5%) in the middle, and the lowest concentration (10%) in the bottom left hand corner. Subtract the concentrations in a diagonal manner and place the number opposite the remaining concentration. Subtract the concentrations in a diagonal manner and place the number opposite the remaining concentration. Calculate the proportions of each needed and multiply by the quantity to be prepared. 20%: (2.5 parts/10 parts) × 500 mL = 125 mL; 10%: (7.5 parts/10 parts) × 500 mL = 375 mL.

84. **Answer = 120 g.** This is an alligation problem to prepare an ointment. Draw a tic-tac-toe table, placing the highest concentration (2.5%) in the upper left hand corner, the desired concentration (1%) in the middle, and the lowest concentration (0.25%) in the bottom left hand corner. Subtract the concentrations in a diagonal manner and place the number opposite the remaining concentration. Calculate the proportions of each needed. Set up a proportion to calculate the total weight of the preparation by using the 240 g of 0.25% ointment: 1.5 parts/2.25 parts = 240 g/X, where X = 360 g. To calculate the amount of 2.5% needed, subtract the amount of the 0.25% from the total weight of the compound: 360 g (total weight) − 240 g (wt of 0.25%) = 120 g (wt of 2.5%).

85. **Answer = 600 mL.** This problem can be solved by multiplying the rate (25 mL/hr) by the amount of time (24 hr): (25 mL/hr) × (24 hr) = 600 mL.

86. **Answer = 12.5 mL/hr.** Rate = volume/time (hr) or 1,000 mL/8 hr = 125 mL/hr.

87. **Answer = a. 41 mL/hr.** Rate = volume/time or 1,000 mL/24 hr = 41 hr. Whenever an individual has a number less than a whole, it is rounded down in flow rates.
    b. 10 gtt/min. The problem can be solved by the following formula: (rate) × (drop factor) × (conversion factor) = gtt/min: (41 mL/hr) × (15 gtt/mL) × (1 hr/60 min) = 10 gtt/min.

88. **Answer = 0500 hr on the next day.** Calculate the amount of time the IV will last (time = volume/time) or 1,500 mL/75 mL/hr = 20 hr. The first bag was hung at 0900 hours and it will last 20 hours: 0900 hr + 2000 hr − 2400 hr/day = 0500 hr on the next day.

89. **Answer = 62.5 mL/hr.** Rate = volume/time or 250 mL/4 hr = 62.5 mL/hr. **62.5 mg/hr.** Rate = amount of drug/time. 250 mL/4 hr = 62.5 mg/hr.

90. **Answer = 420 mL.** Volume = (rate) × (time) or (120 mL/hr) × (3½ hr) = 420 mL.

91. **Answer = 31 gtt/min.** Solve by using: (rate) × (drop factor) × (conversion factor) = gtt/min: (1,000 mL/8 hr) × (15 gtt/mL) × (1 hr/60 min) = 31 gtt/min.

92. **Answer = 80 mL/hr.** Solve by using: Rate = (gtt/min)/(drop factor) × (conversion factor): (20 gtt/min)/(15 gtt/mL) × (1 hr/60 min) = 80 mL/hr.

93. **Answer = 5 mL/min.** Calculate the amount of time 0.1 g (100 mg) would be infused into the body if the patient is receiving 1 mg/min using a proportion: 1 mg/min = 100 mg/X min, which is 100 min. 100 mg is contained in 500 mL, which will take 100 minutes to infuse. The flow rate = volume (500 mL)/time (100 minutes) = 5 mL/min.

94. **Answer = 3.82 mL.** Convert the patient's weight from pounds to kilograms (280 lb × 1 kg/2.2 lb = 127.27 kg). Calculate the dose needed: (127.27 kg) × (150 units/kg) = 19,095 units. Solve using a proportion: 5,000 units/mL = 19,095 units/X mL, where X = 3.82 mL.

95. **Answer = 16 gtt/min.** Calculate the rate (100 mL/1.5 hr) = 66 mL/hr. Calculate gtt/min by multiplying the rate by the drop factor by the conversion factor: (66 mL/hr) × (15 gtt/mL) × (1 hr/60 min) = 16 gtt/min.

96. **Answer = 25 gtt/min.** Calculate the rate (150 mL/2 hr = 75 mL/hr). Calculate gtt/min by multiplying the rate by the drop factor by the conversion factor: (75 mL/hr) × (20 gtt/mL) × (1 hr/60 min) = 25 gtt/min.

97. **Answer = 12 gtt/min.** Calculate gtt/min by multiplying the rate by the drop factor by the conversion factor: (50 mL/hr) × (15 gtt/mL) × (1 hr/60 min) = 12 gtt/min.

98. **Answer = 62 gtt/min.** Rate = 125 mL/hr; drop factor (DF) = 30 gtt/ mL and 1 hour/60 min (conversion factor [CF]). Solve using the following formula: (rate) × (DF) × (CF) = gtt/min: (125 mL/hr) × (30 gtt/mL) × (1 hr/60 min) = 62.gtt/min. **Remember gtt/min are always rounded downward when one has a fraction of a drop.**

99. **Answer = $3,377,865.** Overhead is the sum of all the expenses a business experiences. In this problem, because there are two pharmacists, multiply the pharmacist salary by 2 and the pharmacy technician's salary by 3 to calculate the total salaries. Add up all of the expenses to obtain the overhead.

100. **Answer = $8.00.** Gross profit can be calculated by subtracting the cost, which in this case is the same as the average wholesale price (AWP) or from the retail price. $67.99 – $59.99 = $8.00.

101. **Answer = $4.00.** Markup is another term for gross profit. In this problem the markup is equal to retail price (13.99) – the drug cost (9.99), which is $4.00.

102. **Answer = 30%.** Markup rate is the markup dollars divided by the cost times 100. Calculate the markup: retail price ($25.99) – cost ($19.99) = $6.00. Divide the markup dollars ($6.00) by the cost ($19.99) and multiply by 100: ($6.00/$19.99) × 100 = 30%.

103. **Answer = $8.75.** Net profit is the retail price ($112.99) minus the cost of product or the actual acquisition cost ($99.99) minus any expenses ($4.25) associated with the product: ($112.99 – $9.99) – $4.25 = $8.75.

104. **Answer = $94.68.** Add the cost of the test strips ($67.50) to the overhead costs ($3.50) to obtain the total cost ($67.50 + $3.50 = $71.00). To calculate the selling price, add the total cost and net profit together to obtain the selling price: $71.00 + $23.68 = $94.68.

105. **Answer = $1,911.** The pharmacy will receive a 2% discount off the total bill if the bill is paid in full within 30 days. $1,950.00 – (0.02)(1,950.00) = $1,911.00

106. **Answer = 11.76.** Inventory turns can be calculated by dividing total sales by the inventory value or the average inventory value. Sales (3,000,000)/inventory ($255,000) = 11.76 inventory turns.

107. **Answer = 10.95.** The average inventory can be calculated by adding the initial inventory ($225,000) and the final inventory ($250,000) and dividing the sum ($475,000) by 2, resulting in an average inventory of $237,500. Divide total sales ($2,600,000) by average inventory ($237,500) = 10.95 inventory turns.

108. **Answer = a. 8.33 mg/capsule.** You have been given a formula that will yield 24 capsules. Divide the amount of hydrocodone bitartrate (0.2 g) by the number of capsules one is to prepare. 0.2 g/24 capsules = 0.00833 g/capsule. Convert 0.00833 g to milligrams by multiplying 0.0833 g × 1,000 mg/g = 8.33 mg/capsule.

   b. **430 mg per capsule.** Add up the total weight of all of the ingredients (10.4 g) and divide by 24 capsules. Each capsule will weigh 0.43 g. Convert grams to milligrams. 0.43 g × 1,000 mg/g = 430 mg.

   c. **75 mg.** 0.6 g of caffeine/24 capsules = 0.025 g of caffeine/capsule. Convert the grams to milligrams. 0.025 g × 1,000 mg/1 g = 25 mg. The directions state that the patient is to take one capsule three times per day. 25 mg of caffeine/capsule × 3 capsules = 75 mg.

109. **Answer = 10-1 g Carafate tablets.** Calculate the amount of Carafate needed for the compound; this can be done through the use of a proportion: 400 mg/5 mL = X mg/125 mL, where 10,000 mg of

Carafate is the entire quantity. One can calculate the number of grams needed by using a proportion. 1 g/1,000 mg = X g/10,000 mg, where X = 10 − 1 g tablets of Carafate.

110. **Answer = 43.2 g of iodine; 51.84 g of sodium iodide.** You have been asked to prepare 12 dozen 15-mL bottles, which is equal to (12)(12 bottles/1 dozen bottles)(15 mL) = 2,160 mL of solution. The formula will make 1,000 mL of solution. Calculate the amount needed of each ingredient by using the following formula: [total quantity needed of compound (TQN)/quantity required for original formula (QRF)] × amount of ingredient in original formula: (2,160 mL/1,000 mL) × 20 g of iodide = 43.2 g of iodide and (2,160 mL/1,000 mL) × 24 g of sodium iodide = 51.84 g of sodium iodide.

111. **Answer = Benzoyl benzoate   30 mL**
     Triethanolamine   0.6 mL
     Oleic acid   2.4 mL
     Purified water to make   120 mL
     This problem needs a smaller quantity to be made than is called for in the original formula. Use the following formula: (TQN/QRF) × amount of each ingredient. (120 mL/500 mL) × 125 mL = 30 mL of benzoate; (120 mL/500 mL) × 2.5 mL = 0.6 mL of triethanolamine; (125 mL/500 mL) × 10 mL = 2.4 mL of oleic acid.

112. **Answer = Dextromethorphan   5,760 mg (5.76 g)**
     Guaifenesin   76,800 mg (76.8 g)
     Flavored syrup to make   3,840 mL
     This problem is enlarged from the original formula and can be calculated using the following formula: (TQN/QRF) × amount of each ingredient. (3,840 mL/5 mL) × 7.5 mg = 5,760 mg (5.76 g) of dextromethorphan; (3840 mL/5 mL) × 100 mg = 76,800 mg (76.8 g) of guaifenesin.

113. **Answer = Coal tar   9.08 g**
     Precipitated sulfur   13.62 g
     Salicylic acid   4.54 g
     Lidex ointment   108.96 g
     Aquabase   317.80 g
     This formula is going to be enlarged. One pound is equal to 454 g. This problem is not qs (or brought) to a final weight; therefore, one must add up all of the ingredients to determine the weight in the original formula which is 100 g. The following formula can be used: (TQN/QRF) × amount of each ingredient. (454 g/100 g) × amount of each ingredient × 2.0 g = 9.08 g of coal tar; (454 g/100 g) × 3.0 g = 13.62 g of precipitated sulfur; (454 g/100 g) × 1.0 g = 4.54 g of salicylic acid; (454 g/100 g) × 24 g = 108.96 g of Lidex ointment; and (454 g/100 g) × 70 g = 317.8 g of Aquabase.

114. **Answer = Estriol   5 g**
     Estrone   0.625 g
     Estradiol   0.625 g
     Polyethylene glycol   14,500.5 kg
     Polyethylene glycol   33,500.5 kg
     This formula is being enlarged. The following formula can be used: (TQN/QRF) × amount of each ingredient. (2,500 capsules/100 capsules) × 200 mg = 5 g of estriol, (2,500 capsules/100 capsules) × 25 mg = 0.625 g of estrone; (2,500 capsules/100 capsules) × 25 mg of estradiol; (2,500 capsules/100 capsules) × 20 g = 0.5 kg of PEG 1450; and (2,500 capsules/100 capsules) × 20 g = 0.5 kg of PEG 3350.

CHAPTER 3 ANSWERS TO REVIEW QUESTIONS

1. a—Group Purchasing Organizations (GPO) negotiate the best possible prices for hospitals; they do not purchase the medications for a hospital. The purchasing department of the hospital makes the purchases.
2. b—Some patients may experience difficulty swallowing capsules, caplets, and tablets. Solid dosage forms are extremely convenient for self-medication and are easy to package and dispense. Solid oral dosage forms lack taste or smell, which can prevent a patient from taking a medication.
3. a—Capsules are contained in a gelatin shell, and the size of the shell can vary based on the amount of medication it will contain.
4. d—Tablets are prepared by compressing; capsules may be prepared using the "punch method."

5. a—Effervescent salts release carbon dioxide when dissolved in water; plasters adhere to the skin; powders may administered either externally or internally; a troche, also known as lozenge or pastille, dissolves in the mouth.

6. b—Liquids are easier to swallow than solid oral dosage forms.

7. b—Elixirs are a clear, sweetened, flavored hydroalcoholic containing water and alcohol and may or may not be medicated. Aromatic waters are solutions of water containing oils, which have a fragrance and are volatile; a suspension is a dispersion with two phases that has solid particles dispersed in the liquid. A syrup contains sucrose (sugar).

8. a—An emulsion is a liquid dispersed in another. Emulsions can be either oil/water or water/oil. A gel is a dispersion with extremely fine particles and when mixed is a semisolid dosage form. A lotion is a topical dispersion that contains insoluble substances; an ointment is a semisolid topical dispersion.

9. a—The date of the repackaging does not need to appear on the label, but it does need to be entered into the repackaging log. A repackaged medication must contain the generic name of the medication, the manufacturer's name and lot number, and the expiration date after packaging. The repackaging date can be either 6 months from the date it is repackaged or one quarter of the manufacturer's time, whichever is less.

10. a—The expiration date after repackaging does not need to be on the label.

11. c—Either the drug manufacturer or the FDA can issue a medication recall. Medication recalls can be one of three types, depending on the severity of the situation.

12. b—A modified unit dose can be known as a punch card, bingo card, or blister card.

13. b—A prime vendor agreement occurs between a pharmacy and a wholesaler in which the pharmacy agrees to purchase the majority (80–95%) of their products from the wholesaler. In return, the wholesaler agrees to provide the pharmacy with a range of services, which may include electronic order entry devices, bar-coded labels, emergency service, and competitive pricing.

14. c—Syrups contain sucrose (sugar).

15. b—Liniments are considered a solution rather than a dispersion because the solute is dissolved in a solvent. Liniments may be either an alcoholic or oleaginous solution.

16. b—Emulsions possess a solute dispersed through a dispersing vehicle. Emulsions can either be oil-in-water or water-in-oil.

17. c—A pastille is also known as a troche or lozenge that dissolves in the mouth.

18. a—A collodion contains pyroxylin (tiny particles of cellulose) and can be dissolved in either alcohol or ether.

19. a—Suspensions are considered dispersions and have two phases.

20. d—A paste is a dispersion similar to an ointment, but it contains more solid material.

21. d—The Pharmacy and Therapeutics Committee (P&T), composed of physicians, nurses, pharmacists, and hospital administrators, develops the formulary for an institution.

22. b—Six months is the maximum amount of time that can be assigned to a repackaged medication.

23. a—The subscription contains special instructions to the pharmacist; the signa indicates directions to be typed on the label; the inscription is the name, strength, and quantity of medication; and the Rx symbol means recipe or take.

24. a—Hazardous drugs and chemicals require the purchaser to receive a Material Safety Data Sheet (MSDS) from the manufacturer, distributor, or importer.

25. b—Ophthalmic products must be isotonic or else damage can occur to the eye.

CHAPTER 4 ANSWERS TO REVIEW QUESTIONS

1. a—Glass mortars and pestles are used to mix liquids, Wedgwood is used for crystals, and porcelain is used for powders.

2. a—The Department of Transportation (DOT) is responsible for the transportation of hazardous materials.

3. b—High-efficiency particulate airflow (HEPA) filters need to be certified every 6 months unless they become wet.

4. c—Radioactive Yellow III has the highest concentration, Radioactive Yellow II has the second highest, and Radioactive White I has the lowest concentration. Radioactive Orange IV does not exist.

5. b—Laminar flow hoods need to be certified every 6 months.

6. d-The USP-NF consists of drug monographs and standards. Approved Drug Products with Therapeutic Equivalence Evaluations is what is known as the Orange Book. Drug Facts and Comparisons and the PDR (Physician's Drug Reference) provide valuable information about drug products.

7. b-Class A balances must have a minimum sensitivity of 6 mg.
8. c-Rubber Spatulas are used because corrosive materials may react with the steel.
9. a-70% Isopropyl alcohol is used to clean laminar flow hoods. Rubbing alcohol will leave a film on the top of a laminar flow hood.
10. c-The lumen is the name of the opening of a needle. The bevel is the angled tip of the needle where the lumen is found. The hilt of the needle attaches to the hub of the barrel of the syringe. The shaft is the length of the needle.
11. a—Laminar flow hoods should be a Class 100 area, where there are no more than 100 particles that are 0.5 micron and larger per cubic foot of air. The number indicates the number of particles 0.5 micron and larger per cubic foot of air.
12. c—Pipettes should be used to measure volumes less than 1.5 mL.
13. d—Disease management services are reimbursed through the submission of an HCFS 1500 form.
14. d—The seller is responsible for the product during transportation.
15. a—Institutional pharmacies process medication orders instead of prescriptions. Ambulatory pharmacies process prescriptions.
16. c—Professional samples are frowned on because they may create a bias in purchasing.
17. b—Class B balances can weigh between 650 mg and 120 g and can be used for compounding.
18. d—A laminar flow hood must be on a minimum of 30 min before it is used to prepare an admixture.
19. a—A Type A hood can be converted to a Type B3 hood. A Type A1 hood does not exist.
20. d—Pharmacy balances must be certified every year by the Department of Taxation.
21. c—Finished radiopharmaceuticals are stored in the packaging area; the breakdown room is used to store empty or used radiopharmaceuticals before they are returned and dismantled for reuse; the compounding area is the compounding or dispensing area; and the storage and disposal area is used to store radioactive waste.
22. b—Face to face is the most effective way to communicate; the least effective way of those mentioned is a memo.
23. d—JCAHO does not certify retail pharmacies.
24. a—All pharmacies must have a Class A balance.
25. c—The air velocity of a laminar flow hood is 90 linear feet per minute (±20%).

CHAPTER 5 ANSWERS TO PRACTICE EXAMINATIONS

Practice Examination I Answers

1. a—ACE inhibitors have a potassium sparing effect, which, if taken with potassium-sparing diuretics, may result in hyperkalemia
2. b—The first letter maybe either an A or B. The second letter is the first letter of the prescriber's last name. Next, one adds the numbers in the first, third, and fifth position. Next, one adds the numbers in the second, fourth, and sixth positions; multiply this sum by two. Add both sums together and the correct number should be the last number.
3. c—Use the following equation: (IS)(IV) = (FS)(FV), where IS (initial strength or 25%) IV (initial volume is being calculated); FS (final strength or 10%), and FV (final volume, which is 4 fl oz or 120 mL). This calculation yields 48 mL. Subtract the initial volume (48 mL) from the final volume (120 mL), which will yield the amount of diluent (72 mL).
4. a—The Controlled Substance Act of 1970 allows 0 refills for Schedule II medications.
5. b—An elixir is a mixture of alcohol and water.
6. b—The Drug Listing Act of 1972 provided a unique numbering system for each product. This 11-digit number identifies the manufacturer, the product, and its package.
7. c—Nifedipine is a calcium channel blocker. Beta-blockers are easily identified by the nomenclature syllable of -olol.
8. d—i (Roman numeral for 1); gtt (drop); ou (each eye); tid (three times per day) ud (as directed).
9. c—The "hypo-" prefix means low, and the root word "kalemia" means potassium.
10. d—The smaller the number, the weaker or more dilute the substance.
11. d—UTI is an acronym for urinary tract infection
12. b—Imitrex is taken at the onset of a migraine headache.
13. d—There are 480 mL in a pint solution, and a teaspoon dose is equal to 5 mL. 480 mL/5 mL/dose = 96 doses.

14. a—Overhead is the sum of all the expenses in a business. Examples of overhead in a pharmacy include all the salaries of the employees, cost of inventory, the expense-associated utilities, supplies, licenses, and computer hardware/software.

15. b—Food and Drug Administration.

16. a—Oxycodone + APAP is the same as Percocet and Tylox. Under the Controlled Substance Act of 1970, these products have a extremely high potential for abuse, but they have a medicinal use in the United States.

17. d—Vitamin K is a warfarin antagonist. It will increase the clotting factors II, VII, IX, and X.

18. b—In compliance with the Accutane Prescribing Law of 2002, all Accutane prescriptions must be handwritten by the prescriber and filled within 7 days of being written with the approved yellow seal attached and having no refills authorized.

19. c—The patient is taking 2 tablets twice per day for a total of 4 tablets per day. 40 tablets divided by 4 tablets per day will last 10 days.

20. d—A minidrip or microdrip system yields 60 drops per milliliter.

21. c—According to the Controlled Substance Act of 1970, the maximum number of authorized refills for a Schedule III-V drug is 5.

22. a—Doxycycline is the only tetracycline that can be taken with dairy products.

23. b—There are 24 hr in a day, and, if the drug is taken every 6 hr, it will require 4 doses in a day's time.

24. d—Multiply the cost ($2.00) by the desired profit (0.3), which will yield a profit of $0.60. Adding the profit ($0.60) to the cost ($2.00) will result of a selling price of $2.60.

25. c—"Nephro" is the Latin root word for kidney.

26. d—Using the formula:
    Final weight × percent (express as a decimal) = amount of active ingredient
    Both the percent (20%) and the amount of active ingredient (10 g) are provided in the problem. Placing this information in the equation, one finds that the:
    Final weight = amount of active ingredient/percent (as a decimal)
    Final weight = 10 g/0.02 or 50 g.

27. c—1 mg of protamine sulfate will neutralize 90–120 units of heparin.

28. c—Scurvy is a deficiency of vitamin C; deficiencies of vitamin A result in night blindness; B1 in beriberi; and vitamin D in rickets.

29. b—"od" is derived from the Latin term "oculo dextro," which is translated to right eye.

30. a—Bupropion is generic name for the antidepressant Wellbutrin and the generic name for the smoking cessation product Zyban.

31. b—The generic name for Lodine is etodolac.

32. c—Using the formula IS × IV = FS × FV, the initial strength is 25%, the initial volume is 600 mL, the final volume (initial volume)(600 mL) + amount of diluent (100 mL) is 700 mL. Inserting these values in the equation yields a final strength of 21.4%.

33. b—An individual must determine how long the bag will last (1,000 units/hr = 20,000 units/X hr). The bag will last 20 hr. The rate of infusion can be calculated by dividing 500 mL by 20 hr, resulting in 25 mL/hr. Then, use the following formula: rate × drop size × 1 hr/60 min = gtt/min. Therefore, using (25 mL/hr)(15 gtt/mL)(1 hr/60 min) will yield 6 gtt/min.

34. c—Using Young's rule [age(years)/age(years) + 12] × the adult dose will give the appropriate dose for the child. 5 months is approximately 0.42 years: (0.42/0.42 +12) × 200 mg = 6.67 mg.

35. c—Using Clark's rule [weight (lb)/150] × adult dose will provide the child with the correct dose: [(70 lb)/150] × 250 mg = 16 mg.

36. c—"Hepato" is the Latin root word meaning liver.

37. d—According to the FDA, an X rating indicates that the medication is contraindicated in pregnant women.

38. c—Food aids in the absorption of nitrofurantoin in the body. Amoxicillin (penicillin) is best taken on an empty stomach; minocycline and tetracycline (both tetracyclines) work best if taken on an empty stomach and should not be taken within 1 hr of all dairy products because of chelation.

39. d—AWP and capitation + dispensing fee are both types of third-party reimbursement formulas; a copayment is a predetermined amount of money or a percentage of money that one is responsible for paying on every prescription. A deductible is a yearly, predetermined sum of money payable before the insurer will begin making payments to an individual or institution.

40. c—The Poison Prevention Act of 1970 permits certain medications (i.e., nitroglycerin) not to be dispensed in a child-resistant container.

41. d—30 tablets are dispensed, but 1 tablet is being taken every other day; therefore it will last 60 days.
42. d—Tuberculosis most often affects the lungs, because *M. tuberculosis* prefers an area of high oxygen content.
43. b—A printer is an output device.
44. b—Meperidine is a Schedule II drug that must be stored in a safe per the Controlled Substance Act of 1970.
45. a—The Accutane Law of 2002 does not permit refills on prescriptions of Accutane. The prescription must be handwritten by the physician and dispensed within 7 days of being written.
46. a—An auxiliary label provides additional information to the patient: PPIs are required for products containing estrogens; patient profiles provide the pharmacist information about the patient, such as illness, both OTC and Rx medications being taken, drug allergies, and demographic and payment information; a prescription label provides information to the patient containing the name, strength, quantity of drug, and directions for usage as prescribed by the physician.
47. a—Otic refers to the ear.
48. b—Antitussives are used in the treatment of a dry, nonproductive cough, whereas expectorants are used if a patient has mucus or phlegm.
49. d—Ibuprofen is available OTC as Motrin and Nuprin; naproxen sodium is Aleve; and ranitidine is Zantac. Tramadol is the prescription product known as Ultram.
50. b—Using a proportion, calculate the amount found in 4 fl oz (120 mL): 50 g/1,000 mL = X g/120 mL, where X = 6 g.
51. a—The smaller the number in the denominator, the larger the value of the number.
52. c—Glyburide is the generic for Micronase. The brand names for the following generics are: Amaryl (glimepiride), Glucotrol (glipizide), and Actos (pioglitazone).
53. d—Imipramine (Tofranil) is used to prevent bedwetting in small children.
54. c—Even though both Wellbutrin and Zyban contain the same ingredient, bupropion, Wellbutrin is indicated only for the treatment of depression.
55. b—Itraconazole is the generic drug name for Sporanox, which is available only by prescription.
56. b—Coreg is the brand name for carvedilol.
57. a—Only registered pharmacists are allowed by law to counsel patients.
58. c—The Kefauver-Harris Amendment requires that all drugs be pure, safe, and effective as a result of the thalidomide incident.
59. d—Ultralente insulin has a duration of 18–20 hr. Regular insulin lasts 5–6 hr; NPH insulin lasts 10–16 hr; and Lente insulin has a duration of 12–18 hr.
60. d—Answer A is incorrect because it stated that tsp was tablespoonful instead of teaspoon; qod is every other day instead of 4 times per day; and answer C states penicillin G, whereas the prescription indicates Pen G. There is a difference between penicillin and penicillin G.
61. a—Cardio is derived from the Greek term "kardia," meaning heart.
62. a—One of the ingredients of a compound must be a legend drug.
63. b—One needs to use alligation to solve the problem. When subtracting the desired concentration from the higher concentration and subtracting the lower concentration from the desired concentration, one sees that we will be using equal quantities of each strength.
64. c—Corticosteroids, loop diuretics, and thiazide diuretics have an adverse effect on lipid profiles.
65. b—Itraconazole is the antifungal agent known as Sporanox.
66. c—The Physicians' Desk Reference contains information from the package inserts of more than 4,000 prescription drugs.
67. a—Butorphanol was upgraded from the prescription drug, Stadol, to a controlled substance in 1997.
68. c—The Controlled Substance Act of 1970 allows for an individual age 18 to purchase a 4-oz bottle of an exempt narcotic every 48 hr.
69. d—Sulfisoxazole is a sulfa antibiotic.
70. a—According to the FDA classification system, AA shows that the medication meets bioequivalence requirements.
71. b—Class A balances are used in extemporaneous compounding, not in the preparation of intravenous preparations.
72. a—Acetaminophen. Acetylsalicylic acid (aspirin), ibuprofen (Motrin), and naproxen sodium (Aleve or Anaprox) have the potential to irritate or ulcerate the stomach.

73. b—100 units of insulin are found in 1 mL of liquid.

$$\frac{100 \text{ units}}{1 \text{ mL}} = \frac{40 \text{ units}}{\text{mL}}$$

Cross-multiplying and dividing yields 0.4 mL.

74. d—A specific disease state, such as angina, requires a prompt response, resulting in nitroglycerin being taken sublingually and bypassing the digestive system. Oral medications do not require specific skills of the patient, unlike injectable medications where specific skills are necessary. The rate of action may be affected by the amount of time in which a therapeutic response needs to occur. An example would be an IV injection; IVs provide a quicker response because the medication is administered into the bloodstream and gets to the site of action much more quickly than does an oral or topical dose. The shape, color, or taste of a medication does not affect the route of administration. The shape, color, or taste may affect the patient's compliance in taking a medication.

75. d—Beakers and graduates are not precise enough to measure a small volume such as 1.5 mL. A measuring device cannot have a capacity greater than five times the amount of volume to be measured.

76. c—GMP stands for Good Manufacturing Practices and is adhered for compounding prescriptions. The DEA is responsible for the Controlled Substance Act; the FDA for ensuring the food and medications are pure, safe, and effective; whereas OBRA 90 discusses Drug Utilization Review and counseling patients.

77. d—Glucosamine has been shown to be helpful in treating arthritis, whereas feverfew may be used for migraines, ginger as an antiemetic, and ginkgo for circulatory issues.

78. c—Metformin is the generic name for Glucophage. The following generic names are for the following proprietary drugs: glipizide (Glucotrol), glyburide (Micronase or DiaBeta), and pioglitazone (Actos).

79. a—Zithromax is the brand name for azithromycin; Biaxin (clarithromycin), Minocin (minocycline), and Floxin (ofloxacin).

80. c—AWP stands for Average Wholesale Price and is a term used in determining costs and calculating profitability of a product.

81. d—Even though both lotions and suspensions are dispersions, lotions are dissolved particles, whereas suspensions contain solid particles.

82. d—0.4 g is the same as 400 mg.

83. b—Durham-Humphrey Amendment.

84. b—Narcotics have a tendency to sedate (CNS depression) an individual. CNS stimulation would have the opposite effect.

85. b—Calculate the amount of active ingredient by multiplying the final volume by the percent of clindamycin expressed as a decimal (480 mL × 0.02 = 9.6 g). Convert 9.6 g to grams by multiplying 9.6 g × 1000 mg/g = 9,600 mg. Divide the total weight of clindamycin by the weight of each capsule (9,600 mg /150 mg per capsule = 64 capsules).

86. b—Capsules have a gelatin shell as an outer covering, unlike the other products mentioned.

87. b—AWP + dispensing fee is a common method of reimbursing pharmacies for medications. Calculate the cost of 30 tablets (100 tablets/$120.00 = 30 tablets/X), where X is $36.00 and the AWP for this medication; $3.25 is added to the AWP ($36.00), yielding $39.25.

88. a—The problem can be solved using the following formula: (IS)(IV) = (FS)(FV), where IS = 65%, IV = 1200 ml and FS = 45% or (65%)(1200 ml)/(45%) = 1733 ml. The amount of diluent added is equal to FV-IV, which is 1733 ml-1200 ml = 533 ml.

89. b—Convert 10 g to milligrams (10 g × 1,000 mg/g = 10,000 mg). Divide the total weight by the weight per dose (10,000 mg/500 mg per dose = 20 doses).

90. c—The Controlled Substance Act requires that a partially filled Schedule II prescription be filled within 72 hr if the pharmacy did not have the entire quantity for the patient. If it is not filled within 72 hr, the remaining quantity will become void.

91. c—Parchment paper may be used if an ointment slab is not available. After use, the parchment paper is discarded.

92. b—For patients who are allergic to penicillin, there is a 10% chance they will be allergic to a cephalosporin.

93. c—Oral medications are the most commonly used because of the ease of administration

94. b—One must be at least 6 inches inside of the laminar airflow hood to use proper aseptic technique.

95. c—Any errors made on a Form 222 cannot be corrected. This form must be retained in the pharmacy for at least 2 years.

96. a—Absorption is the process of taking the drug from the administration site to the bloodstream; distribution is the process of taking the medication to organs and tissues; metabolism transforms the medication in the liver; and elimination (excretion) is the process by which the drug is removed from the body.

97. d—D10W stands for 10% dextrose dissolved in water. w/f% is the number of grams dissolved in 100 mL of solution. Using the following proportion, one can solve the problem: (10 g/100 mL = X g/1,000 mL), resulting in 10 g.

98. a—Decongestants may cause CNS stimulation, which may cause the heart to beat harder, thus pushing more blood through the circulatory system and resulting in increased blood pressure. Decongestants do not decrease blood pressure.

99. c—Calculate the total number of doses required (2 tablets/dose × 2 doses/day × 25 days = 100 tablets). Calculate the cost of 100 tablets ($321.66/500 tablets = X/100 tablets, where X = $64.33). Look for the fee on the table that corresponds to an AWP of $64.33, which would be $10.00. AWP + fee ($64.33 + $10.00 = $74.33).

100. b—Normal saline is 0.9%; therefore, ½ NS would be 0.9%/2 or 0.45%. Solve using the following equation: (IS)(IV) = (FS)(FV), substituting the following values (0.9%)(250 mL) = (0.45%)(X mL), where X = 500 mL, which is the final volume. FV – IV = amount of water to be added. 500 mL – 250 mL = 250 mL of water.

101. a—

$$\frac{1 \text{ gr}}{60 \text{ mg}} = \frac{\frac{1}{4} \text{ gr}}{X \text{ mg}}$$

Cross-multiplying and dividing will yield X = 15 mg.

$$\frac{15 \text{ mg}}{1 \text{ tablet}} = \frac{15 \text{ mg}}{X \text{ tablet}}$$

$$X = 1 \text{ tablet}$$

102. a—This is a proportion problem. 25,000 units/500 mL = X units/1 mL; where X = 50 mL).

103. b—One liter contains 1,000 mL and 2 teaspoons is equal to 10 mL: 1,000 mL/10 mL per dose will yield 100 doses.

104. c—An advantage of parenteral medication is that it is injected directly into the patient and the patient does not need to be conscious.

105. b—The Justice Department set up the Drug Enforcement Agency (DEA) to enforce the Controlled Substance Act of 1970.

106. a—An emulsion is a dispersion in which one liquid is dispersed into another immiscible liquid. Emulsions can be either water/oil or oil/water. Emulsions contain a third phase, which is an emulsifying agent used to prevent the emulsions from separating.

107. a—Presently, only pharmacists are allowed to accept new prescriptions being telephoned into a pharmacy from a physician's office according to federal law.

108. d—The subscription is instructions to the pharmacist. These instructions may include the following information: compounding, packaging, labeling, refills, and allowing a generic drug to be dispensed.

109. d—Medications can be degraded by light, temperature, and moisture. Amber containers are used to block ultraviolet rays from breaking the medication down.

110. a—Amino acids, dextrose, and lipids are used to prepare a total nutrient admixture.

111. a—The Americans with Disabilities Act prohibits discrimination against an individual with either a physical, mental, or emotional disability. The employer must make a reasonable accommodation for the employee. If the disability does not interfere with the individual's ability to perform a particular task, he or she must be considered for employment.

112. c—Doxycycline is in the tetracycline family of antibiotics.

113. a—IV is an approved pharmacy abbreviation for intravenous.

114. c—Pharmacies purchase their medications either directly from the manufacturer or from a secondary vendor such as a wholesaler. Chain pharmacy warehouses are a secondary vendor for a particular chain; GPO's negotiate prices for hospitals.

115. d—The Pharmacy and Therapeutics Committee, which is composed of physicians, pharmacists, nurses, and administrative personnel, develops the formulary for a hospital.

116. b—Methyldopa (Aldomet) is the only approved antihypertensive agent for pregnant women.

117. c—"qsad" is an abbreviation for a sufficient quantity to make.

118. d—USP-NF stands for United States Pharmacopoeia-National Formulary.

119. a—Group Purchasing Organizations (GPO) negotiate prices for hospitals. They do not make the actual purchase of medications for hospitals.

120. c—The Federal Controlled Substance Act requires that all pharmacy records be maintained for a minimum of 2 years.

121. a—The hypothalamus regulates the body and its goal is to maintain homeostasis within the body.

122. d—Antifungal agents such as Sporanox have been found to be as effective as taking the medication daily and are cheaper for the patient.

123. b—The Pure Drug Act introduced the terms "adulteration" and "misbranding," but the Food, Drug, and Cosmetic Act of 1938 clearly defined these terms. Adulteration deals with the condition of the product, whereas misbranding discusses the labeling aspect of the product.

124. a—The word part -pril is found in the nomenclature of ACE inhibitors.

125. b—Penicillin does not cause drowsiness; it should not be taken with juices or soft drinks because the acid in the beverages may break down the drug. It is best if penicillin is taken on an empty stomach because of absorption reasons. Water is the best vehicle for taking medication.

126. d—The problem can be solved using the following formula: FV × strength (expressed as a decimal) = amount of active ingredient (g) or 100 mL × 1/10,000 = 0.01 g.

127. b—The patient would be receiving 500 mg daily instead of 250 mg per daily, which is twice the amount prescribed by the physician.

128. d—Multiply 500 g by 5% (500 g × 0.05 = 25 g).

129. c—The term 3% net means that a purchaser can reduce a purchase by 3% if he or she pays within a stated period (30 days in this case). Multiply $500.00 by 0.03 = $15.00 (amount of discount). Invoice – discount = amount to be remitted ($500.00 – $15.00 = $485.00).

130. c—A flow rate is a volume of liquid infused per period of time (hr). Calculate by dividing 1 L (1,000 mL)/24 hr = 41.67 mL/hr. Flow rates are rounded downward instead of upward; therefore, 41.67 mL/hr = 41 mL/hr.

131. d—The Controlled Substance Act states that controlled substance prescriptions and invoices containing controlled substances must be stamped with a red 1-inch C.

132. a—Glass mortars and pestles are best used for mixing liquids because of the smooth surface and they will not stain like porcelain or Wedgwood.

133. b—Selling price – cost = markup ($50.00 – $35.00 = $15.00). Markup/cost × 100% = markup rate ($15.00/$35.00) – 100% = 43%.

134. b—Calculate rate/hour and then divide by 60 min/hr (800 mL/12 hr = 66 mL/hr; 66 mL/hr/60 min/hr = 1.1 mL/min).

135. d—%w/v is defined as the number of grams/100 mL. Calculate using the following formula: final volume × percent (expressed as a decimal) = amount of active ingredient; (500 mL × 0.1 = 50 g).

136. b—Solve using the following formula: final volume × fraction (expressed as a decimal) = amount of active ingredient; 650 mL × 1/200 = 3.25 g. Convert grams to mg (3.25 g × 1,000 mg/g = 3,250 mg). 1 gr/65 mg = X gr/X mg, where X = 325 mg. Next calculate the number of tablets needed by using the following proportion: 325 mg/1 tablet = 3,250 mg/X tablets, where X = 10 tablets needed to prepare the solution.

137. c—%w/v is the number of grams/100 mL; 4 fl oz = 120 mL. Solve using a proportion 5 g/100 mL = X g/120 mL, where X = 6 g.

138. c—Calculate the rate (1,000 mL/4 hr = 250 mL/hr). Next solve using the following formula: (rate)(kit size)(1 hr/60 min) = gtt/min or (250 mL/hr)(10 gtt/mL)(1 hr/60 min) = 41 gtt/min.

139. b—Two tablespoons = 30 mL. Solve using the following formula: (IS)(IV) = (FS)(FV); (30 mL)(85%) = (10%)(FV), where the FV = 255 mL. To calculate the number of 3 fl oz (90 mL) bottles, divide the final volume by the volume per bottle (255 mL/90 mL per bottle = 2 full 3 fl oz bottles prepared).

140. d—According to the United States Pharmacopoeia, Syrup USP contains sucrose (sugar) dissolved in water.

PRACTICE EXAMINATION II ANSWERS

1. d—30 mL (1 oz) MOM (Milk of Magnesia) po (by mouth) ac (before meals) hs (bedtime) prn (as needed).

2. c—2.79 kg = 2,790 g; and 5 pints × 2 cups/pint × 8 fl oz/pint × 30 mL/fl oz = 2,400 mL. 1 mL of water weighs 1 g. Specific gravity = weight of substance/weight of an equal volume of water or 2,790 g/2,400 g = 1.16.

3. b—Inflammation is an indication for the use of steroids rather than a side effect.

4. d—Sulfamethoxazole/trimethoprim DS (Bactrim DS), amoxicillin/clavulanate (Augmentin), cephalexin (Keflex), sulfamethoxazole/trimethoprim (Bactrim or Septra).

5. c—The suffix "-ectomy" means removal (e.g., appendectomy, thyroidectomy).

6. a—This is an alligation problem, where the 2.5% is the highest concentration, 0.25% is the lowest concentration, 1% is the concentration of the final product. 2.5 − 1 = 1.5 parts of the 0.25%; 1.0 − 0.25 = 0.75 parts of 2.5%. The total number of parts is 2.25 (0.75 + 1.5 = 2.25). Set up a proportion to calculate the total weight: 1.5 parts of 0.25%/2.25 total parts of compound = 240 g of 0.25%/total weight of compound, where the total weight is 360 g. Total weight of compound − weight of 0.25% = weight of 2.5% (360 g − 240 g = 120 g).

7. c—The maximum number of refills allowed for a Schedule III medication if approved by the prescriber is 5 refills within 6 months of the date the prescription was written.

8. d—"qid" means 4 times per day. 40 capsules/4 capsules per day would yield 10 days.

9. d—ii (Roman numeral for 2) gtt (drops) os (left eye) bid (twice per day).

10. b—Pharmacy technicians may accept new and refill prescriptions from a patient, input data into the pharmacy terminal, count medication, process labels, and order medications, but presently they are *not* allowed to counsel patients.

11. d—Premarin is conjugated estrogens, unlike the other three products, which are different dosage forms of estradiol.

12. d—Laminar airflow hoods are used to prepare sterile products. Extemporaneous compounds are not sterile products. A Class A balance, a compounding slab, graduate cylinders, spatulas, mortar and pestle are a few of the pieces of pharmacy equipment used in extemporaneous compounding.

13. d—"Gram" is the basic unit of weight in the metric system.

14. c—Diuretics have a tendency to remove potassium from the body: hypo- (low) kalemia (potassium).

15. d—"DUR" is an acronym for Drug Utilization Review, which is mandated under OBRA-90.

16. d—1 quart is equal to approximately 0.96 L or 1 L.

17. b—The maximum number of different Schedule II medications legally allowed on a Form 222 is 10, which is found in the Controlled Substance Act of 1970.

18. c—Cocaine is a Schedule II drug under the Controlled Substance Act of 1970. Cocaine does have a medical use in the United States, but has a high potential for abuse.

19. d—"Hypo" means low, "gly" means sugar, and "emia" means blood. Low blood sugar.

20. c—"qid" (four times a day) indicates how many times per day a medication would be taken. The terms "ac and hs" tell the patient when during the day the medication is to be taken.

21. b—The Controlled Substance Act allows for one 4-oz bottle of an exempt narcotic to be purchased by an individual older than age 18 every 48 hr.

22. b—This problem can be solved using alligation, where 20% is the highest concentration, 3% is the concentration to be prepared, and petrolatum has a concentration of 0%. For the 20%, subtract the 0% from the 3%, which will require 3 parts of 20%; for the 0%, subtract 3% from 20%, which will give 17 parts of the 3%.

23. b—Solve using the following formula (IS)(IV) = (FS)(FV); (2%)(120 mL) = (FS)(480 mL), where the FS is 0.5%.

24. d—Solve using the following formula: (rate)(kit size)(1 hr/60 min) = gtt/min, where (100 mL/0.5 hr)(10 gtt/mL)(1 hr/60 min) = 33 gtt/min.

25. a—"au" means each ear.

26. b—Solve using Clark's rule: [weight (lb)/150] × adult dose = amount of medication patient should receive. Convert kilograms to pounds (8 kg × 2.2 lb/kg = 17.6 lb). Substitute the given information: 17.6/150 × 10 mL = 1.2 mL.

27. b—Solve using Clark's rule: [wt (lb)/150] × adult dose; (25/150) × 100 mg = 16.67 mg (17 mg).

28. a—Atorvastatin is the generic name for Lipitor, which is used in the treatment of hyperlipidemia (high cholesterol).

29. b—Guaifenesin is an expectorant, whereas the other three products are bronchodilators.

30. d—Young males receiving trazodone should be warned of experiencing priapism (a prolonged erection).

31. c—A liter is equal to 1,000 mL. Solving the following proportion:

$$1,000 \text{ mL}/8 \text{ hr} = X \text{ mL/hr, where } X = 125 \text{ mL}$$

32. c—A synergistic effect is a joint action of drugs in which their combined effect is more intense or longer in duration than the sum of their individual effects.
33. b—Using Young's rule: Age of child in years/(age of child in years + 12) × adult dose will yield 3.3 mg.
34. b—Cascara sagrada is used as a laxative; American ginseng is used to provide energy for the body, goldenseal is used for the immune system; and melatonin is used to induce sleep.
35. b—Inventory is the amount of product or goods available for sale.
36. a—A proper size syringe should not contain more than twice the volume to be measured.
37. c—Specific gravity = weight of a substance/weight of an equal volume of water or 170/150 = 1.13.
38. c—Pills, tablets, and capsules should be counted in multiples of fives.
39. c—1 gr is equal to approximately 65 mg; therefore 2 gr would weigh 130 mg.
40. b—One teaspoon is equal to 5 mL. "tid" means three times per day. The patient will be receiving 1 tsp three times per day or 15 mL. The total amount of medication to be dispensed is 75 mL. 75 mL/15 mL per day = 5 days.
41. a—Disulfiram (Antabuse) is used to treat patients suffering from alcohol abuse. Disulfiram stops the metabolism of alcohol at the aldehyde stage, which causes aldehyde to accumulate in the body. If alcohol is consumed, the patient becomes extremely sick. This sickness is characterized by symptoms of blurred vision, confusion, difficult breathing, intense throbbing in the head and neck, chest pain, nausea, severe headache, severe vomiting, thirst, and uneasiness.
42. a—"-osis" means abnormal condition and is found in words such as nephrosis or halitosis.
43. b—There are two types of emulsions, oil-in-water or water-in-oil. Emulsions are dispersions, in which one liquid is dispersed in another immiscible liquid.
44. b—1 kg is equal to 2.2 lb; therefore, 4.4 lb is equal to 2 kg.
45. a—Outside air flows into the back of the horizontal airflow hood and through the hood's HEPA filter and out toward the opening and the air is recirculated into the room. A vertical airflow hood is similar to the horizontal except that the air cannot be recirculated into the room. This air goes through two HEPA filters and is released into an open area or is vented to the outside.
46. d—Using the formula (IV)(IS) = (FV)(FS); where 5% is the initial strength, 1 pint (480 mL) is the initial volume and 1:50 (2%) is the final strength, the final volume would be 1,200 mL.
47. c—The FDA is responsible for ensuring that all medications are pure, safe, and effective. If a product is adulterated or misbranded, the FDA may issue a product recall if the manufacturer does not voluntarily issue one.
48. c—The following are the approved DAW codes used in pharmacy; DAW 0: Generic allowed by physician; DAW 1: Brand name required by MD; and DAW 2: Generic allowed, but patient requested brand name drug.
49. b—Military time begins at 12:01 AM and ends at midnight, which is 24:00 hours. 0800 is the same as 8 AM.
50. b—Suppositories are inserted into body orifices such as the rectum, urethra, and vagina. PR is an abbreviation meaning "per rectum."
51. b—Norflex is a skeletal muscle relaxant.
52. d—A medication is guaranteed by the manufacturer to be effective until the last day of the month.
53. b—Inderal can be used prophylactically for migraines; Imitrex, Midrin, and Stadol are used as abortive therapies for migraine headaches.
54. b—Clotrimazole is an antifungal agent.
55. a—The inscription is the name, strength, and quantity of the medication to be dispensed; Rx means to take a particular drug, the signa means "write on label" and is direction to the patient, and the subscription contains instructions to the pharmacist such as refills, packaging, and generic substitution.
56. c—Convert milligrams to a gram (24 mg = 0.024 g) and solve the problem using proportions. $250.00/1 g = $X/0.024 g, where X = $6.00.
57. d—Calculate how long the bag will last (volume/rate or 1,000 mL/100 mL per hour), which is 10 hr. Using military time, add 10 hr to 0800 hr to get 1800 hr.
58. b—A fentanyl patch or Duragesic is a transdermal patch that will provide the patient with continuous medication for 3 days (72 hr).

59. b—An LCSW is a Licensed Clinical Social Worker, who works with individuals with affective disorders. They cannot prescribe medications.

60. b—A PCA is a patient-controlled analgesia device used to infuse analgesics into the patient.

61. c—MedWatch is a program instituted by the FDA that involves a voluntary reporting of adverse health events and medical products.

62. c—The lumen is the opening in the needle by which medication is expelled from a syringe.

63. d—All of the above except answer D are required on a Controlled Substance Administration Record, which is used to document controlled substance usage in a hospital or long-term care institution.

64. b—All pharmacies wishing to dispense controlled substances must register with the DEA by submitting a DEA Form 224.

65. c—Controlled dose (CD), controlled release (CR), and sustained release (SR) are time or extended-release dosage forms. The abbreviation ERF does not exist in the practice of pharmacy.

66. d—The number size is inversely proportionate to the amount it will contain; the smaller the number, the greater the capacity of the capsule.

67. a—Atenolol (Tenormin), carisoprodol (Soma), nadolol (Corgard), and propranolol (Inderal).

68. b—Both federal and state law do not allow for a patient to call a new prescription into the pharmacy. A patient may refill a prescription by telephone.

69. c—International units are a form of measure to indicate activity of a biological product. Vitamin B is measured in milligrams.

70. a—Policies are rules, procedures are involved with processes, protocol is concerned with appropriate behavior, and standards are expectations.

71. b—70% isopropyl alcohol is used to clean both horizontal and vertical laminar flow hoods.

72. a—BS is an approved abbreviation meaning blood sugar.

73. c—Enalapril is the same as Vasotec. The generic name for Accupril is quinapril; Monopril is fosinopril; and Zestril is lisinopril.

74. a—Acetaminophen should be taken because it does not thin the blood like aspirin, NSAIDs, or narcotic analgesics. A person could hemorrhage to death if his or her blood is too thin.

75. a—Benztropine (Cogentin) is used to minimize the effects by responding to the excess muscle activity of antipsychotics.

76. d—Solve by using the following formula: Final volume × % (expressed as a decimal) = amount of active ingredient. Final volume × 0.2 = 40 g, where the final volume will be 200 mL.

77. d—Antihistamines should not be used; beta blockers may constrict the bronchi; and many patients are sensitive to aspirin, and NSAIDs.

78. a—Tessalon Perles (benzonatate) are used as an antitussive because they anesthetize the stretch receptors in the airway, lungs, and pleura, but not the respiratory center.

79. b—Lansoprazole (Prevacid) is not an OTC product.

80. b—The generic name for Pepcid is famotidine.

81. d—An owner, a pharmacist, or a pharmacy supervisor who has been given the power of attorney is authorized to sign a DEA Form 222.

82. d—Flow rate is a specific volume/unit of time (1,000 mL/8 hr = 125 mL/hr).

83. c—Convert 154 lb to kilograms (154 lb/2.2 lb per kg = 70 kg). Calculate the amount of drug the patient will receive per day (12 mg/kg/day × 70 kg = 840 mg). Multiply the amount per day times 5 days (840 mg/day × 5 days = 4,200 mg). Convert milligrams to grams (4,200 mg/1,000 mg per g = 4.2 g).

84. b—ii (2) caps (capsules) stat (immediately) then i (one) cap (capsule) q (every) hr (hour), max (maximum) 5 caps (5 capsules)/(per or in) 12 hr (hours).

85. c—Joint.

86. c—MAC stands for maximum allowable cost and is used in reimbursement of multisource drugs by third-party insurance plans. Generic drugs are nonproprietary, whereas brand or trade drugs are proprietary drugs that are covered by a patent.

87. b—MAOIs inhibit the activity of enzymes, which break down catecholamine; therefore, the buildup of transmitters occurs at the synapse. Because of this buildup, they must be washed out of the system before continuing with another antidepressant.

88. c—DEA numbers are required only on the hard copy of a prescription for a controlled substance.

89. b—Using the formula (IS)(IV) = (FS)(FV), where the initial strength is 30%, the final volume is 2.5 L (2,500 mL) and the final strength is 5%; the initial volume will be 417 mL. The problem is asking for

the amount of water (diluent) to be added. Use the equation of final volume − initial volume = amount of diluent to be added to get 2,083 mL.

90. c—One pair of gloves is worn underneath the cuffs of the protective clothing and the second pair of gloves goes over the top of the cuffs of the protective clothing.

91. b—Amoxicillin is used prophylactically whenever a patient has a heart prosthesis, congenital heart disease, or mitral valve prolapse.

92. b—NS is an abbreviation for normal saline (0.9%), which is one of the vehicles used in IV admixtures.

93. a—Desyrel may cause a young male to experience priapism.

94. c—Lorazepam is a Schedule IV drug.

95. c—Ranitidine (Zantac) is not among the drugs to be excluded from using child-resistant containers under the Poison Control Act of 1970.

96. d—Sublingual tablets are absorbed directly into the bloodstream by being placed under the tongue, and therefore bypassing the digestive system.

97. c—The Drug Topics Red Book is a good source of drug costs. Information found in the Red Book includes emergency information, clinical reference guides, practice management and professional development, pharmacy and health care organizations, drug reimbursement information, manufacturer/wholesaler information, product identification, Rx product listings, OTC/nondrug product listings and complementary/herbal product referencing.

98. c—Set the problem up as proportion using 3 mg/1 lb = X mg/60 lb, where X = 180 mg.

99. c—Noncompliance reports are a tool used to monitor savings/losses of a pharmacy, when a Group Purchasing Organization (GPO) has negotiated specific prices for pharmaceutical products with a specific vendor.

100. b—A nonproprietary drug is another name for a generic drug; a proprietary or trade name is another name for a brand name drug; investigational drugs have not obtained FDA approval; and an OTC is an over-the-counter medication that does not need a prescription from a physician to purchase.

101. b—According to the Controlled Substance Act of 1970, an individual must be at least 18 years of age to purchase exempt narcotics.

102. c—A patient taking milk with their tetracycline is a drug-food interaction. Milk chelates (binds) with tetracycline, resulting in a loss of effectiveness of the medication. Adverse effects are undesirable effects of a medication; a synergistic effect occurs when the sum of the effects of two drugs is greater than taking them separately.

103. c—1800 hours is the same as 6 PM. Military time begins at midnight and each hour of the day corresponds to a specific time. Military time does not reset at noon. Military time does not consider AM or PM.

104. c—A Code Blue is a system to communicate to hospital staff that a patient is experiencing a life-threatening situation, such as his or her heart or breathing has ceased. A Code Blue allows the hospital staff to respond with appropriate emergency procedures.

105. b—Histamine 2 receptor agonists would aggravate a gastrointestinal problem rather than cure it or alleviate the symptoms.

106. c—Chewing benzonatate (Tessalon Perles) would result in the patient having excessive salivation.

107. d—Zidovudine is the generic name for Retrovir.

108. a—A pharmacy is to prepare a "stat order" as quickly as possible, within 5–15 minutes of receiving the order.

109. a—Body surface area is the most accurate method because it takes into consideration both the height and weight of the patient.

110. d—Solving the problem using the formula 9C = 5F − 160 will yield an answer of 50 degrees.

111. c—This problem can be solved by using a proportion. 4.4 mEq/1 mL = 45 mEq/X mL, where X = 10.2 mL.

112. b—A deficiency in vitamin B1 causes beriberi; deficiencies in vitamin A result in night blindness, dry corneas, and inability of the epithelial cells to shed; vitamin C deficiency causes scurvy; and a vitamin D deficiency causes rickets.

113. c—A subscriber is the policyholder. A beneficiary is the individual who may receive a cash payout on the death of the subscriber; the dependent is an individual covered under an insurance plan. The patient may either be a subscriber or a dependent on an insurance plan.

114. b—Side effects of anti-cholinergic drugs include drying up of body fluid, which may cause a dry mouth, difficulty urinating or defecating, an inability to perspire, or the eye lens to become dry.

115. b—Convert the patient's weight in pounds to kilograms (13.2 lb × 1 kg/2.2 lb = 6 kg). Multiply the patient's weight in kg by the dose (6 kg × 25 mg/kg = 150 mg).

116. c—Multiply the percentage (expressed as a decimal) of talc by the total weight (120 g × 0.02 = 2.4 g or 2,400 mg).

117. b—One of the first things to be done in lowering hypertension is to modify the person's lifestyle, which includes reducing sodium intake, eliminating excess calories from the diet, increasing physical activity levels, and reducing alcohol and nicotine consumption. Increasing the amount of sleep an individual receives has no effect on reducing hypertension.

118. a—Hydrochlorothiazide is one of the ingredients found in all of the following medications: Diovan HCT, Dyazide, Hyzaar, and Zestoretic. Diovan HCT is valsartan and hydrochlorothiazide; Dyazide is triamterene and hydrochlorothiazide; Hyzaar is losartan and hydrochlorothiazide; and Zestoretic is lisinopril and hydrochlorothiazide.

119. c—Phytonadione (vitamin K) is the antidote to the anticoagulant, warfarin. Both heparin and enoxaparin are used to dissolve clots in the body and their antidote is protamine sulfate.

120. d—To convert a ratio to a percent, divide the first number by the second number and then multiply the answer by 100.

121. d—The first five digits of an NDC number refer to the drug manufacturer, the next four digits identify the drug product, and the final two digits identify the packaging of the product.

122. c—MDI is an abbreviation meaning metered-dose inhaler.

123. c—A solvent is the vehicle that contains the dissolved drug. A solute is the drug that is dissolved into the solvent; a solution contains both the solvent and solute; syrup is an example of a solvent.

124. a—Arrhythmias are an abnormal heart beat. Bradycardia, flutter, and tachycardia are examples of various arrhythmias.

125. c—%w/w is defined as the number of grams of a solute dissolved in 100 g. 30 g = 1 oz. Using a proportion of 1 g/100 g = X g/30 g, X = 0.3 g.

126. d—Each state has a Board of Pharmacy, which is responsible for determining the licensing requirements of pharmacists in that state. The State Board of Pharmacy can suspend or revoke the license of a pharmacist in that particular state. The Board of Pharmacy is responsible for the practice of pharmacy in a state, which includes pharmacy technicians.

127. b—"fibro-" means muscle; "-algia" means pain.

128. a—120 mg is the minimum weighable amount on a Class A or Class III balance.

129. a—Capsules can be prepared using the "punch method."

130. c—Material Safety Data Sheets are required by OSHA and must be provided by the manufacturer, importer, or distributor of a hazardous chemical in the workplace. They must be in English and must contain the following information: chemical and common names; if a mixture, the chemical and common names of the ingredients; physical and chemical characteristics; physical hazards; health hazards; route of entry into the body; OSHA permissible exposure limit; precautions for safe handling and use; procedures for cleanup of spills; emergency and first aid procedures; date of preparation of MSDS or date of latest revision; and the name, address, and telephone number of the manufacturer, importer, or distributor.

131. c—Most liquid antibiotics including amoxicillin need to be stored in a refrigerator after they are reconstituted. Reconstituted antibiotics are good for 10 days after reconstitution.

132. a—Can be solved by using the following formula: Cost + [(markup rate)(cost)] = retail price or $4.50 + [(0.30)(4.50)] = $5.85.

133. a—Depakote (divalproex), Neurontin (gabapentin), Mysoline (primidone), and Depakene (valproic acid).

134. b—Color of ingredient does not need to be noted on the Master Formula Sheet.

135. b—"-oculo" means eye, "ultro" means each.

136. c—Laminar flow hoods used in the preparation of IV admixtures are a critical component of aseptic technique. The class of the HEPA filter used will determine the number of particles allowed per given area.

137. a—A closed formulary is a limited list of medications that may be used in filling prescriptions in an institution or allowed by a managed care third party; an open formulary allows for any medication to be dispensed; and a restricted formulary is a hybrid of both an open and closed formulary system.

138. c—Variable copayment may be affected by the cost of the prescription or if it is considered a lifestyle drug. Variable copayments may occur if a patient requests the brand name drug when the physician has given permission for a generic to be used. A fixed copayment means that a patient pays the same amount of copay regardless of the cost of the prescription; percentage copay indicates that a patient will pay a given percentage on every prescription regardless of the cost.

139. d—The Physicians' Desk Reference is a compilation of monographs submitted by the manufacturers and is published yearly.

140. b—A prescription taken "po" is taken by mouth and would be an oral preparation.

PRACTICE EXAMINATION III ANSWERS

1. b—Both horizontal and vertical laminar airflow hoods must be on for at least 30 min before being used in the preparation of aseptic products.

2. a—"hs" means at the hour of bed or hour of sleep.

3. b—Lorabid is a macrolide antibiotic

4. a—Colchicine is used in the treatment of gout and is not an NSAID.

5. d—Nitrofurantoin is better absorbed into the body if it is taken with food.

6. c—"os" means left eye.

7. a—A buccal tablet is placed between the gum and cheek. It is absorbed directly into the bloodstream and bypasses the digestive system.

8. a—A dosage schedule states exactly when a medication is to be administered to the patients such as 8 AM or 4 PM.

9. d—Warfarin is contraindicated because it would prevent the blood clotting or coagulating.

10. c—"-ectomy" means removal and is found in words such as tonsillectomy, vasectomy, and mastectomy.

11. c—According to the Controlled Substance Act of 1970, the maximum numbers of refills allowed by a physician is five refills within 6 months of the date of the prescription being written.

12. b—To solve this problem, the following formula should be used: (IS)(IV) = (FS)(FV), and substitute the following: (50%)(120 mL) = (FS)(300 mL), where the final volume is calculated by adding 6 oz (180 mL) to the initial volume of 120 mL. The final strength is 20%.

13. c—Post monitoring of medications is a tool for quality assurance to ensure medications are pure, safe, and effective. Adverse side effects are monitored and any potential for harm is noted. If the medication may have detrimental effects on an individual, it may be pulled from the market by the manufacturer or the FDA. Recent examples include Rezulin, Redux, and Pondimin.

14. d—Hyperthyroidism—overproduction of the thyroid gland—may result in a goiter.

15. d—Regular insulin is the only type of insulin that may be added to an IV solution.

16. c—A monograph is literature on a specific drug by the drug manufacturer that may include a description, indications, contraindications, adverse effects, and warnings. The PDR is an example of a collection of drug monographs.

17. d—OBRA mandated that both a Drug Utilization Review and an offer to counsel must be made to every patient. A Drug Utilization Review is a technical task that a technician may perform, whereas counseling must be performed by a pharmacist.

18. a—1 cubic centimeter (cc) = 1 milliliter (mL).

19. c—A combination of alcohol in any form or concentration may interact with metronidazole, causing extreme, unpleasant side effects from processes occurring in the liver.

20. b—A patient would receive a maximum of six doses of (5 cc = 5 mL)/day for 5 days. The pharmacy would need to dispense 150 mL (5 fl oz) to fill the prescription.

21. d—A corticosteroid ointment is more potent than a cream, gel, or lotion, assuming they are of the same concentration.

22. d—A biennial inventory is required of all controlled substances by the DEA every 2 years.

23. a—MAOIs, SSRIs, and TCAs are used to treat depression. Antipsychotics are used to treat a different affective disorder.

24. d—There are 30 mL to a fluid ounce. 240 mL/30 mL per fluid ounce = 8 oz.

25. a—A unit dose is the amount of medication required for one dose of the medication. The order is for 40 mg. To solve for the volume desired, use: 10 mg/mL = 40 mg/X mL or 4 mL.

26. c—The patient is receiving 10 mg per dose and will receive three doses in 1 day. 3 doses × 10 mg/dose will equal 30 mg.
27. d—Olopatadine is the generic name for Patanol. Brimonidine is Alphagan, ciprofloxacin is Ciloxan, and latanoprost is Xalatan.
28. a—According to the DEA and the Controlled Substance Act, medications placed in Schedule I have no medicinal use in the United States and have the highest potential for abuse.
29. b—Ease of administration is an advantage of an oral dosage form. There are no special skills required to administer this form.
30. c—The Pharmacy and Therapeutic Committee, composed of physicians, nurses, pharmacists, and administrators, determines the formulary based on the advantages/disadvantages of a medication and its cost-effectiveness.
31. a—Young's rule calculates a dose based on a child's age and uses the following formula: [Age (years)/[age (years) + 12] × adult dose; 10/(10+12) × 30 mg = 13 mg.
32. d—On-line adjudication (electronic) is the method most commonly used to submit payments to insurance carriers. In certain situations, a hard copy of the claim form (Universal Claim Form) may be required to be submitted for payment.
33. a—A month is considered to have 30 days in it. Because the patient is only taking the medication every other day, they would be taking 15 tablets in 30 days.
34. c—2.4 g = 2,400 mg (1 g = 1,000 mg); therefore, 600 mg/1 tablet = 2,400 mg/X tablets each day.
35. b—A generic drug must contain the same active ingredients as the original brand name drug; be identical in strength, dosage form, and route of administration; have the same use indications; meet the same batch requirements for identity, strength, purity, and quality; and yield similar blood absorption and urinary excretion curves for the active ingredient.
36. c—Solve using the following equation: Final volume × strength (expressed as a decimal) = amount of active ingredient (g); 600 mL × 1/5,000 = 0.12 g; convert 0.12 g to mg (0.12 g × 1,000 mg/1 g = 120 mg). Calculate the number of tablets to dispense by dividing the total dose/dose per tablet: 120 mg/30 mg per tablet = 4 tablets.
37. d—Solve by calculating the amount of medication the patient is to receive daily weight of child × dose × frequency (30 kg × 10 mg/kg × 3 doses per day = 900 mg per day). To calculate the volume, solve using a proportion: 50 mg/mL = 900 mg/X mL, where X = 18 mL.
38. d—"NPO" means that the patient is not to receive anything by mouth, which means no food, liquid, or medication to be taken orally.
39. c—Zyprexa (olanzapine), Aricept (donepezil), Skelaxin (metaxalone), and Risperdal (risperidone).
40. d—MS (morphine sulfate) IM (intramuscularly) q (every) 4 h (4 hr) prn (as needed) for pain. The verb "inject" was chosen because of the route of administration.
41. b—"prn" means as needed for a particular condition.
42. c—1 L = 1,000 mL. Solve using the following formula: (IS)(IV) = (FS)(FV); (70%)(1,000 mL) = (30%)(X mL), where X = 2,333 mL. To calculate the amount of water to be added, subtract the initial volume from the final volume (2,333 mL − 1000 mL = 1,333 mL).
43. d—"i tab tid" means take 1 tablet three times per day. 30 tablets/3 tablets/day = 10 days' supply.
44. d—This is an alligation problem. Draw a tic-tac-toe table and place the highest concentration (10%) in the upper left hand corner; the lowest concentration (1%) in the lower left hand corner; and the quantity to be prepared in the middle (45 g of 2%). Perform the following: 10 − 2 = 8 parts of the 1% solution and 2 − 1 = 1 part of the 10%. Add the parts together (8 + 1 = 9 parts); calculate the amounts of each by concentration (10%:1/9 × 45 g = 5 g; 1%:8/9 × 45 g = 40 g).
45. c—Itraconazole (Sporanox) is an antifungal agent, which is prescribed using "pulse dosing." Pulse dosing requires that the patient take one capsule daily for 1 week, skip 3 weeks, and resume. This form of dosing is effective therapeutically and is cost-effective.
46. d—i (1) cap (capsule) qid (four times per day) ac (before meals) and hs (bedtime).
47. b—"DAW 1" means the physician is requesting that the patient receive the brand name drug.
48. a—Capitation is a form of reimbursement used by insurance companies. This form of reimbursement favors the insurance company when the cost of the prescriptions exceeds the capitation being paid.
49. a—"Non rep" means do not repeat and is used to indicate that no additional refills are authorized.
50. c—Ciprofloxacin (Cipro) is a quinolone antibiotic.

51. a—"AAC" means actual acquisition cost, which means the pharmacy is reimbursed for what they actually paid for the medication after receiving discounts from either the manufacturer or wholesaler.

52. d—Fexofenadine is available only as an oral preparation. The following are transdermal names for the following products: clonidine (Catapres TTS), estradiol (Estraderm or Climara), and fentanyl (Duragesic).

53. c—Zestril is the brand name for lisinopril; enalapril (Vasotec), fosinopril (Monopril), and quinapril (Accupril).

54. c—Solve using the following formula: (IS)(IV) = (FS)(FV); (10%)(100 mL) = (0.9%)(X mL), where X = 1,111 mL. To calculate the amount of diluent, subtract the initial volume from the final volume (1,111 mL − 100 mL = 1,011 mL of diluent).

55. d—If tetracycline is taken after it has passed its expiration established by the manufacturer, the patient may die. If the other products are taken after they have expired, the effectiveness will not be guaranteed by the manufacturer and the patient may experience side effects.

56. a—An aseptic technique is the process of preparing sterile product to be injected into the body. Extemporaneous compounding, geometric dilution, and levigation are terms used in the production of nonsterile compounds.

57. c—Procedures are a way to avoid errors in performing a specific task.

58. a—Osteo is the root word for bone. The following root words are for the other terms; cell (cyte), lymph (lymph), and muscle (myo).

59. b—Solve using Clark's rule: [wt (lb)/150] × adult dose; [40/150] × 25 mg = 6.66 mg.

60. c—GERD is an acronym for gastroesophageal reflux disease, describing symptoms commonly referred to heartburn.

61. c—"tid" means three times per day.

62. d—Pharmacy technicians perform technical tasks; responding to a potential contraindication is a judgment decision, which only pharmacists can perform.

63. c—Salicylates have the tendency to irritate the stomach and affect blood platelets before an overdosage occurs. Tinnitus is a ringing in the ears and is a symptom of salicylate overdosage.

64. d—NSAIDs are indicated for use as an analgesic, an anti-inflammatory agent, or to reduce fever as an antipyretic.

65. a—Atenolol is the generic name for Tenormin; metoprolol (Lopressor or Toprol XL), nadolol (Corgard), and propranolol (Inderal).

66. c—Class I recalls result in serious adverse health consequence or death; Class II recalls may cause temporary or medically reversible adverse health consequences; Class II recall is not likely to cause an adverse health consequence.

67. b—Look at the bottom of the meniscus or the lowest point of the liquid when a liquid is being measured.

68. c—A used needle should be disposed in a red plastic sharps container to prevent an individual from being injured by a needle.

69. c—Room temperature is 15–30°C (59–86°F).

70. b—The first five digits of an NDC identify the drug manufacturer, the next four digits indicate the drug product, and the last two digits refer to the packaging of the drug.

71. b—Calculate by using the following formula: Final volume × strength (expressed as a decimal = amount of active ingredient (g); 5 mL × 0.15 = 0.75 g or 750 mg.

72. a—Benzocaine is a topical local anesthetic.

73. a—The Controlled Substance Act of 1970 requires that a pharmacy submit a DEA Form 41 in triplicate before the destruction of any controlled substances.

74. d—This is an alligation problem. Set the problem up with 10% in the top left corner, 5% in the center, and 2% in the bottom left corner. Calculate the number of parts of each strength to be used: 10% requires 3 parts (5 − 2) and the 2% requires 5 parts (10 − 5). To calculate the quantities of each, multiply ratio of parts by the total quantity to be prepared (10%: 3 parts/8 parts × 25 g = 9.4 g; 2%: 5 parts/8 parts × 25 g = 15.6 g).

75. d—Venlafaxine is the generic name for Effexor and is an SSRI.

76. b—Methylphenidate (Ritalin) is a Schedule II drug according to the Controlled Substance Act.

77. a—A Class A balance is a piece of required equipment for all pharmacies. Class A balances have a sensitivity of 6 mg.

78. c—Nifedipine is generic name for both Procardia and Adalat, which are calcium channel blockers.

79. c—A dry, non-productive cough may occur as a side effect for patients taking ACE inhibitors.

80. a—A prefix occurs before the root word, which is followed by a suffix. Vowels combine the prefix, root word, and suffix together.

81. c—10 mg/mL is the same as 0.01 g/mL, which is equal to 1%. Solve using the following formula: (IS)(IV) = (FS)(FV), where (10%)(IV) = (1%)(120 mL), where IV = 12 mL.

82. d—An adverse reaction may occur if alcohol is consumed in any strength or form; stomach irritation is less likely to occur if it is taken with food; and because metronidazole is an antibiotic, metronidazole should be taken until completion to ensure the infection has been eradicated.

83. a—The patient would take a maximum of 2 tablets per dose with a maximum of 6 doses per day. 60 tablets/2 tablets/dose/6 doses/day will last 5 days.

84. b—Ciprofloxacin (Cipro) should not be given because it will affect the formation of the tendons in the body and may result in temporary damage.

85. d—Syrup contain sucrose (sugar).

86. c—Solve using the following formula: Final volume × strength (expressed as a decimal) = amount of active ingredient (g); 1,000 mL × 1/1,000 = 1 g. Convert grams to milligrams (1 g × 1,000 mg/g = 1,000 mg). 10 gr = 650 mg. Next calculate the number of tablets by dividing the total weight by the weight per tablet (1,000 mg/650 mg per tablet = 1½ tablets).

87. d—The Occupational Safety and Health Act was enacted to protect the employee in the workplace and reduce the possibility of an employee being injured at work.

88. c—Reye syndrome may develop if a child who has been exposed to the virus causing chickenpox takes aspirin. Tylenol is highly recommended for children instead of aspirin.

89. d—D5W means 5% dextrose in water. 1 L = 1,000 mL. %w/v is defined as the number of grams per 100 mL of solution. Can be solved using the following proportion: 5 g/100 mL = X g/1,000 mL, where X = 50 g.

90. b—Calan and Isoptin are brand names for verapamil.

91. a—Elixirs contain alcohol.

92. c—"ac" means before meals.

93. a—Oxycodone + acetaminophen is the generic name for Percocet, which is a Schedule II drug under the Controlled Substance Act. Schedule II drugs cannot be refilled. The physician must write a new prescription if the patient requires additional medication.

94. d—"Intra" means within, whereas "hypo" means below, "iso" means equal, and "inter" means between.

95. b—50 mg/1 mL = 75 mg/X mL, where X = 1.5 mL.

96. c—Inunction refers to the process of rubbing a substance into the skin. Inunction is used when applying creams, lotions, ointments, and pastes.

97. d—An individual may experience a severe rash as a result of photosensitivity to the sun if the patient is taking tetracycline. A patient should take tetracycline 1 hour before or 2 hours after a meal, which will prevent food and the medication from binding together. Antibiotics should be taken until they are completed.

98. a—The Durham-Humphrey Amendment of 1951 requires that the Federal Legend (Federal law prohibits the dispensing of this medication without a prescription) appear on all prescription medication containers. Answer B is required by the Controlled Substance Act of 1970 to appear on all prescriptions of controlled substances; answer C is required on any OTC product that is not in a child-resistant package as a result of the Poison Control Act of 1970; and answer D is a warning required by the Food, Drug, and Cosmetic Act of 1938.

99. a—JCAHO stands for the Joint Commission on Accreditation of Healthcare Organizations. Pyxis, Robot Rx, and SureMed are automated dispensing systems.

100. b—D5W means 5% dextrose dissolved in water.

101. b—A list price is a synonym for suggested retail price. Discounted price, net price, and sale price reflect a reduction in price.

102. c—Readily retrievable is being able to provide the necessary information to a third party, such as the DEA or representatives from a particular state board of pharmacy, within 72 hr.

103. d—Beta 2 agonists, cromolyn, and corticosteroids are treatments for asthma.

104. d—The State Board of Pharmacy will investigate all reported claims of medication error and will consider appropriate sanctions against all providers. The State Board of Pharmacy is concerned with the practice of pharmacy in a particular state, which includes the behavior of pharmacists. The DEA is

concerned about adherence to the Controlled Substance Act; the FDA's priorities are to ensure that food and medications are pure, safe, and effective; Med Watch is concerned with adverse effects of medications.

105. b—H2 antagonists do not have an interaction with phenobarbital. Beta-blockers, TCAs (tricyclic antidepressants), and warfarin have a negative drug interaction with phenobarbital.

106. a—"prn" means as needed for a particular indication. Also, it may refer to unlimited refills for a specific period as determined by either federal or state laws, whichever is the more stringent.

107. b—A solution contains both a solute and a solvent.

108. d—A person's age will affect the physical condition of his or her organs. A person's disease state can influence other organ systems, such as the liver and kidney, and whether a medication may be contraindicated with a specific disease. An individual's gender can affect how a medication is absorbed, distributed, metabolized, or excreted from the body.

109. d—The Controlled Substance Act allows for certain controlled substances to be purchased without a prescription under specific conditions. These substances are Schedule V drugs. The medications involve products containing specific amounts of codeine and paregoric. To purchase a container, the individual must be at least 18 years of age, the product must be packaged in the manufacturer's original container (4-oz bottle), the exempt narcotic log must be signed, it must be sold by a pharmacist, and the patient may only purchase one 4-oz bottle in 48 hr.

110. c—An anaphylactic reaction is an extremely serious allergic reactions, which may be fatal. A person undergoing an anaphylactic reaction will find his or her trachea constricting and will experience difficulty breathing.

111. d—Taking fluoxetine, oral contraceptives, or theophylline with phenytoin will result in a drug interaction.

112. b—Nosocomial infections are hospital-derived infections.

113. d—Computers do all of these activities.

114. d—A red C stamped on a prescription indicates that the medication is a controlled substance. All filled controlled substance prescriptions must be stamped with a red, 1-inch C.

115. a—Capoten (captopril), Coreg (carvedilol), Catapres (clonidine), Plavix (clopidogrel).

116. d—Glaucoma is a chronic disorder characterized by abnormally high internal eye pressure that destroys the optic nerve and can cause partial to complete blindness.

117. c—Fexofenadine (Allegra) requires a prescription. Chlorpheniramine (Chlor-Trimeton), diphenhydramine (Benadryl), and loratadine (Claritin) are all antihistamines available OTC.

118. d—Antihypertensives do not exhibit a drug-drug interaction with oral contraceptives. Antibiotics, anticonvulsants, and antifungal agents will reduce the effectiveness of oral contraceptives.

119. d—Type II (adult onset) diabetes can be controlled through behavior modification, which will result in a reduction of body weight. Type I requires insulin injections because of the body's inability to produce insulin; gestational diabetes will normally be reversed after pregnancy. Secondary diabetes is caused by various medications.

120. a—A "crash cart" is synonymous with a Code Blue cart. A Code Blue is announced whenever a patient undergoes a serious condition, which may result in death. Serious situations involving the heart or the lungs are the more common causes for calling a Code Blue.

121. a—"MAR" stands for Medication Administration Record.

122. c—I-9s must be completed on all new employees. An employee must provide specific identification to prove his or her identity. Failure to provide documentation will result in not being hired. A business can face extremely high fines for not maintaining properly completed I-9s.

123. d—Prescriptions are medication orders written by a physician to be obtained through a community or mail-order pharmacy.

124. b—A modified unit dose is a drug distribution system that combines unit-dose medications blister-packaged onto a multiple-dose card, instead of being placed into a box. They are referred to as punch cards, bingo cards, or blister cards and may contain 30, 60, or 90 units on one card.

125. b—A HEPA filter is a high-efficiency particulate air filter found in a laminar flow hood to remove contaminants.

126. d—SMZ-TMP DS is the generic for either Bactrim DS or Septra DS, which are sulfa drugs used to treat a urinary tract infection.

127. d—Celebrex is an NSAID, whose mechanism of action is a COX-2 inhibitor.

128. b—Prevacid (lansoprazole), Nexium (esomeprazole), Prilosec (omeprazole), Protonix (pantoprazole).

129. d—Troches, lozenges, and pastilles are solid dosage forms that are administered buccally.
130. b—FDCA 1938 is the Food, Drug, and Cosmetic Act of 1938, which clearly defined adulteration and misbranding. Preparing prescriptions under unsanitary conditions is an example of adulteration.
131. b—Azactam (aztreonam) is a cephalosporin.
132. c—Drug Topics Orange Book.
133. b—25% means that there are 25 g in 100 mL of solution. Solve using a proportion 25 g/100 mL = X g/200 mL, where X = 50 g. To calculate the kcal, solve using the following proportion: 1 g/3.4 kcal = 50 g/ X kcal, where X = 170 kcal.
134. c—Insurance companies prefer that generic medications are dispensed because of the potential savings to both the insurance company and the patient.
135. b—A bevel is the slanted part of the needle; the hub is the place of attachment of a needle, and the lumen is the opening of the needle. Coring refers to the fragments of a vial that contaminate a parenteral solution.
136. a—Ativan (lorazepam), Dalmane (flurazepam), Klonopin (clonazepam), and Valium (diazepam).
137. c—The subscription on a prescription are directions to a pharmacist, and may include compounding, packaging, labeling, refills, and use of generic medication.
138. c—The gauge of a needle is inversely proportional to the diameter of the needle.
139. c—A deductible is an amount an individual must pay before the insurance company begins to make a payment; coinsurance occurs when two parties are responsible for the payment; copay means the insured party must pay a given amount of money each time before the insurance company begins to pay; and maximum allowable cost is the most the insurance company will pay for a generic medication.
140. b—i is the Roman numeral for one; gtt means drop; ou means each eye; and bid means twice per day. Instill one drop in each eye twice a day.

PRACTICE EXAMINATION IV ANSWERS

1. b—Calculate the volume of medication required to deliver the prescribed amount of drug per hour: 1 g (1,000 mg)/250 mL = 250 mg/ X mL, where X = 62.5 mL. To calculate the flow rate, solve using the following formula: Rate (mL/hr) × drop size (drop/mL) × 1 hr/60 min = gtt/min (62.5 mL/hr)(10 gtt/mL)(1 hr/60 min) = 10 gtt/min.
2. b—A Class II drug recall is one in which the probability exists that the use of the product will cause adverse health events that are temporary or medically reversible. A Class I drug recall shows that there is a reasonable probability that use of the product will cause or lead to serious adverse events or death; a Class III recall will probably not cause an adverse health event.
3. c—Lisinopril is the generic name for Zestril and Prinivil.
4. c—The basic formula for medication reimbursement is drug cost + dispensing fee. There are many variations of this formula taking into consideration AWP, AAC, MAC, and percentages.
5. c—"Milli" is a prefix meaning 1/1,000. There are 1,000 mL in 1 L.
6. d—Nitroglycerin should be taken sublingually because of the urgency of obtaining relief from an angina attack. Sublingual medications bypass the digestive tract and are rapidly absorbed into the bloodstream by being placed under the tongue, which has a large blood supply.
7. d—The half-life of a medication is the amount of time required to eliminate one half of the amount of the drug from the body. Half-life is a tool used to determine dosing frequency of a medication.
8. d—Counseling is a judgmental task that only pharmacists are permitted to perform. Pharmacy technicians are allowed to perform technical tasks only at the current time.
9. d—Tricyclic antidepressants such as amitriptyline may be used in the treatment of chronic pain.
10. d—Using the following formula: Rate (mL/hr) × drop factor (gtt/mL) × (1 hr/60 min) = gtt/min. Substituting the following (500 mL/6 hr) × (15 gtt/mL) × (1 hr/60 min) = 20.83 gtt/min. 20.83 gtt/min is rounded down to 20.
11. d—Tablets are a solid dosage form, whereas creams, ointments, and suspensions are dispersions.
12. d—The problem can be solved using a proportion: 125 mg/5 mL = 500 mg/X mL, where X = 20 mL.
13. c—Diltiazem (Cardizem) is a calcium channel blocker. Atenolol and carvedilol are beta-blockers and lisinopril is an ACE inhibitor.
14. d—"os" means left eye, which is the only difference among all of the interpretations.

15. d—Singulair is a montelukast. Advair is a combination of fluticasone and salmeterol; Allegra D is fexofenadine and pseudoephedrine; and Combivent is albuterol and ipratropium.

16. b—A side effect of antianxiety medications, antidepressants, and anticonvulsants is drowsiness.

17. b—During the process of geometric dilution, an individual is combining more than one ingredient. One begins by using the most potent (normally the smallest quantity) first in the mortar, then an equal amount of the next most potent drug is added. This process continues until all quantities have been added and mixed. During geometric dilution, the total quantity of drug being prepared is approximately doubling with each ingredient added.

18. a—Compliance is an act of adhering to particular directions. The ease of administration is a factor in a patient's compliance in taking a medication. Both first and second pass are components of pharmacokinetics.

19. c—A physician's DEA number is required only on the hard copy of a prescription or controlled substances; the DEA number is not required on the prescription label of controlled substances.

20. b—Comminution is the act of reducing a substance to small, fine particles; blending is the act of combining two substances; sifting is used to combine powders; and tumbling is accomplished by combining powders in a bag.

21. b—Tylenol 3 contains 325 mg of APAP and 30 mg (½ gr) of codeine in it.

22. c—Glyburide is the generic name for both Micronase and DiaBeta.

23. a—Alendronate is the generic for Fosamax. The other medications' brand names are calcitonin-salmon (Miacalcin), etidronate (Didronel), and raloxifene (Evista).

24. a—Pharmacokinetics is the study of the absorption, distribution, metabolism, and elimination of a drug from the body. Pharmacognosy is the study of natural products; pharmacology describes how a drug works on the body; and pharmacopeia is a listing of drugs.

25. d—A dispersion is not dissolved in a vehicle, but rather distributed throughout it. Suppositories are solid dosage forms, whereas dispersions are a liquid dosage form. Emulsions and lotions are liquid dosage forms. An ointment is a type of emulsion.

26. c—Phenytoin is the generic name for Dilantin, an anticonvulsant. Divalproex (Depakote), gabapentin (Neurontin), valproic acid (Depakene).

27. a—An URI is an acronym for upper respiratory infection.

28. c—Using the formula, $9C = 5F - 160$, substitute 98.6 with the F and the answer will be 37°C.

29. b—Using Young's rule [Age (years)/age (years) + 12] × adult dose, the child will need a dose of 21.4 mg.

30. b—Glipizide is the generic name for Glucotrol.

31. c—Risperidone (Risperdal) is an antipsychotic used to relieve symptoms but not cure the disease.

32. d—St. John's wort has been used in the treatment of depression.

33. c—Olanzapine is the generic name for Zyprexa, olopatadine is the generic for Patanol, nefazodone is Serzone, and trazodone is Desyrel.

34. c—One dose is equal to 1 tsp (5 mL), which is taken three times per day for 10 days. The pharmacy will need to dispense 150 mL to the patient.

35. c—A DAW 2 means that a physician approved the dispensing of a generic drug, but the patient requested the brand name drug. A DAW means that the physician approved the dispensing of a generic drug; a DAW 1 indicates that the physician wants the patient to receive the brand name drug only. A DAW 5 means that the pharmacy has designated this drug as their generic drug of choice.

36. b—Class A balances, which are used to measure solid ingredients in compounding in a pharmacy, must have a minimum sensitivity of 6 mg.

37. b—Forceps are used to prevent oils from the hands from being deposited on the weight, which may alter the composition of the weight.

38. d—Tablets are produced by compression, capsules may be made by using the "punch method," and suppositories are made by compression and molding.

39. d—Melatonin has been shown to be effective in assisting individuals falling asleep, especially when travelers in different time zones.

40. b—The Controlled Substance Act of 1970 allows for a maximum of five refills for Schedules III–V within 5 months of the date the prescription was written.

41. d—A potential side effect of ibuprofen is stomach irritation. To reduce this possibility, food should be taken to act as a buffer against stomach irritation.

42. b—Ipecac is an emetic to induce vomiting; Emetrol is an antiemetic, PEG is used as a bowel evacuant, and simethicone is an antiflatulent.

43. d—"qs ad" are directions to the pharmacist in compounding a prescription "to make up to" a given weight or volume of a substance.

44. c—A loading dose of a medication is a greater than normal dose of a medication, which enables the drug to obtain a therapeutic level in the body sooner than normal.

45. b—w/v shows the concentration of a solid dissolved in a liquid. It is the number of grams dissolved in 100 mL of liquid.

46. d—Insulin is administered subcutaneously above and below the waist, in the buttocks, and upper arms.

47. c—HCTZ is an abbreviation for the diuretic hydrochlorothiazide.

48. c—To convert a ratio to a percent, write the ratio as a fraction, divide the numerator by the denominator, and multiply by 100. 1:20 is the same as 1/20. 1/20 = 0.05; 0.05 × 100 = 5.0%.

49. b—According to the Controlled Substance Act, an individual may only purchase one 4-oz bottle of an "exempt narcotic" every 48 hr.

50. a—Aspirin does not have the ability to reduce the level of cholesterol in the body. Fibric acid derivatives and HMG-CoA reductase inhibitors are classifications used to treat hyperlipidemia. Metamucil has been shown to lower cholesterol in the body.

51. a—Set up the following proportion: 25,000 units/500 mL = X units/1 mL, where X = 50 units.

52. d—Rickets is caused by a deficiency of vitamin D. Deficiencies of vitamin A result in night blindness, vitamin B1 in beriberi, and vitamin C in scurvy.

53. a—CSAR means Controlled Substance Administration Record. CSARs are used in hospitals and other institutional facilities to acknowledge the administration of a controlled substance to a patient. The administrator must sign his or her name and the time of administration.

54. c—Sulfasalazine does not require monitoring through blood work. Patients taking lithium, phenytoin, and warfarin need to have frequent blood samples tested to ensure they are receiving the appropriate dose of medication.

55. d—Regular insulin should be drawn up first if mixing with NPH insulin. Regular insulin does mix with Lente insulin; and glargine does not mix with any insulin.

56. d—Lamivudine is the generic name for Epivir (3TC); ddi (didanosine) is the generic for Videx.

57. d—The Controlled Substance Act requires that a pharmacy perform a biennial inventory of all controlled substances stocked in a pharmacy. An exact count must be performed on Schedule II medications and an estimated count must be done on Schedules III–V. An institution may perform an inventory more frequently if required by either state law or organizational policy

58. c—Specific gravity is a ratio of the weight of a substance to the weight of an equal volume of water (SG = weight of substance/weight of an equal volume of water): SG = 6,565 g/5,000 g: SG = 1.31.

59. c—Rx means to take a given product of a given strength and quantity.

60. d—U&C means the charge is the usual and customary charge, which a patient would pay if their third-party payer were not involved in the transaction.

61. d—An individual who recommends a product to a patient is performing a judgmental duty, which only a pharmacist may do.

62. b—"derm" means skin, "cerebr" (brain), "cranio" (skull), and "dent" (tooth).

63. c—Midrin is a combination product used to abort a migraine headache but is not a selective 5-HT receptor agonist. Imitrex, Maxalt, and Zomig are 5-HT receptor agonists.

64. c—Medicare is a federal program for individuals older than age 65; Medicaid is a federal program administered by the state for individuals (families) who meet specific income guidelines; Worker's Compensation is for individuals who are injured while working.

65. a—The Drug Topics Orange Book provides USP and NF drug standards and dispensing requirements.

66. a—An individual undergoing "dig toxicity" may experience the following: arrhythmias, nausea, and vomiting. They may see yellow-green halos around objects.

67. b—Nurses administer medication to patients and therefore would document the MAR. Physicians diagnose and prescribe, pharmacists dispense, and pharmacy technicians assist pharmacists in performing their duties.

68. d—One teaspoon is equal to 5 mL, and the patient is receiving 4 doses per day for 10 days: (5 mL/dose × 4 doses/day × 10 days = 200 mL).

69. d—The fluffy precipitate indicates the precipitation of dextrose and needs to be shaken to ensure that dextrose is thoroughly distributed throughout the bag.

70. c—Solve using proportions. 1 L = 1,000 mL. 100,000 units/1,000 mL = X units/50 mL, where X = 5,000 units.

71. c—All prescriptions containing estrogens require the pharmacy to provide the patient with a Patient Product Insert (PPI).

72. d—An individual taking Lasix as a diuretic may lose potassium and require a potassium supplement. Aldactone, Dyazide, and Dyrenium are potassium-sparing diuretics.

73. c—Isoniazid (INH) is used to treat tuberculosis. Albuterol, ipratropium, and salmeterol are used to treat asthma.

74. c—%w/v is defined as the X g/100 mL. Calculate the number of grams in 100 mL by using the following proportion: 40 mg/1 mL = X mg/100 mL, where x = 4,000 mg. Convert milligrams to grams (4,000 mg × 1 g/1,000 mg = 4 g). 4 g/100 mL = 4% w/v.

75. c—5 mL/tsp × 3 tsp/tbsp × 2 tbsp/ fl oz × 8 fl oz / cup × 2 cups/ pt = 480 mL.

76. d—Glyburide, an oral hypoglycemic agent, used in the treatment of diabetes.

77. c—iss is a Roman numeral indicating 1½ gr. 65 mg/gr × 1½ gr = 97.5 mg.

78. b—Days supply = total quantity dispensed/quantity taken per day (40 capsules/4 capsules/day = 10-day supply.

79. d—"ung" is a Latin abbreviation meaning ointment. Ointments are a dosage form applied externally on the skin unless otherwise directed.

80. c—1.5 mEq/1 mL = 30mEq/X mL, where X = 20 mL.

81. c—m/100 mL = 100 g/X, where X = 1,000 mL or 1 L.

82. d—Unit dose labels require the name and strength of the medication, expiration date of the medication, manufacturer's name, and lot number.

83. c—A potassium supplement is taken when there is a deficiency of potassium in the body. "Hypo" means below, "kalemia" means potassium.

84. b—Anticholinergics have a tendency to dry up all bodily secretions of the body as a side effect.

85. b—Oxycodore with acetaminophen is a Schedule II drug and, according to the Controlled Substance Act, Schedule II drugs need to be kept in the pharmacy safe when not in use.

86. b—Calculate the number of units per hour (20 units/1 min = X units/60 min (1 hr), where X = 1,200 units). Calculate the volume to be infused per hour (100,000 units/1,000 mL = 1,200 units/X mL, where X = 12 mL in 1 hr). Calculate the number of gtt/min by using the following formula: (mL/hr)(drop size)(1 hr/60 min) = gtt/min. (12 mL/hr)(60 gtt/mL)(1 hr/60 min) = 12 gtt/min.

87. d—Plastic is less expensive than glass; the pliability of the bag requires less storage space, and the bags are transparent.

88. c—An 80/20 Report, also known as a Velocity Report, shows a detailed summary of your purchasing history. It lists those products that reflect 80% of your purchasing dollars.

89. c—A copy of the Controlled Substance Act, National Formulary, and US Pharmacopeia are required texts in all pharmacies by the State Boards of Pharmacy. All pharmacies must maintain a library for reference.

90. c—Procardia (nifedipine) is a calcium channel blocker.

91. d—Amino acids, dextrose, and lipids are use in preparing a total nutrient admixture, which is a parenteral form of nutrition for patients with specific conditions. Proteins are not used in this preparation.

92. a—Electrolytes refer to substances necessary to carry out the electrical activity of nerves and muscles in the body. A mEq is 1/1,000 of an equivalent weight and is used to measure replacement of electrolytes in the body.

93. b—Generic drugs are nonproprietary drugs.

94. a—Hazardous drugs are prepared in a biological safety hood, IVs in a horizontal flow hood, antineoplastics in a vertical flow hood, and various extemporaneous products are prepared using an ointment slab.

95. c—Convert pounds to kilograms (180 lb × 1 kg/2.2 lb = 81.82 kg). Calculate daily dosage (81.82 kg × 1.75 mg/kg/day = 143 mg/day).

96. a—The Controlled Substance Act requires that all prescriptions for controlled substances have the physician's DEA number on them.

97. a—"Hyper" means greater than, "hypo" less than, and "iso" the same as.

98. d—240 mL of the prescription is to be prepared. The patient is to receive four doses of 5 mL daily or a total of 20 mL. To calculate the amount of Tussin to be taken daily, solve using a proportion (30 mL of Tussin/240 mL of total solution = X mL of Tussin/20 mL of total solution, where X = 2.5 mL of

Answers **317**

Tussin). Calculate the amount of guaifenesin (100 mg of guaifenesin/5 mL of Tussin solution = X mg of guaifenesin/2.5 mL, where X = 50 mg).

99. b—"pr" means per rectum.
100. d—A TPN must be isotonic to the blood or else the blood cells will either expand or collapse in the blood vessel. A hypotonic solution will cause the blood cells to collapse, whereas a hypertonic solution will cause the cell to expand.
101. d—"Rhinitis" means a runny nose.
102. a—A small volume parenteral contains less than 100 mL of solution.
103. b—Inhibition is the process whereby an agent can slow or block enzyme activity, which impairs the metabolism of drugs and as a result may increase their concentration. Additive effects are the combined effects of two drugs. Potentiation is an effect that increases or prolongs the action of another drug and the total effect is greater than the sum of the effects of each drug taken alone. Synergism is the joint action of drugs in which their combined effects is more intense or longer in duration than the sum of their individual effects.
104. c—Solve using the following formula: Final volume × % strength (expressed as a decimal) will yield the amount of active ingredient in grams: 250 mL × 0.25 = 62.5 g.
105. b—Elixirs, spirits, and syrups contain either alcohol or sugar; diabetics should not receive either of them; emulsions do not contain alcohol or sugar.
106. b—A flutter is a type of arrhythmia in which the patient's heart is experiencing 200–350 beats per minute.
107. c—Sulfasalazine may cause photosensitivity to an individual if he or she is exposed to direct sunlight; one should drink plenty of water to prevent crystals from developing in the kidneys. Sulfasalazine has the tendency to change the color of one's urine from a yellow to an orange-brown color.
108. c—Solve by using the following formula: (Initial volume)(initial strength) = (final volume)(final strength): (300 mL)(50%) = (300 mL + 200 mL = 500 mL)(final strength), where the final strength is 30%. 30% means that there are 30 g in 100 mL. To calculate the number of grams in 500 mL, a proportion is used: 30 g/100 mL = X g/500 mL, where X = 150 g.
109. c—This is an alligation problem requiring an individual to make a 40% dextrose solution from both 60% and 10% dextrose solution. Place the 60% in the upper left hand corner, the 40% in the middle, and the 10% in the lower left hand corner. 60%-40% = 20 parts of the 10% solution. 40%-10%= 30 parts of the 60% solution. The total number of parts is equal to 50 parts. To calculate the required quantities of each solution use a proportion. 30 parts of 60% solution/50 parts of 40 solution = Xml of 60% solution/ 1,000 ml of 40% solution, where X = 600 mL of 60%. 20 parts of 10% solution/50 parts of the 40% solution = XmL of 10% solution/ 1,000 mL of 40% solution, where X = 400 ml of the 10% solution.
110. a—The gauze swab will protect the finger from being cut by fine pieces of glass.
111. b—Inventory turnover rate is calculated by dividing the total sales by the average inventory value. $2,750,000/[($225,000 + $250,000)/2] = 11.58 turns.
112. c—1 pint = 480 mL. Solve by using a proportion: 2 mg/1 mL = X mg/480 mL, where X = 960 mg. Convert milligrams to grams (960 mg × 1 g/1,000 mg = 0.96 g).
113. c—Catapres TTS is changed weekly.
114. c—Percocet is oxycodone + acetaminophen; Tylenol C Codeine (acetaminophen + codeine), Vicodin and Lortab (hydrocodone + acetaminophen), and Darvocet N (propoxyphene + acetaminophen).
115. a—Convert pounds to kilograms (44 lb × 1 kg/2.2 lb = 20 kg). Next calculate amount the patient is to receive each day (4 mg/kg × 20 kg = 80 mg/day). Next, calculate the volume to be given to the patient (30 mg/5 mL = 80 mg/X mL, where X = 13.3 mL).
116. d—OSHA stands for the Occupational Safety and Health Administration which is concerned with employee safety; HIPAA stands for the Health Insurance Portability and Accountability Act, which is concerned with patient confidentiality; JCAHO is the Joint Commission on Accreditation of Healthcare Organizations, which is responsible for establishing standards for hospitals, nursing homes, and long-term care facilities, and ensuring that the standards are maintained; OBRA is the Omnibus Budget Reconciliation Act requiring drug utilization review and that an offer to counsel is to be made to every customer.
117. b—Elixirs are a clear, sweetened, flavored hydroalcoholic solution containing both water and ethanol; collodions are a liquid dosage form for topical application with pyroxylin dissolved in alcohol and

ether; suspensions are a dispersion in which small particles of a solid are distributed throughout a liquid; syrup is an aqueous solution thickened with sugar.

118. b—"ou" means each eye.
119. c—Convert grams to milligrams (2 g × 1,000 mg/g = 2,000 mg). Set up a proportion: 2,000 mg/30 mL = X mg/5 mL, where X = 333 mg.
120. d—Hyperalimentation and total parenteral nutrition are synonymous terms that describe the process of feeding patients who are unable to eat solids and liquids.
121. d—Latanoprost (Xalatan) needs to be refrigerated after opening.
122. b—Irbesartan (Avapro), candesartan (Atacand), losartan (Cozaar), and valsartan (Diovan).
123. a—Air flows in only one direction in a laminar flow hood, away from the hood in a horizontal flow hood and upward in a vertical flow hood.
124. b—During Phase 2, a final review is done on the ingredients of the agent in question. The public is able to give feedback. All data are taken into account. In Phase 1, advisors evaluate the agent in question as to whether it is safe and effective when taken by the consumer or patient. During Phase 3, all the final evidence is presented and all aspects of the agent exhausted, and the final monograph is published.
125. d—Glucophage (metformin), Amaryl (glimepiride), glipizide (Glucotrol), and Micronase (glyburide).
126. d—As a patient ages, his or her ability to hear properly is reduced; the patient may begin to develop multiple disease states; as a result of multiple disease states, the patient is required to take multiple medications.
127. d—Vasotec is available as both an oral and intravenous dosage form.
128. d—Griseofulvin may cause photosensitivity in an individual, resulting in a severe sunburn or rash. Because it is a suspension, it should be shaken to prevent precipitation and needs to be stored at room temperature.
129. d—Tegretol is available as a chewable tablet, an oral tablet, and a suspension. As a transdermal dosage form, Catapres is known as Catapres TTS and needs to be changed weekly; Duragesic is a Schedule II medication, which provides fentanyl as a narcotic analgesic and lasts for 3 days; and Nitroglycerin is known as Nitro-Dur or Nitrodisc.
130. d—Prednisone is the generic name for Deltasone; lithium (Eskalith); methylprednisolone (Medrol); prednisolone (Pediapred).
131. a—The sale of an "exempt narcotic" requires that an individual be at least 18 years of age, a resident of the community, and that no more than one 4-oz bottle be sold in the original manufacturer's bottle every 48 hr. The patient must complete the exempt narcotic log (record), which includes the date of the purchase, their name and address. The pharmacist must see that the name, quantity of the product, and the selling price of the product are entered in the "Exempt Narcotic Book." The pharmacist must sign their name in the book as the seller of the "exempt narcotic."
132. d—Etoposide needs to be prepared in a biological safety cabinet because it is a plant alkaloid used in the treatment of cancer.
133. a—Bupropion (Wellbutrin or Zyban) is not an MAO inhibitor. MAO inhibitors include phenelzine (Nardil), selegiline (Eldepryl), and tranylcypromine (Parnate).
134. d—Convert grams to milligrams (1.2 g × 1,000 mg/g = 1,200 mg). Use a proportion to calculate the volume to be infused (50 mg/1 mL = 1,200 mg/X mL, where X = 24 mL).
135. c—Evista is used to treat osteoporosis.
136. c—The Master Formula Sheet, also known as a Pharmacy compounding log, indicates the amount of each ingredient used, the procedures used in the preparation and the labeling instructions.
137. c—"hepat" means liver.
138. a—At bedtime (hs), if needed (prn).
139. b—ASHP is an acronym standing for American Society of Health System Pharmacists.
140. b—A Type II (cytolytic) reaction occurs because of the reactions of circulating antibodies of the immunoglobulin (Ig)G, IgM, or IgA class with an antigen associated with a cell membrane. Type I (anaphylactic) reactions are produced when the antigen has stimulated the production of the antibody, which then becomes fixed to basophils and mast cells in the tissues. A Type III (toxin-precipitin) reaction occurs when the precipitin complex is removed from the bloodstream by the reticuloendothelial cells in the spleen. A Type IV (cell-mediated hypersensitivity) reactions depends on the presence of T-cell lymphocytes that combine with the antigen.

Bibliography

American Pharmacists Association. (2000) *Handbook of Non-prescription Drugs*. Washington, D.C.

American Society of Health-System Pharmacists. (1996–1997) ASHP statement of the pharmacy and therapeutics committee. *Practice Standards of ASHP* 1996–1997. Bethesda, MD.

American Society of Health-System Pharmacists. (2003) *Practice Standards of the American Society of Health-System Pharmacists*. Bethesda, MD.

American Society of Health-System Pharmacists. (2004) ASHP technical assistance bulletin on handling cytotoxic and hazardous drugs. *Practice Standards of ASHP*.

American Society of Health-System Pharmacists. (2004) ASHP technical assistance bulletin on quality assurance for pharmacy-prepared sterile products. *Practice Standards of ASHP*.

Ansel, H., Allen, L., and Popovich, N. (2000) *Pharmaceutical Dosage Forms and Drug Delivery Systems* (7th ed). Baltimore: Lippincott Williams & Wilkins.

Ansel, H.C., and Stoklosa, M.J. *Pharmaceutical Calculations*. (2001) Philadelphia, PA: Lippincott Williams & Wilkins.

Automeds, 875 Woodlands Parkway, Vernon Hills, IL 60061: 888-537-3102. http://www.automedrx.com

Barker, K.N., Felkey, B.G., Flynn, E.A., et al. (1998) White paper on automation in pharmacy. *Consulting Pharmacists* 46, 2346.

Bryan, D., and Marback, R.C. (1984) Laminar-airflow equipment certification: what the pharmacist needs to know. *American Journal of Hospital Pharmacy* 41, 1343–1349.

Blumenthal, M., Goldberg, A., and Brickman, J. (Eds.) (2000) *Herbal Medicine: Expanded Commission E Monographs*. Newton, MA: Integrative Medicine Communications.

Cohen, M.R. (Ed.) (1999) *Medication Errors*. Washington, D.C.: American Pharmaceutical Association.

Davis, N. M., Cohen, M.R., and Teplisky, B. (1992) Look-alike and sound-alike drug names. *Hospital Pharmacy* 27, 96–106.

Garrelts, J.C., Koehn, L., and Rich, D.S. (2001). Automated medication distribution systems and compliance with Joint Commission Standards. *American Journal Hospital Pharmacist* 51, 1193–1196.

Gennaro, A.R. *Remington: The Science and Practice of Pharmacy* 20th edition. Philadelphia, PA: Lippincott Williams & Wilkins.

Heller, W.M. (1980). Time limits on the use of opened multiple dose vials. *American Journal of Hospital Pharmacists* 37, 1610–1613.

Hicks, W.E. (Ed.) (1999) *Practice standards of ASHP, 1998-99*. Bethesda, MD: ASHP.

Joint Commission on Accreditation of Healthcare Organizations. (2002). *Comprehensive Accreditation Manual for Hospitals*. Oakbrook Terrace, IL: JCAHO.

Jonsen, A.R. (2002). *Clinical Ethics*. New York: McGraw-Hill.

Kimmel, P.D., Weygandt, J.J., and Kieso, D.E. (2000) *Accounting and Finance: Managerial Use and Analysis*. New York: John Wiley and Sons, Inc.

Kocher, K. (1994). *Pharmacy Certified Technician Calculations Workbook*. Lansing, MI: Michigan Pharmacists Association Education Center.

Lesar, T.S., Briceland, L., and Stein, D.S. (1997) Factors related to errors in medication prescribing. *JAMA* 277, 312–317.

Mckesson Automation, 700 Waterfront Drive, Pittsburgh, PA 15222; (412) 209-1400; http://www.robot-rx.com.

Neuewnschwander, M., Cohen, M.R., Valda Patchett, A.J., Kelley, J., and Trohimovich, B. (2003). Practical guide to bar coding for patient medication safety. *American Journal of Health-System Pharmacists* 60, 768–779.

Omnicell, 1101 East Meadow Dr., Palo Alto, CA 94303, 800-850-6664; http://www.omnicell.com.

Pyxis Corporation, 3750 Torrey View Ct., San Diego, CA 92130, 858-480-6000; http://pyxiscorp.com.

Rich, D.S. (1996). Expiration dating of pharmacy packaging. *Hospital Pharmacy 31,* 1159–1160.

Schermerhorn, J.R., Jr., Hunt, J.G., Osborn, R.N. (2000) *Organizational Behavior.* New York: John Wiley & Sons, Inc.

Shrewsburg, R. (2001) *Applied Pharmaceutics in Contemporary Compounding.* Englewood, CO: Morton Publishing

United States Pharmacopeial Convention. (1995) General notices and requirements: Preservation, packaging, storage, and labeling. *The United States Pharmacopeia XXIII/The National Formulary XVIII.*

STATUTES

Alcohol Tax Law. 26 U.S.C. SS5214, 5217.

Controlled Substances Act of 1970, P.L. No. 91-513, 84 Stat. 1236 (codified in scattered sections of 18, 19, 21, 31, 40, 42, and 49 U.S.C.).

Federal Food, Drug and Cosmetic Act 21 U.S.C. SS301-392.

Health Maintenance Organization Act of 1973. U.S. Statute 914.

Poison Prevention Packaging Act of 1970. P.L. No. 91-601, 84 Stat. 1670 (codified in 15 U.S.C. SS1471-1476, and scattered sections of 7 and 21 U.S.C.).

Social Security Amendments of 1965 (Medicare and Medicaid). U.S. Statutes at Large 286.

REGULATIONS

Consumer Product Safety Commission (Poison Prevention Packaging Act). 16 C.F.R. SS 1700–1704.

Drug Enforcement Administration. 21 C.F.R. SS1301–SS1316.

Food and Drug Administration, 21 C.F.R. SS1–SS1230.

Social Security Administration (Medicare); Health Care Financing Administration (Medicaid). Hospitals-20 C.F.R. SS 405: Skilled Nursing Facilities-20 C.F.R. ss405; HMOs-42 C.F. R.SS 110.

Index

Pellets, 126
Penicillin
 liquids to be taken with, 2, 273
 pharmacology considerations, 35, 171, 175, 300, 302
Pentosan polysulfate sodium, 53
Per diem, 103, 155
Percentage strength, 5, 12, 86-87, 164, 274, 276, 298
Percentages
 calculating, 5, 86-87, 274
Performance evaluations, 157
Periodic automatic replacement (PAR value), 128
Peripheral acting agents, 58
Perpetual inventories, 23
Personal digital assistants (PDAs), 29
Personal protective equipment (PPE), 131
Pharmaceutical Research Journal (AAPR), 34
Pharmaceuticals
 conversion charts, 235-236
  abbreviations, 237-242
  amounts, 237
  body conditions, 240-241
  dosage forms, 237-238
  medications, 239-240
  miscellaneous pharmacy, 241
  pharmaceuticals, 235-236
  sites and time of administration, 238-239
  solutions, 238
 drug classifications
  list of top 200 prescriptions, 249-253
  and nomenclature, 35-72
 manufacturers, 103
 professional standards, 132-134
 recalls, 129, 132, 139, 296
Pharmacies
 abbreviation charts, 237-241
 administration and management of, 114-157
 calculations, 83-90
 communication, 141, 142, 173, 301
 drug, medical and legal issues affecting, 29
 informational sources available in, 144-146
 missions, goals and structure of, 141
 organizational journals, 34-35
 physical areas devoted to functions, 147
 preventing prescription errors, 135, 136t, 137t
 quality improvements in, 144-146
 regulatory agencies for, 28
 resource allocation, 141-142
Pharmacists
 allowing prescription-writing by, 29
 assistance of
  in serving patients, 19-124, 278-295
 counseling by, 103
 regulatory agencies for, 28
Pharmacokinetics, 34, 129

Pharmacology
 drug nomenclature, 35-72
 review questions and answers, 115-119, 283-288
Pharmacy and Therapeutics Committee (P&T), 128, 140, 174, 196, 296, 301, 309
Pharmacy calculations
 alligation method, 87-88
 children's doses, 88-89
 commercial math, 90
 concentration/ dilution, 87
 conversion charts, 235-241
 doses, 86
 flow rates, 88
 math review, 119-124, 289-295
 metric/ household/ apothecary conversions, 85-86, 235-236
 powder volume, 87
 ratios/proportions, 84
 reducing/enlarging formulas, 85
 roman numerals, 83
 specific gravity, 88
 temperature conversions, 90
 units/ MEQ, 86
Pharmacy laws, 19-28
Pharmacy Technician Certification Examination (PTCE)
 absences and emergencies, 231
 admission to, 229-230
 candidate attestation, 228
 examination checklist and schedule, 230
 format and breakdowns of, 233-234
 information concerning, 127-234
 preparation for, 234
 procedures to follow, 230-231
 scoring, 231-233
 test taking skills, 1
Pharmacy Technicians Certification Board (PTCB)
 examination information, 227-234
 making provisions for disabilities, 228-229
Pharmacy technicians (CPhT)
 aseptic techniques for, 92, 94, 99, 100f, 101f
 assisting pharmacists
  in serving patients, 19-124, 278-295
 code of ethics for, 19
 definition of, 19
 learning monitoring and screening equipment, 75-76
 preventing prescription errors, 135, 136t, 137t
 professional membership organizations, 271
 PTCE examination information, 227-234
 regulatory agencies for, 28
 roles and responsibilities of, 142-143, 167, 299
Phenazopyridine, 53
Physician order sheets (POS), 156